MW00514521

Introduction to
DIALYSIS

Introduction to
DIALYSIS

Edited by

Martin G. Cogan, M.D. and Marvin R. Garovoy, M.D.
University of California, San Francisco

With Contributions by:

Nephrology
Frank A. Gotch, M.D.
Patricia Schoenfeld, M.D.

Vascular Surgery
William C. Krupski, M.D.
Ronald L. Webb, M.D.
David J. Effeney, B.S. M.B.

Nephrology Nursing
Marcia L. Keen, R.N., B.S.N.
Margaret Devney-Bruks,
R.N., M.S.N.

Renal Pharmacology
Donald P. Alexander, Pharm. D.
John G. Gambertoglio, Pharm. D.

Pediatric Nephrology
Donald E. Potter, M.D.

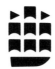

Churchill Livingstone
New York, Edinburgh, London, and Melbourne 1985

Acquisitions editor: *Lynne Herndon*
Production editor: *Charlie Lebeda*
Production supervisor: *Kerry A. O'Rourke*
Compositor: *Maryland Composition Company, Inc.*
Printer/Binder: *The Maple-Vail Book Manufacturing Group*

Distributed in the United Kingdom by Churchill Livingstone,
Robert Stevenson House, 1–3 Baxter's Place, Leith Walk,
Edinburgh EH1 3AF and associated companies, branches
and representatives throughout the world.

First published in 1985

Printed in U.S.A.

ISBN 0–443–08305–3

9 8 7 6 5 4 3 2 1

Printed in U.S.A.

Library of Congress Cataloging in Publication Data

Main entry under title:

Introduction to dialysis.

   Includes bibliographies and index.
   1. Hemodialysis.   2. Artificial kidney.
I. Cogan, Martin G.   II. Garovoy, Marvin R.
III. Gotch, Frank A.   [DNLM: 1. Hemodialysis.
WJ 378 I618]
RC901.7.H45I59   1985   617'.461059   84-17513
ISBN 0-443-08305-3

Manufactured in the United States of America

CONTRIBUTORS

Donald P. Alexander, Pharm. D.
Assistant Clinical Professor of Pharmacy, School of Pharmacy, University of California, San Francisco; Presently, Assistant Professor of Pharmacy, Department of Pharmacy Practice, College of Pharmacy, University of Utah

Martin G. Cogan, M.D.
Assistant Professor of Medicine, University of California School of Medicine, San Francisco; Medical Director, Acute Hemodialysis Unit, Moffitt Hospital, University of California, San Francisco

Margaret Devney-Bruks, R.N., M.S.N.
Assistant Clinical Professor of Nursing, University of California School of Nursing, San Francisco; Clinical Specialist in Nephrology, Moffitt Hospital, University of California, San Francisco

David J. Effeney, B.S., M.B.
Associate Professor of Surgery, University of California School of Medicine, San Francisco; Chief, Vascular Surgery Section, Veterans Administration Medical Center, San Francisco

John G. Gambertoglio, Pharm. D.
Adjunct Associate Professor of Clinical Pharmacology, University of California School of Pharmacy, San Francisco; Clinical Pharmacist, Kidney Transplant Service, Moffitt Hospital, University of California, San Francisco

Marvin R. Garovoy, M.D.
Associate Professor of Surgery and Medicine, University of California School of Medicine, San Francisco; Director, Immunogenetics and Transplantation Laboratory, Moffitt Hospital, University of California, San Francisco

Frank A. Gotch, M.D.
Associate Clinical Professor of Medicine, University of California School of Medicine, San Francisco; Director, Dialysis Treatment and Research Center, Franklin Hospital, San Francisco

Marcia L. Keen, R.N., B.S.N.
Research Supervisor, Dialysis Treatment and Research Center, Franklin Hospital, San Francisco

William C. Krupski, M.D.
Assistant Professor of Surgery, University of California School of Medicine, San Francisco; Assistant Chief, Vascular Surgery Section, Veterans Administration Medical Center, San Francisco

Donald E. Potter, M.D.
Associate Clinical Professor of Pediatrics, University of California School of Medicine, San Francisco; Director, Pediatric Dialysis, University of California, San Francisco

Patricia Schoenfeld, M.D.
Associate Clinical Professor of Medicine, University of California School of Medicine, San Francisco; Director, University of California Renal Center, San Francisco General Hospital, San Francisco

Ronald L. Webb, M.D.
Associate Clinical Professor of Surgery, University of California School of Medicine, San Francisco; Attending Surgeon, Merritt Hospital, Oakland

PREFACE

At this time, the kidney is the only human organ whose function can be artificially replaced on a reliable and chronic basis. Dialysis cannot claim to duplicate the intricate transport and endocrine processes inherent in normal renal function. Nevertheless, dialytic technology has advanced to the point that a tolerable homeostatic level of existence can be routinely achieved for patients with renal failure.

The purpose of this text is to acquaint those charged with the care of renal failure patients to principles of sound dialytic therapy. As one of the most quantifiable of all medical therapies, the transport processes of a dialysis procedure can be described rigorously. As such, one of our aims is to convey how a quantitative understanding of the dialysis process can be translated into good, rational clinical care. Equally important is the thorough understanding of the other, complex clinical problems that arise during and between dialyses. Where possible, a description of the "state of the art" is given. When national consensus does not exist, some recommendations regarding optimal care inevitably reflect local, San Francisco opinion and represent the way we would hope dialysis be performed. Since the art and science of dialysis and the accepted guidelines for the care of the patient with renal disease are dynamic entities, the authors have attempted to "freeze the action," and have portrayed the way dialytic care should be best rendered currently. Emphasis has been placed on the practical and the clinically relevant aspects of dialysis and of drug kinetics in renal failure. Space constraints required that many other relevant issues be deferred.

This ambitious attempt to present a condensed, practical but hopefully lucid overview of the marvelous technological breakthrough that dialysis represents was the synthesis of effort by many talented people. We would especially extend thanks to the authors for their superb and often prescient contributions, to Gail Feazell for the excellent medical illustrations, to John R. Collins, Ph.D. for expert editorial assistance, to Donald Potter, M.D. and Michael Weiner, M.D. for critical review of portions of the book, and to Lynne Herndon for publishing assistance.

This book is dedicated to the important people in our lives: to Ralph Cogan, Floyd Rector and Jack Collins and to Nathan Garovoy; and, of course, to our dialysis patients.

M.G.C.
M.R.G.

CONTENTS

Pediatric Sections:
Donald E. Potter

ABBREVIATIONS

AV	arteriovenous
BUN	blood urea nitrogen
C	solute concentration
$\quad C_B$	blood solute concentration
$\quad C_D$	dialysate solute concentration
$\quad C_s$	systemic concentration
Cr	creatinine
$\quad Cr_u$	urine creatinine concentration
D	dialysance
D_L	heparin loading dose
ER	extraction ratio
f	fractional removal
G	generation rate
$\quad G_U$	generation of urea
$\quad G_{Cr}$	generation of creatinine
H	hematocrit
Ir	heparin infusion rate
J	flux
K_1, K_0	flux coefficients
$\quad K$	clearance (urea)
$\quad\quad K_r$	residual renal clearance
$\quad\quad\quad K_{rU}$	residual renal urea clearance
$\quad\quad\quad\quad K_{rE}$	effective renal urea clearance
$\quad\quad\quad K_{rCr}$	residual renal creatinine clearance
$\quad\quad K_T$	total fractional urea clearance
$\quad K_e$	heparin elimination rate constant
$\quad K_{UF}$	ultrafiltration coefficient
k	dialyzer-specific proportionality constant
NBW	normalized body weight
P	hydraulic pressure
$\quad P_B$	blood pressure
$\quad P_D$	dialysate pressure

PCR	protein catabolic rate
pcr	(normalized for body weight) protein catabolic rate
PD	peritoneal dialysis
CPD	chronic peritoneal dialysis
CAPD	continuous ambulatory peritoneal dialysis
CCPD	continuous cycling peritoneal dialysis
IPD	intermittent peritoneal dialysis
Q	flow
Q_B	blood flow
Q_D	dialysate flow
Q_F	ultrafiltrate
Q_P	plasma flow
QP	pumped dialysate
Q_{UF} Pump	ultrafiltrate pump
R	anticoagulation response
R_d	desired anticoagulation response
R_s	steady-state anticoagulation response
R_{K_r}	ratio of urea to creatinine clearances
RO	reverse osmosis
S	sensitivity
S_a	apparent sensitivity
t	time
θ	interdialytic interval
t_{dc}	discontinuation time for heparin infusion
TMP	transmembrane pressure
U	urea
U_u	urine urea nitrogen
V	volume (urea distribution volume)
V_u	urine volume
WBPTT	whole blood partial thromboplastin time
$WBPTT_{BL}$	baseline WBPTT
$WBPTT_{3\,min}$	WBPTT 3 minutes following heparin dose

Subscripts

i	in
o	out
1	initial
2	second
3	third
t	end

Introduction to
DIALYSIS

1

DIALYZERS AND DELIVERY SYSTEMS

Frank A. Gotch   Marcia L. Keen

THE ARTIFICIAL KIDNEY

The artificial kidney is designed to provide controllable transfer of solutes and water across a semipermeable membrane separating flowing blood and dialysate streams. The transfer processes are dialysis and ultrafiltration; the device is a dialyzer; and the three basic structural elements of all dialyzers are the blood compartment, the membrane, and the dialysate compartment.

Structural and Design Requirements

Several fundamental material and design requirements must be met in the construction of efficient dialyzers suitable for clinical therapy. The blood-contacting surfaces and flow geometry must be relatively nonthrombogenic. The materials used must be nontoxic and free of leachable toxic substances. The blood and dialysate flow paths must result in the distribution of blood and dialysate in thin films uniformly flowing across the membrane; consequently, the ratio of membrane surface area to contained volume must be high. The hydraulic resistance to blood and dialysate flow should be low and predictable. Three basic dialyzer designs have evolved in attempts to achieve these goals, consisting of coil, parallel plate, and hollow fiber configurations.

Coil Dialyzer. The coil dialyzer is an early design in which the blood compartment is comprised of one or two long membrane tubes placed between support screens and then tightly wound with the screens around a plastic core. This results in a coiled tubular membrane, laminated between support screens, which is then enclosed in a rigid cylindrical case to minimize increase in contained volume with increase in coil pressure. Dialysate flows vertically through the multiple support screen layers sandwiched between the coils of membrane.

1

This is a cross-flow dialyzer because the dialysate flow path is across and at right angles to blood flow through the tubular membrane. This design has serious performance limitations, which have gradually restricted its use as better designs have evolved. The hydraulic resistance to blood flow is very high because of the long single-channel blood compartment with a small cross-sectional area for flow. Consequently, the minimal blood compartment mean pressure is quite high and results in substantial obligatory ultrafiltration.

The coil design does not produce uniform dialysate flow distribution across the membrane at the 500-ml/min dialysate flow rate used with other designs. To compensate for this inadequacy, much higher dialysate flow rates (~20 L/min) can be applied to scrub stationary dialysate film off the membrane by using a recirculating single pass flow configuration. A small volume of dialysate (8–10 L) is recirculated across the membrane at a high flow rate (20 L/min) with simultaneous flow of fresh dialysate at ~450 ml/min through the 8- to 10-L reservoir. This procedure improves efficiency, but, due to increased solute concentration in the recirculating reservoir, the net clearance of solute is still substantially below that achieved with single pass flow at 20 L/min,

Parallel Plate Dialyzer. In the parallel plate dialyzer, sheets of membrane are mounted on plastic support screens, and then are stacked in multiple layers ranging from 2 to 20 or more (Fig. 1-1). This design allows multiple parallel blood and dialysate flow channels with much lower hydraulic resistance to flow. At the inlet and outlet, blood and dialysate manifolds distribute these streams to their respective compartments.

In recent years the physical size of parallel plate dialyzers has been greatly reduced and the efficiency improved. These improvements have resulted from better membrane supports, which provide (1) thin blood and dialysate channels with highly uniform dimensions, (2) minimal masking or blocking of membranes on the support, and (3) minimal stretching or deformation of membranes.

Early plate designs (such as the Kiil artificial kidney widely used 25 years ago) utilized parallel ridge membrane supports oriented along the length of the cast membrane. Consequently, there was substantial membrane stretching between the support ridges because the crosswise tensile strength of cellulosic sheet membranes is only 1/10 of the lengthwise strength. This constraint predetermined a variable channel height with nonuniform flow distribution, thick channels with long diffusion distances due to sagging of the membrane with draping over the support ridges, and variable membrane masking. These design defects resulted in low-efficiency devices with large contained blood volumes and variable performance with respect to solute transport and ultrafiltration.

Modern plate dialyzers contain molded membrane supports produced with very tight dimensional tolerances. As shown in Figure 1-1, the membrane is typically supported on tiny pyramidal excrescences molded onto the plastic support surfaces. There is much less membrane deformation and masking, since the membrane stress is bidirectional. The resulting thin and uniform channel heights afford good distribution of blood and dialysate flow and high ratios of surface area to contained volume. The secondary flow paths around the support points

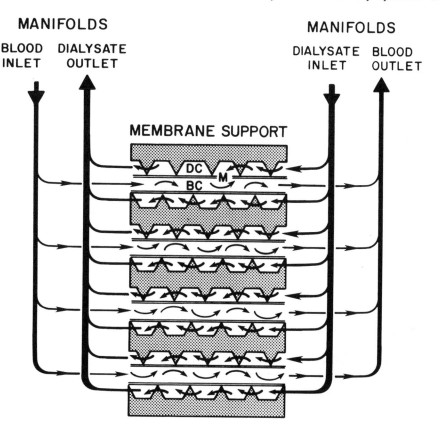

BC - BLOOD COMPARTMENT
DC - DIALYSATE COMPARTMENT
 M - MEMBRANE

Fig. 1-1. Structure of a typical parallel plate dialyzer.

break up laminar flow profiles and promote mixing in the blood and dialysate streams, which also improves efficiency.

Hollow Fiber Dialyzer. The hollow fiber dialyzer is the most effective design for providing low-volume high-efficiency devices with low hydraulic resistance to flow. The essential structural elements are shown schematically in Figure 1-2. The membrane is comprised of tiny cellulosic hollow fibers approximately the size of a human hair, with an internal diameter of $\sim$200 μm, wall thickness 8–40 μm, and length $\sim$20 cm. The total membrane area ranges from 0.8 to 2.0 m^2 and is determined by the number of fibers in the device. The aggregate fibers, numbering 7,000 to 15,000, are termed the "fiber bundle," which is enclosed in a cylindrical jacket. The fibers are potted in polyurethane at each end of the fiber bundle in the tube sheet, which serves as the membrane support. The blood inlet and outlet manifolds—shallow cylindrical caps covering the tube sheets—

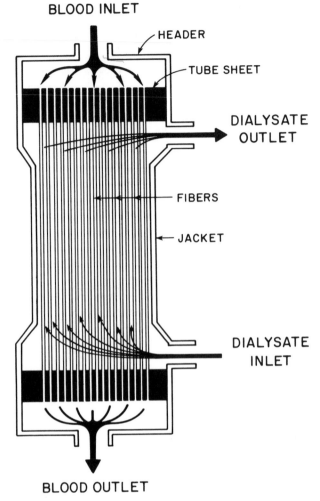

BLOOD INLET

HEADER

TUBE SHEET

DIALYSATE OUTLET

FIBERS

JACKET

DIALYSATE INLET

BLOOD OUTLET

Fig. 1-2. Structure of a typical hollow fiber dialyzer.

are termed "headers." The inlet and outlet dialysate manifolds are simply expanded sections of the dialysate jacket adjacent to the tube sheets.

Very small hollow tubes are dimensionally stable over a wide range of pressure, which creates a noncompliant blood compartment in the hollow fiber dialyzer. This unique property of these dialyzers permits quantitative assessment of the magnitude of thrombus formation when hollow fiber dialyzers are reused. The amount of volume needed to fill the blood compartment of a dialyzer (priming volume) in successive uses provides a simple method for predicting the remaining unclotted volume in reprocessed hollow fiber dialyzers. Since the blood compartments of plate and coil dialyzers are compliant, performance cannot be predicted from measurement of priming volume.

Uniform distribution of blood flow through the fiber bundle is achieved by maintaining the inner diameter constant during fiber spinning, a remarkable technical feat, considering that total fiber length is between 1 and 2 miles in each device. Uniform dialysate flow distribution over the outside fiber surface is achieved by controlling fiber packing density and by using baffles in the inlet and outlet dialysate ports.

The blood and dialysate flows may be in the same direction (concurrent) or in opposite directions (countercurrent) in plate and hollow fiber dialyzers. Typical flow geometry is countercurrent, which is about 20% more efficient than concurrent flow.

Ultrafiltration

Mechanism of Ultrafiltration. Virtually all interdialytic fluid intake must be removed from the bloodstream flowing through the dialyzer during dialysis. It is essential to prescribe and control the fluid removal rate so that total fluid removed during treatment will equal total fluid gain since the previous treatment.

The process of water removal from the bloodstream is called ultrafiltration, and the amount of fluid removed is the ultrafiltrate (Q_F). The driving force for ultrafiltration is the hydraulic pressure difference across the membrane, that is, the transmembrane pressure (TMP), expressed in millimeters of mercury (mmHg). The TMP is determined by the average or mean pressure in the blood compartment ($\overline{P_B}$) minus the mean dialysate compartment pressure ($\overline{P_D}$); thus, TMP $= \overline{P_B} - \overline{P_D}$. Although plasma protein oncotic pressure also influences Q_F, the effect is small relative to the hydrostatic pressure, so the level of Q_F can be considered directly proportional to TMP, as

$$Q_F = k(TMP) \qquad (1\text{-}1)$$

where k is a dialyzer-specific proportionality constant.

Ultrafiltration represents the bulk flow of water across the membrane in ultramicroscopic streams and is analogous to water flow in pipes, where the rate of flow is dependent on the pressure and cross-sectional area for flow. The ultrafiltrate stream is termed "convective flow," and the mechanism of water transfer across the membrane is "convective transport."

The relationship of Q_F to TMP is entirely dependent on membrane properties and is independent of blood and dialysate flow rates over a wide range in parallel plate and hollow fiber dialyzers. It is apparent that k in Equation (1-1) represents Q_F/TMP, and when expressed per square centimeter of membrane area, it defines the hydraulic permeability of the membrane. Hydraulic permeability is determined by the thickness of the membrane and its physical structure, which consists of a loose network of branching, interlocking polymerized molecules. Virtually all dialysis membranes currently in clinical use are cellulosic and comprised of polymerized glucose. The void spaces between the polymer structure are operationally considered to be cylindrical water-filled pores. The pore corss-sectional area and total number of pores determine the hydraulic permeability of the membrane. A typical technique to increase the cross-sectional area of pores is to incorporate other substances within the cellulosic formulation used to cast or spin the membrane. When these substances are subsequently leached out, larger voids in the membrane structure result.

The solute content of the ultrafiltrate streams is considered to be convectively transported across the membrane. The actual solute composition of ultrafiltrate is determined both by the solute concentration difference across the membrane (which will be considered later) and pore size relative to solute molecular size. As solute molecular size approaches pore size, the solute is reflected or sieved out at the membrane edge and excluded from the convective stream of ultrafiltrate. With conventional cellulosic membranes, low molecular weight solutes such as urea are freely convected across the membrane, while ~40% of solutes with mol wt 1000 and 100% of proteins (mol wt $\geq$ 60,000) are sieved out of the convective stream at the membrane edge.

Hydraulic permeability increases as a function of the pore radius raised to the fourth power. It is thus apparent that if membranes are opened up by increasing pore size to increase transfer of larger molecules, the hydraulic permeability increases enormously, resulting in far more difficult control of prescribed Q_F. Such membranes are in limited clinical use as hemofiltration membranes employed in pure convective transport devices with specialized equipment to control the ultrafiltration rate. In conventional dialysis therapy convective transport contributes little to solute removal (except in the case of certain solutes considered in detail in the Appendix), since tighter membranes are used with more readily controlled Q_F.

Clinical Control of Ultrafiltration. The total capacity of a dialyzer for ultrafiltration is given by the ultrafiltration coefficient (K_{UF}) of the dialyzer and has clinical units of ml/h · mmHg. The K_{UF} is a specific value for the proportionality constant in Equation (1-1), which combines hydraulic permeability and membrane area and operationally relates Q_F to TMP in a specific dialyzer in accordance with

$$Q_F = K_{UF}(\text{TMP}) \tag{1-2}$$

Since TMP $= \overline{P_B} - \overline{P_D}$, Equation (1-2) can also be written as

$$Q_F = K_{UF}(\overline{P_B} - \overline{P_D}) \tag{1-3}$$

Equation (1-3) provides the basis for prescribing Q_F in clinical therapy. The K_{UF} is specified by the manufacturer for each dialyzer and ranges from 1.5 to 5.0 ml/h · mmHg in most currently used devices. Examples of the relationship of Q_{UF} to TMP for two dialyzers with different values of K_{UF} are shown in Figure 1-3. In clinical use it is not convenient to determine $\overline{P_B}$ and $\overline{P_D}$; typically pressures are monitored at the outlet of the blood compartment (P_{Bo}) and dialysate compartment (P_{Do}). If the pressure drops across the compartments are small and similar, $P_{Bo} - P_{Do}$ will closely approximate $\overline{P_B} - \overline{P_D}$, and the operational clinical expression to prescribe Q_F becomes

$$Q_F = K_{UF}(P_{Bo} - P_{Do}) \tag{1-4}$$

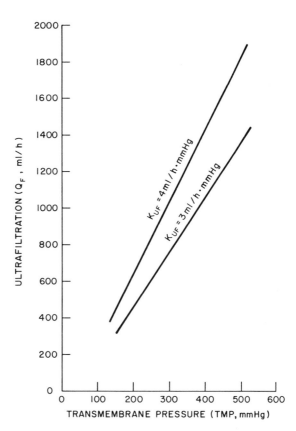

Fig. 1-3. Relationship of ultrafiltration rate (Q_F) to transmembrane pressure (TMP) for two prototypical dialyzers with ultrafiltration coefficients (K_{UF}) of 3 and 4 ml/(h · mmHg).

Equation (1-4) is used to determine the P_{Bo} and P_{Do} values required to achieve a prescribed Q_F during dialysis. In clinical use, the Q_F to be prescribed is calculated by dividing the total fluid to be removed by the length of dialysis. The value of $P_{Bo} - P_{Do}$ is then determined by rearranging Equation (1-4) to give

$$P_{Bo} - P_{Do} = \frac{Q_F}{K_{UF}} \qquad (1\text{-}5)$$

The P_{Bo} is usually not manipulated in clinical therapy and left at the ambient value determined by blood flow and fistula resistance to flow. Thus Equation (1-5) is solved for P_{Do}:

$$P_{Do} = P_{Bo} - \frac{Q_F}{K_{UF}} \qquad (1\text{-}6)$$

and P_{Do} calculated. With substantial required Q_F, the calculated value of P_{Do} is negative, and suction is required on the dialysate side of the membrane. It should be noted that Equation (1-5) could just as easily be solved for P_{Bo}. The desired

TMP could then be achieved by leaving P_{Do} at ambient levels and by increasing P_{Bo}, using a clamp on the venous blood line. If the precision of the pressure control system for the blood compartment is better than the dialysate compartment (not infrequently the case), better control can be achieved by increasing P_{Bo} to achieve the required TMP. The clamp used should be 2 inches or more in length to achieve adequate precision of pressure control.

The precision of Q_F control is dependent on the accuracy of TMP control, the reproducibility of manufacturing specifications on K_{UF}, and the magnitude of clotting in the device. With current state-of-the-art equipment, TMP is controlled to ± 50 mmHg, while the accuracy of manufacturing K_{UF} varies $\pm 15\%$. The effect of this variability in the control parameters results in a strong dependence of Q_F error on dialyzer K_{UF} with error increasing as K_{UF} increases. These relationships are depicted in Figure 1-4, where the error in total fluid removed is plotted as a function of the total fluid targeted for removal at two different values for K_{UF}. For example, if the total ultrafiltrate over the course of a dialysis is 2.5 L, the error increases from a maximum of ± 0.5 L at $K_{UF} = 1.5$ ml/h · mmHg to 1.38 L at $K_{UF} = 5.0$ ml/h · mmHg. Thus, with TMP control of ± 50 mmHg, the low K_{UF} devices will provide much more precise control of Q_F than high K_{UF} devices.

Effect of clotting on K_{UF}. Dialyzers are frequently cleaned and reused. This practice has been shown to improve membrane biocompatibility and is cost-effective. Safe dialyzer reuse requires that the ultrafiltration capacity of the reused device be predictable and not substantially reduced below that for the new dialyzer.

The major reason for retirement of a used dialyzer is clotting in the device, which results in occluded fibers and loss of effective membrane area. The magnitude of clotting is readily assessed in the hollow fiber dialyzer, which has a noncompliant blood compartment, by measuring the change in priming volume. The decrease in priming volume or, more precisely, decrease in fiber bundle

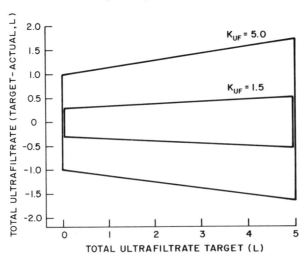

Fig. 1-4. Error in total ultrafiltrate (target − actual) as a function of total ultrafiltrate targeted for two dialyzers with ultrafiltration coefficients (K_{UF}) of 5.0 and 1.5 ml/(h · mmHg).

volume, is a measure of the fraction of fibers occluded and fractional loss of area. Although blood will not flow through the clotted fibers, the porous thrombus material provides a negligible barrier to ultrafiltration. Consequently, at the start of dialysis ultrafiltration will readily occur across the clotted fibers, resulting in plasma flow into the fibers from both ends, which replaces the protein-free ultrafiltrate leaving the fibers. This results in rapidly increasing protein concentration in the fiber lumen. Within a few minutes the protein oncotic pressure will equal TMP and ultrafiltration will cease. Through this mechanism the fractional loss of ultrafiltration capacity will be directly proportional to the fractional decrease in fiber bundle volume and effective membrane area. A generally accepted criterion for reuse is $\leq 20\%$ loss of fibers, which will assure that K_{UF} is $\geq 80\%$ of the original value.

Recently, automated dialyzer reprocessing devices have been developed which provide for measurement of K_{UF} in the reused device; these devices use protein-free water to perfuse the blood and dialysate compartments. The K_{UF} measured in this way provides no information on the functional capacity of the reused device for either ultrafiltration or solute transport. As discussed above, thrombus is highly permeable to water so that the ultrafiltration of protein-free aqueous solution will be virtually unchanged even with extensive clotting of the device.

Solute Transport

Mechanistic Basis of Transport. If a solute is added to a container of water, it will distribute itself at uniform concentration throughout the water. This process, inherent in all solutions, is called diffusion. Diffusion results from random movement of solute molecules driven by the thermal energy of solute and water molecules. Diffusion can also be considered as simply chemical mixing, whereby any local differences in concentration disappear as the solution approaches diffusion equilibrium. The time required for complete mixing to occur depends on solute molecular size, temperature, and the length of the diffusion path or size of the container. The dialyzer can be considered in this context as a triple laminated solution consisting of flowing blood and dialysate with stationary membrane water interposed between the two streams.

For solutes such as urea the inflowing blood concentration is high, while inflowing dialysate concentration is usually zero, resulting in a concentration gradient for diffusion from blood to dialysate. In a perfect dialyzer design, diffusion equilibrium would result in the blood and dialysate streams during their passage through the device. Thus in a completely efficient dialyzer with countercurrent, single pass blood and dialysate flows at equal velocity, urea concentration equilibrium would be reached between the blood inlet and dialysate outlet streams; hence virtually all urea contained in the inflowing bloodstream would be transferred to the outflowing dialysate stream. This level of efficiency is never achieved in clinical dialyzers. At best, efficiency is about 50%, requiring dialysate flow 2 to 2.5 times blood flow.

The rate at which solute diffuses through or permeates the triple laminate of blood, membrane, and dialysate is termed the overall permeability of the device and is expressed by overall transport coefficient (K_o, cm^2/min), which is a physical constant experimentally measured that describes the efficiency of any specific dialyzer design. The K_o is a proportionality constant defined as the rate of solute transfer or flux (J) divided by the membrane area (A) and an appropriately defined mean concentration difference driving force (ΔC) between blood and dialysate, and is given by

$$K_o = \frac{\text{flux/membrane area}}{\text{concentration gradient}} = \frac{J/A}{\Delta C} \qquad (1\text{-}7)$$

which can be arranged to give

$$J = K_o \cdot A \cdot \Delta C \qquad (1\text{-}8)$$

Equation (1-8) gives a mechanistic definition of diffusive transport across the dialyzer. It is apparent that flux is directly proportional to ΔC and can be increased only by increasing K_o or A. The transport coefficient K_o is an analog of k in Equation (1-1), in that K_o defines solute flux per unit area of membrane divided by the concentration gradient driving force, while k describes water flux per unit of area divided by the pressure gradient driving force. Similarly, the product of $K_o \cdot A$ (or K, as discussed below) describes total solute transport capacity of a specific dialyzer, while K_{UF} (which is the product $k \cdot A$) describes total water transport capacity.

The value of K_o or transport efficiency of a dialyzer, is determined by the physical properties of the membrane and the geometry of the blood and dialysate flow paths. The overall solute diffusion path is schematically depicted in Figure 1-5 to be comprised of three discrete segments. Solute is shown in this figure diffusing down a blood-to-dialysate concentration gradient from the center of the blood channel to the membrane edge, across the membrane, and then to the center of the dialysate channel. A concentration gradient from blood to dialysate applies to waste solutes such as urea, creatinine, uric acid, and phosphate. The concentration gradient is reversed for acetate with net diffusion from dialysate to blood, and at times for other electrolytes (Na, K, Ca) and glucose when blood levels are below dialysate levels.

The design requirements to maximize solute permeability or K_o have been alluded to in the discussion of dialyzer structure. The length of the blood and dialysate diffusion paths must be minimized by distributing blood and dialysate as thin films flowing over the membrane surfaces. Channeling or nonuniform flow distribution of either blood or dialysate reduces efficiency in a manner similar to the effect of ventilation-perfusion mismatch on pulmonary function. Secondary flow around the multiple point supports in plate dialyzers results in some convective mixing in the blood and dialysate streams and augments diffusive transport. Membrane pore size has a powerful effect on solute permeability, which decreases to zero as solute molecular size approaches pore size.

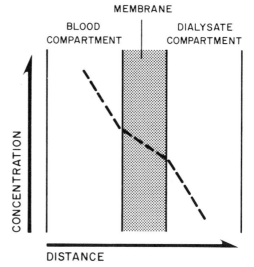

MEMBRANE

BLOOD
COMPARTMENT

DIALYSATE
COMPARTMENT

CONCENTRATION

DISTANCE

Fig. 1-5. Solute diffusion path in a dialyzer.

The design must be relatively nonthrombogenic, since local thrombus formation will block blood flow across the membrane and decrease efficiency.

Since the mechanism of solute transport is diffusion, driven by a concentration gradient, it follows that there is a unique K_o for each solute, which is dependent on its molecular size because the diffusion rate is inversely proportional to molecular size. In general, molecular size correlates well with molecular weight, although some solutes become hydrated in solution, resulting in increased size relative to their molecular weight and slower diffusion rates. The strong relationship of solute transport or clearance to molecular weight for a typical dialyzer is shown in Figure 1-6. For comparison, a similar relationship is illustrated for a normal kidney, which shows no molecular weight dependence of clearance for solutes of up to 10,000 daltons.

The total dialyzer capacity for transport of a specific molecular species is given mechanistically by $K_o \cdot A$, ml/min. The $K_o \cdot A$ represents the total flux divided by the concentration driving force, ΔC (see Eq. 1-7). The ΔC in this expression is defined as the log mean concentration gradient, which is derived from dialysate and blood inlet and outlet concentrations and flow rates. Consequently, $K_o \cdot A$ is a constant intrinsically independent of blood and dialysate flow rates. The $K_o \cdot A$ is a very useful parameter because, if this value is known, the clinically used transport parameters to be discussed below can be calculated for any set of blood and dialysate flow rates and can also be used to predict performance if there is clotting in the device.

Dialysance and Clearance. Since the dialyzer is clinically operated by adjusting inlet blood and dialysate flow rates (Q_{Bi} and Q_{Di}), it is clinically more relevant to describe transport by clearance (K) and dialysance (D), which are blood and dialysate flow-rate-dependent transport parameters. These two clinical parameters differ from each other and from $K_o \cdot A$ only with respect to the

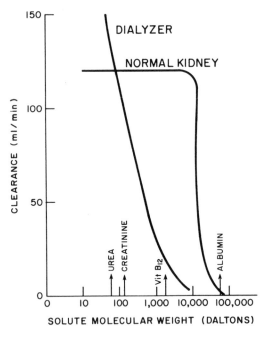

Fig. 1-6. Clearance of solutes as a function of molecular weight in a typical dialyzer and, for comparison, in a normal kidney.

definitions of the concentration gradient driving force. The definitions of K and D are given by Equations (1-9) and (1-10).

$$K = \frac{\text{flux}}{\Delta C} = \frac{J}{C_{Bi}} \tag{1-9}$$

$$D = \frac{\text{flux}}{\Delta C} = \frac{J}{C_{Bi} - C_{Di}} \tag{1-10}$$

In the case of K, the concentration driving force is represented by C_{Bi}, the blood inlet solute concentration. For D, the driving force is represented by $C_{Bi} - C_{Di}$; the dialysate inlet concentration is subtracted from the blood concentration to define ΔC. The units of K and D are important for understanding the physical meaning of these clinical transport parameters. The units of J are mass ÷ time. Therefore the units of $J \div \Delta C$ are (mass/time) · (volume/mass), which reduces to volume/time, and the usual clinical units for K and D are ml/min or L/min. Since K is defined as the amount of solute transferred divided by the amount contained in each milliliter of blood flowing into the dialyzer, the value for K represents the volume of blood completely cleared of solute per minute. In the case of D, C_{Di} is subtracted from C_{Bi} to calculate dialysance. D represents the volume of blood that would be completely cleared of solute if C_{Di} were zero. In single-pass dialysate flow geometry, C_{Di} is, in fact, zero, so $K = D$. In devices with recirculating dialysate flow, solute accumulates in dialysate and reduces the concentration driving force. At the start of dialysis with this flow geometry when C_{Di} is zero, dialysance will equal clearance, and subsequently D will remain constant, while K, the actual cleared volume, falls as C_{Di} rises. For simplicity in the following discussion, only the characteristics and clinical utility of K will be discussed. It should be remembered that D is a more appropriate description of the solute transfer process in recirculating dialysate systems.

It is important to appreciate the difference between K and flux (J). K remains constant throughout the dialysis, since it represents flux $\div \Delta C$. In contrast, flux decreases during dialysis as ΔC falls. From Equation (1-9) it can be seen that $J = C_{Bi}(K)$ and is directly dependent on concentration. Although urea *clearance* remains constant, the *amount* of urea removed per minute will be much less at the end than at the beginning of dialysis because C_{Bi} has decreased markedly. This is called a first-order removal mechanism because absolute removal is directly dependent on concentration.

Flow-Related Properties of Clearance. As shown in Equation (1-9), determination of K requires measurement of flux, the amount of solute transferred from blood to dialysate (or the opposite, depending on the concentration gradient) and the inlet blood concentration. Flux can be described from mass balance across the blood compartment as

$$\text{Flux} = \begin{array}{c} \text{solute transferred} \\ \text{from blood} \\ \text{to dialysate} \end{array} = \begin{array}{c} \text{solute content} \\ \text{inflowing} \\ \text{blood} \end{array} - \begin{array}{c} \text{solute content} \\ \text{outflowing} \\ \text{blood} \end{array} \quad (1\text{-}11)$$

$$J = Q_{Bi}C_{Bi} - Q_{Bo}C_{Bo} = Q_{Bi}C_{Bi} - (Q_{Bi} - Q_F)C_{Bo} \quad (1\text{-}12)$$

where Q_{Bi} is the rate of blood flow into the dialyzer and Q_{Bo} is the rate of blood flow out of the device, which in turn is equal to Q_{Bi} minus Q_F, the rate of ultrafiltration.

Since K is defined as J/C_{Bi}, then

$$K = Q_{Bi}\frac{C_{Bi} - C_{Bo}}{C_{Bi}} + Q_F\frac{C_{Bo}}{C_{Bi}} = Q_{Bi}(\text{ER}) + Q_F\frac{C_{Bo}}{C_{Bi}} \quad (1\text{-}13)$$

$$\begin{array}{cc} \text{Diffusive} & \text{Convective} \\ \text{clearance} & \text{clearance} \end{array}$$

where ER is the extraction ratio, defined as $(C_{Bi} - C_{Bo})/C_{Bi}$.

In clinical usage the dialyzer is usually operated as a combined diffusive and convective transport device. The relative net contributions of diffusion and convection to total K are shown in Equation (1-13). These expressions do not rigorously describe the actual mechanisms of transport, but are valid operational expressions that describe the net contribution of diffusion and convection to total transport. The amount of convective transport is usually small; this is treated quantitatively in the Appendix of this chapter.

The extraction ratio (ER) in Equation (1-13) describes the fractional decrease in blood solute concentration occurring across the dialyzer due to diffusive transport. If all solute in the inflowing blood is transferred, C_{Bo} is zero, so the ER = 1.0. The net convective clearance is zero irrespective of Q_F, since C_{Bo} is zero; diffusive clearance is equal to Q_{Bi}, since $K = Q_{Bi}(ER) = Q_{Bi}$. Under these operational conditions the clearance of the dialyzer is said to be blood flow-limited, since clearance is determined by the blood flow rate. The ER essentially reflects dialyzer permeability. At relatively low blood flow rates permeability exceeds the rate of solute delivery in inflowing blood so that ER = 1.0 and $K = Q_{Bi}$. As Q_{Bi} increases, solute delivery exceeds permeability, C_{Bo} increases (reflecting solute in outflowing blood that has not been transferred to dialysate) and, consequently, the ER decreases. K then becomes less than Q_{Bi}. The dialyzer is considered to be permeability-limited in this operational region.

The general relationship of K to Q_{Bi} will be similar for all dialyzers, but the exact relationships will vary and depend on flow geometry, membrane permeability, and total membrane area. These general and specific relationships can be seen in Figure 1-7, where K of urea is depicted as a function of Q_{Bi} for three hollow fiber dialyzers, differing only with respect to total membrane area. In all three devices there is a region of flow-limited clearance at low Q_{Bi}, followed by progressive transition to permeability-limited clearance at high blood flows. It should again be emphasized that total flux under these circumstances is a complex function of flow because of changes in mean solute concentration on the blood side rather than changes in K.

Recalling that in dialyzers transport of a solute is mechanistically determined by its diffusion rate, which is inversely proportional to molecular size, it follows that each solute will have a unique clearance curve as a function of blood flow rate. The family of clearance curves for a typical dialyzer is shown in Figure 1-8 for solutes of increasing molecular size, from urea to albumin.

Clearance versus K_oA. As described above, K is the clinically used parameter of transport capacity and represents the volumetric rate at which blood is cleared of solute at specified Q_{Bi} and Q_D values. In order to prescribe a K for a specific

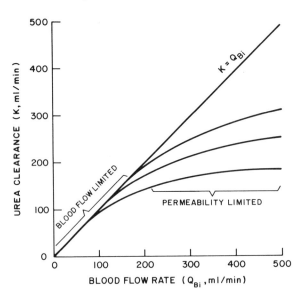

Fig. 1-7. Urea clearance (K) as a function of blood flow (Q_{Bi}) for three typical hollow fiber dialyzers with different surface areas. Clearance limitations due to blood flow and permeability are depicted.

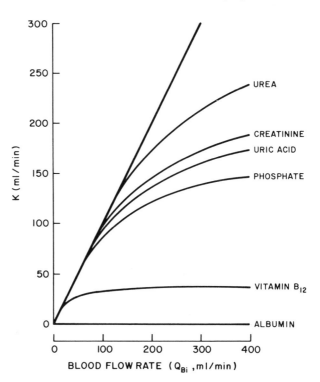

Fig. 1-8. Clearance (K) of solutes of varying molecular weight as a function of blood flow rate (Q_{Bi}) for a typical hollow fiber dialyzer.

solute, such as urea, during dialysis, it is necessary to know the relationship of K to Q_{Bi} and Q_D. Usually Q_D is fixed at 500 ml/min, so that curves such as those in Figures 1-7 and 1-8 are very helpful to find the Q_{Bi} required to achieve a specific K value, or, conversely, to find the K that will be delivered at any specific value of Q_{Bi}. In Figure 1-7, the urea clearance as a function of Q_{Bi} is shown for dialyzers with varying surface area. In Figure 1-8, typical solute clearances are shown again as a function of Q_{Bi}. The diminution in K as molecular weight increases is apparent (see also Figure 1-6). Such curves are available from the manufacturers or from the literature, or they can be generated by measuring K over a wide range of Q_{Bi} values.

The Effect of Clotting on K. In the reprocessed dialyzer it is essential to verify that solute transport capacity is not appreciably less than in the new device. Consequently, the magnitude of clotting assessed from measured change in priming volume as discussed earlier must be correlated with change in K.

In the hollow fiber dialyzer fiber occlusion by thrombus results in higher blood flow rate in open fibers if total Q_{Bi} remains constant. For example, if 20% of fibers are occluded, Q_{Bi} is distributed to the remaining 80% of open fibers, and flow rate per fiber will increase by 25%. Since K is blood flow-dependent, these values will increase in the open fibers and K will not decrease linearly with clotting as is the case with K_{UF}.

The effect of clotting on K can be readily calculated from the K_o and change

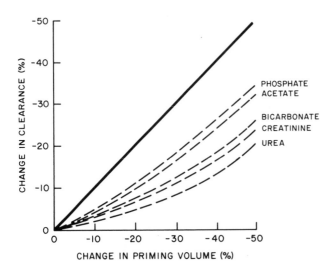

Fig. 1-9. Fractional change in clearance for solutes of varying molecular weight as a function of change in priming volume during reuse of a hollow fiber dialyzer.

in membrane area determined from change in fiber bundle volume. The fractional changes in these parameters as a function of fractional clotting in a typical dialyzer are shown in Figure 1-9. These curves show that K loss relative to clotting increases as molecular size increases. The reason is that permeability or K_o decreases as solute molecular size increases, and in the permeability-limited dialyzer K increases less with increasing blood flow (see Figure 1-7). If the widely used criterion for kidney retirement is adhered to (change in fiber bundle volume >20%), the decrease in K for all solutes depicted in Figure 1-8 will be quite minimal and range from 4 to 11%. The average loss in K over the life of a dialyzer would be even less, in the range of 2 to 5%, since dialyzer clotting reaches 20% only during the last use, after which it is retired.

THE DELIVERY SYSTEM

The delivery system functions are (1) to provide on-line proportioning of water with a dialysate concentrate, (2) to monitor dialysate for temperature, composition, and blood leaks, and (3) to control dialysate pressure and flow rate through the dialyzer. The bloodstream monitors for pressure and air are also incorporated in the delivery system, while the blood pumps may be separate or contained in the delivery system. If the blood pump is separate, it must be electrically tied into the delivery system, which contains the blood circuit monitors.

The composition of the dialysate solution is designed to approximate the normal electrolyte structure of plasma and extracellular water. In the early days of dialysis the dialysate was prepared manually in a 100-L holding tank by dissolving prepackaged dry chemicals. The preparation steps consisted of first mixing NaCl, KCl, and NaHCO$_3$ and then adding a small amount of lactic acid and initiating CO$_2$ flow through the solution to result in pCO$_2 \simeq 40$ mmHg and pH ≃ 7.40. After these steps were completed, $CaCl_2$ and $MgCl_2$ were added. This sequence was critical because the calcium and magnesium salts would precipitate out unless the pH of the bicarbonate solution was brought down to ~7.40.

The sharp increase in patient population in the early 1960s led to the development of systems for on-line preparation of dialysate by proportioning an aqueous dialysate concentrate with water. Acetate, which takes up a hydrogen ion during its metabolism, and therefore restores depleted body buffers, was substituted for bicarbonate because it simplified the proportioning requirements by eliminating the need for acidification.

Twenty years ago there was very little tailoring of dialysate composition for individual patients and nearly all patients were treated with identical dialysate. Under these circumstances it was believed to require less staff time if a large central delivery system was used to proportion and delivery dialysate through a network of piping to each patient station. These systems are still used in many units, although in recent years they have been increasingly replaced by individual delivery systems that provide greater flexibility in the dialysate prescription.

A critical design feature of the central system is the network of dialysate delivery piping. This must be carefully designed to avoid stagnant loops and dead ends that cannot be cleaned, sterilized, and subsequently flushed completely. The staff must be thoroughly familiar with the flow paths in order to develop proper sterilization and flushing procedures. Formaldehyde administration to patients from improperly flushed central systems has had disastrous results.

In recent years there has been increasing use of individual patient delivery systems that provide flexibility for tailoring therapy for individual patient needs. The principles of dialysate preparation and delivery are similar in both systems.

Dialysate Preparation

The delivery system functional components can be logically separated into those before and after the bypass valve. The functional components before or upstream from the bypass valve are depicted in Figure 1-10. The water input to the delivery system is purified by deionization and/or reverse osmosis, which will be considered in more detail below. The first step in the water preparation section is passage through a heat exchanger, in which countercurrent flow of warm spent dialysate transfers a substantial quantity of heat to incoming water and thereby reduces the energy requirements. The water then flows through a heater, which raises its temperature to the specified level, usually 37°C. This is followed by passage through a deaeration vacuum pump, which sharply reduces the content of dissolved air. This step is essential because tap water is invariably pressurized and contains large quantities of dissolved oxygen and nitrogen and typically becomes supersaturated when the temperature is raised to 37°C. This can lead to coating of conductivity probes, resulting in false alarms. It can also result in dialysis of air into the bloodcircuit with air bubbles collecting and filling

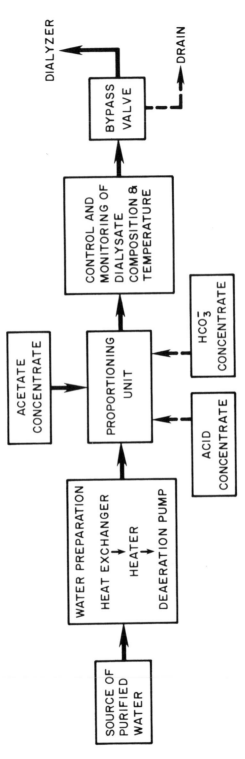

Fig. 1-10. Schematic representation of the functional components of a dialysate delivery system.

the venous drip chamber, so that there is risk of air embolism and of air bubble formation in the dialysate flow path which can disrupt the negative pressure control system.

The proportioning unit is a key section in which warm, deaerated water is proportioned with dialysate concentrate to provide dilute dialysate of specified composition. The concentrated salt solution is usually diluted ~34 parts water to 1 part concentrate, resulting in 35:1 dilution. Several mechanical proportioning designs are in use. In some machines two piston-fitted cylinders with a 34:1 volume ratio and common drive shaft are used. With this design, proportioning is fixed so that different concentrates must be used to vary the dialysate composition.

Separate pumps for water and concentrate are used in many machines and provide the potential flexibility to vary proportioning by controlling the speed of the concentrate pump. In these systems the pumping rate of the water pump is usually constant and Q_D is fixed at 500 ml/min. The capacity to vary the concentrate pumping rate requires a microprocessor-mediated feedback control system using on-line conductivity measurements.

Some proportioning units provide the option of using bicarbonate dialysate. This requires a three-stream system (see Figure 1-10) consisting of prepared water, acid concentrate, and bicarbonate concentrate. The acid stream contains the $CaCl_2$, $MgCl_2$, KCl, part or all of the NaCl, and sufficient HCl or lactic acid to yield a H^+ concentration of ~2 mEq/L (pH = 2.7) after proportioning with water. The water and acid concentrates are proportioned first and then proportioned with the bicarbonate concentrate, which results in dilute dialysate pH ~7.4 and prevents precipitation of the Ca and Mg salts. If the bicarbonate is added first, the addition of calcium will form insoluble salts. The bicarbonate concentrate is not stable in solution, since it gradually decomposes to sodium carbonate and CO_2; consequently, bicarbonate concentrate must be prepared from dry salt immediately prior to dialysis, which requires increased technician time.

Dialysate Composition and Temperature Control

The water preparation and proportioning sections of the delivery system are followed by a control and monitoring section (Figure 1-10). In this section of the flow path, one or two conductivity probes and a temperature thermistor are deployed. The structural requirements for adequate monitoring will be discussed later.

The proportioning unit is monitored (and controlled in feedback systems with capability of on-line varying of proportioning) by measuring total conductivity of the dilute dialysate. The electrical conductance or conductivity of dialysate is dependent on the concentration and mobility of all contained ions. It is usually expressed as mho $\times$ 10^{-3} (millimho) or mho $\times$ 10^{-4} and largely reflects the concentration of sodium salts in the solution, which comprise the bulk of the electrolyte content. The normal conductivity is about 13.5 ± 0.2 mmho. The exact relationship of conductivity to Na^+ concentration varies as a function of the K^+, Ca^{2+}, and Mg^{2+} concentrations, whether the buffer anion is acetate or bicarbonate, and as a function of the concentration of glucose.

The temperature of dialysate must be controlled to avoid both overheating of blood with resultant hemolysis and excessive low temperatures and consequent chilling of the patient. A tolerable temperature range is $37° \pm 3°C$. The dialysate temperature is measured by incorporation of a thermistor in the fluid flow path which serves to control the heater and monitor temperature.

The Bypass Valve. This is a critical component located in the final dialysate flow path prior to delivery to the dialyzer. There must be fail-safe integration of the conductivity and temperature monitors with the bypass valve to ensure that, if these parameters are out of limits, the valve will be activated and dialysate diverted away from the dialyzer to the drain.

Ultrafiltration Control Systems

The function of the delivery system beyond the bypass valve is primarily related to control of ultrafiltration Q_F, usually through control of dialysate pressure and transmembrane pressure (TMP). In addition to this primary function a blood leak detector is always incorporated in the dialysate outflow path (Figure 1-11) in order to monitor for dialyzer blood leaks. These functions are incorporated in each individual delivery system or in individual bedside consoles where a central system is used.

Four types of ultrafiltration control systems shown in Figure 1-11 are currently in clinical use. The simplest and most widely used system is depicted in Figure 1-11A. It relies on the use of an effluent dialysate pump and a manually adjusted variable flow resistance upstream from the dialyzer. The effluent pump often is used to operate an adjustable venturi orifice to control the level of negative pressure. With this system P_{Do} is manually adjusted to provide the TMP required to achieve prescribed Q_F based on the average K_{UF} for the dialyzer, using Equation (1-6). As discussed in the section on ultrafiltration, the error in fluid removal with this system is dependent on the TMP error and variability in K_{UF} such that Q_F error increases directly with these two parameters. The alarm limits on P_{Bo} are usually ± 25 to 50 mmHg; on P_{Do} there may be either no alarm limits or limits set in the range of ± 50 mmHg. This results in Q_F error limits as depicted in Figure 1-4.

In Figure 1-11B a more sophisticated system is depicted, which permits measurement of Q_F during dialysis. During the Q_F measurement, dialysate flow through the dialyzer is stopped by bypassing the dialysate stream around the dialyzer with either the inlet or outlet dialysate port remaining open to the dialysate stream. The dialysate compartment is therefore in equilibrium with the pressure in the dialysate stream. In response to the TMP, ultrafiltrate is formed and flows through a metering section. The dialysate pressure (P_{Do}) can be adjusted in this flow configuration until the Q_F reading is at the prescribed value.

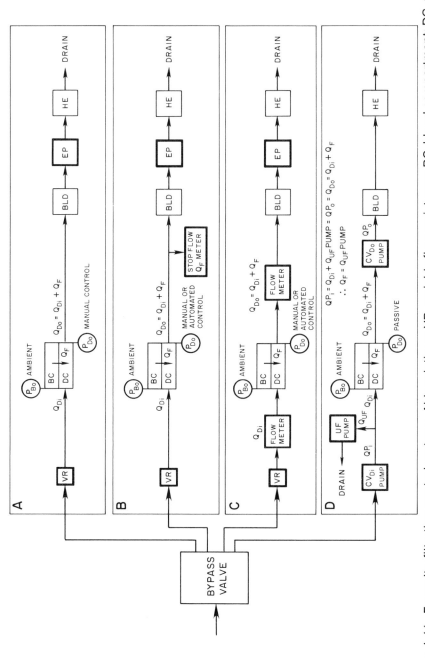

Fig. 1-11. Four ultrafiltration control systems. Abbreviations: VR, variable flow resistance; BC, blood compartment; DC, dialysate compartment; EP, effluent pump; HE heat exchanger; Q_{Di}, dialysate inlet flow; Q_{Do}, dialysate outlet flow; Q_F, ultrafiltrate; P_{Bo}, blood compartment pressure; P_{Do}, dialysate compartment pressure; $CV_{Di}PUMP$, constant volume dialysate inlet pump; $CV_{Do}PUMP$, constant volume dialysate outlet pump; $Q_{UF}PUMP$, ultrafiltrate pump; QP_i, pumped dialysate inlet flow; QP_o, pumped dialysate outlet flow.

21

This system is available in either a manually controlled or microprocessor-controlled design. The manually controlled version probably adds relatively little to the simpler system in Figure 1-11A. Since there is no on-line mechanism to control the TMP and Q_F during dialysis, the manually controlled system is therefore subject to similar errors. With the microprocessor-controlled system there is an algorithm that results in periodic Q_F measurement during dialysis and automatic adjustment of TMP to correct Q_F drift from the programmed value. This system is stated to be accurate to ± 60 ml/h. A potential disadvantage is lost dialysis time during the stop flow measurements, but this is stated to be minimal.

The system depicted in Figure 1-11C provides a mechanism for on-line measurement of Q_F through the use of flowmeters in the dialysate inlet and outlet streams. The difference in flow rates is considered equal to Q_F. It is apparent that the flowmeter must be highly precise, since Q_{Di} is 500 ml/min, while Q_{Do} will range from 500 to 520 ml/min, so the flowmeters must be able to accurately identify flow differentials in the range of 0 to 4%. This system is also available in manual and microprocessor-controlled automated versions and is similar to the stop flow system, in that Q_F is controlled through TMP control. The accuracy of the manual system would be subject to the same errors as the systems in Figure 1-11A, B. The microprocessor-controlled automated system provides very frequent on-line differential dialysate flow monitoring and is stated to provide Q_F accuracy similar to the microprocessor-controlled stop flow system.

The system depicted in Figure 1-11D is available only with microprocessor control and provides continuous on-line control of Q_F. This system differs from the other systems in that Q_F control is volumetric rather than through TMP control. The Q_F control section is a closed system, and dialysate is pumped into (QP$_i$) and out of (QP$_o$) this fixed volume section by matched microprocessor-controlled isovolumetric inlet and outlet diaphragm pumps. A microprocessor-controlled ultrafiltration pump removes fluid (Q_{UF}Pump) from the QP$_i$ stream at the rate programmed. Since it is a closed system with fixed volume and equal inlet and outlet flow rates, ultrafiltrate (Q_F) must flow across the membrane into the dialyzer outlet dialysate stream at the same rate that it is removed from the inlet stream by the ultrafiltrate pump, and thus $Q_F = Q_{UF}$Pump as shown in Figure 1-11D. Transmembrane pressure passively follows the volumetrically controlled Q_F as a function of the dialyzer K_{UF}. This system has the potential to provide highly precise Q_F control subject only to Q_{UF}Pump calibration errors or leakage across valves that need replacement.

The Blood Circuit

The blood circuit is depicted schematically in Figure 1-12. The flow path from the patient to the dialyzer inlet is termed the arterial blood line, and the flow path from dialyzer outlet back to the patient is termed the venous blood line. A blood pump is invariably required with present-day arteriovenous fistulas and grafts to achieve adequate flow through the dialyzer. Roller-type pumps are

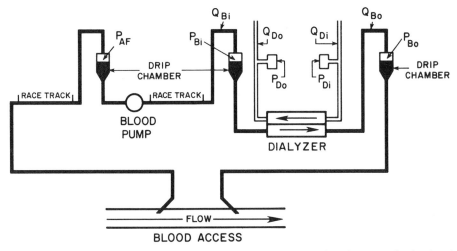

Fig. 1-12. Blood circuit of a hemodialysis delivery system. See Glossary in the front of this volume for abbreviations.

universally used. The occlusion of these pumps must be regularly checked because excessive occlusion can damage red cells, while inadequate occlusion will result in low flow rate.

Since dialyzer clearance is blood flow-dependent, it is important to assure that the prescribed Q_{Bi} is actually delivered by the pump. If pump calibration is checked at regular intervals, the dial setting can be used to establish the desired flow rate with adequate precision. The most precise method for blood flow measurement is the air bubble technique, in which an air bubble is injected into the tubing and its transit time over a specified length of the blood tubing or race track is measured.

As depicted in Figure 1-12, partially air-filled drip chambers are incorporated in the blood circuit at each site of pressure measurement and serve two functions. The provide a site for collection and evacuation of any air that is inadvertently introduced into the blood flow path. They also permit measurement of blood flow path pressures in air rather than in liquid, which simplifies the design requirements of the pressure sensing-blood interface. Ideally, it would be desirable to design an air-free system because the air-blood interface is a powerful stimulus to thrombus formation.

An air bubble detector is always incorporated into the venous blood line to guard against the rare but potentially disastrous consequences of air embolism. Although the drip chambers are effective in trapping the small amounts of air frequently introduced (primarily from bubble time measurements), if massive amounts of air or many microbubbles are introduced the drip chamber will be inadequate. The air bubble detector provides a safeguard by shutting down the blood pump if air is detected in the venous line.

Filters are also frequently incorporated in the venous blood line to trap any thrombus formed in the circuit. There is considerable uncertainty regarding the value of filters because the filter screen itself is a major site of local thrombus formation. Inspection of these screens after dialysis almost invariably shows more thrombus material clinging to the downstream surface than to the upstream surface. It should also be noted that the venous fistula needle provides an effective barrier to any large clots entering the patient. In our experience with more than 100,000 dialyses without venous filter traps, an embolus has never been observed.

Fistula Assessment: Bedside Technique. There is a rapid and simple maneuver that we have routinely employed at the bedside to grossly assess homologous or heterologous graft adequacy. The procedure is used when the patient is on dialysis. Both arterial and venous pressures are recorded. By the use of two fingers and firm pressure, the graft is completely occluded between the two fistula needles. The arterial and venous pressure are noted. With a fully competent graft the arterial pressure becomes less negative or moves toward zero, and the venous pressure will drop or move toward zero. In a graft with compromised arterial inflow, the arterial pressure will become more negative and, depending on the degree of stenosis, may trigger the arterial pressure alarm. The venous pressure will remain the same or rise modestly. If venous stenosis is present, which is more often found with grafts, when the graft is occluded the venous pressure will increase and the arterial pressure will remain unchanged or become slightly more negative. This then provides a rough index of graft patency and is a technique that can be used for each dialysis to monitor the access integrity and detect changes that may warn of impending access failure and recirculation.

Single-Needle Recirculation Assessment. One important aspect of single-needle dialysis that must be assessed is the amount of recirculation occurring with such a device. Significant recirculation (>20%) will affect, obviously, the efficiency of solute removal provided to the patient. The greatest effect will occur with low molecular weight solutes. There will be no influence on ultrafiltration except as pressures fluctuate during the cycle.

The objective of recirculation measurement is to obtain simultaneous pre- and postdialyzer blood samples under clinical operating conditions of the device and a representative sample of the systemic circulation. Accurate measurement of these values provides a reliable estimate of recirculation. Measuring just the arterial blood entering the dialyzer and a simultaneous systemic sample will provide useful information. If the BUN values differ by 0 ± 2 mg/dl, there is little if any recirculation. If the difference exceeds that amount, there is recirculation. However, to actually quantitate the amount of recirculation, one must simultaneously sample from the venous blood line. Knowing the amount of recirculation will allow adjustment of treatment time to provide adequate therapy to a particular patient.

The first method described to reliably assess recirculation requires simultaneous blood sampling from arterial, venous blood lines, and a peripheral venipuncture from the opposite arm. This provides a valid and accurate fractional amount of recirculation.

Recirculation is calculated using the following equation:

$$\frac{C_s - C_{Bi}}{C_s - C_{Bo}} \quad \text{or for urea} \quad \frac{BUN_s - BUN_i}{BUN_s - BUN_o} \tag{1-14}$$

where C_s and BUN_s are the systemic concentrations, mg/dl; C_{Bi} and BUN_i are the blood inlet concentrations, mg/dl; and C_{Bo} and BUN_o are the blood outlet concentrations, mg/dl.

This method, although very accurate, requires venipuncture, which is difficult in some patients and uncomfortable for all patients. Consequently, a modified procedure can be used to obtain a representative systemic sample by using the fistula needle already in place. The procedure is as follows:

1. Establish the desired operating conditions with the device.
2. Verify blood flow rate and dialysate flow rate.
3. Draw simultaneous pre- and postdialyzer blood samples from the injections ports.
4. Immediately stop the pump and apply line clamps on venous fistula tubing (as close as possible to the Y of the tubing set), the arterial blood line and fistula tubing.
5. Separate the arterial fistula line from the arterial blood line.
6. Attach a sterile syringe and withdraw the amount of blood equal to 3 times the volume of the single needle (~20 ml); disconnect and set aside, keeping sterile.
7. Obtain sample for measurement.
8. Return the 20 ml of blood.
9. Reattach all lines and release all clamps.
10. Restart blood flow.

Once blood flow through the dialyzer is stopped, no further change in concentration will occur. Therefore all requirements for accurate measurement are satisfied and result in a technique that is much more acceptable to the patient.

Monitoring

The actual process of dialysis requires the use of equipment and solutions that must be monitored and controlled to ensure safe and effective therapy to the patient. This procedure, which is performed thousands of times each day in the United States, remains potentially lethal. Therefore monitoring of certain parameters is essential to protect the patient. When examining the appropriate monitoring functions in this setting, it is preferable to separate them into the two circuits where they are to be incorporated; consequently, monitoring will be discussed as an integral part of either the blood or the dialysate circuit.

One should not assume that the incorporation of numerous sophisticated safety monitors assures an absolutely safe dialysis environment. The contribution of an informed, knowledgeable, interactive care provider is invaluable to interpreting machine displays and alarms for safe dialytic therapy.

Grimsrud and colleagues in 1967 listed 10 guidelines for safety monitoring of dialysis. Many of these guidelines continue to be germane to our discussion of monitoring:

1. The monitoring sensor should be positioned so that it detects, and can respond to, change before the aberrant condition reaches the patient.

2. Malfunctions should be displayed in user familiar units or terms.

3. Independent tests should be available to verify monitor function and accuracy.

4. Finite limits should be incorporated in some monitors and be resistant to user manipulation or attempts to override.

5. The monitor should be confined to one parameter or function.

6. Audiovisual components should be included in each alarm condition.

7. Activation of certain alarm systems should result in operational changes that are designed to protect the patient and that cannot be circumvented by the user, while an alarm condition continues.

8. Functional stability that prevents the introduction of subjective evaluation by the user should be one of the design considerations.

9. The monitor function is independent of the control function.

10. Monitor failure produces an alarm condition, which must be addressed by the user.

After the delivery system and blood circuit are set up, all monitor systems should be checked. This should be done just prior to dialysis to assure that the audiovisual alarms are operational and that the monitors are controlling the bypass valve, blood pump, and line clamp. A written checklist of the monitors should be contained in the treatment log.

Blood Circuit Monitors. Figure 1-12 portrays the most common configuration of the blood circuit. The segment from the patient to the blood pump will be at negative pressure. As a consequence, any leak in this segment will result in air being drawn into the blood path and through the dialyzer. The remaining segment from the blood pump back to the patient will be at positive pressure and a leak anywhere in this section will result in blood loss from the circuit.

Arteriovenous fistulas and homologous or heterologous grafts are the access modes most commonly employed in chronic hemodialysis patients. It is necessary to employ blood pumps to propel blood through the extracorporeal circuit and back to the patient. When using mechanical assist in this way, the blood compartment pressures should be monitored to avoid the following:

1. Accidental separation at any point in the blood circuit.

2. Continued pumping against an obstruction, either endogenous (clot or vessel wall) or exogenous (a clamp or kinked tubing), which may result in

introduction of air into the blood circuit if obstruction occurs between the patient and the pump (negative pressure section of the circuit) or rupture of the dialyzer or circuit if the obstruction occurs between the dialyzer and the patient.

The most common sites for blood compartment pressure monitoring are the prepump arterial drip chamber (see Figure 1-12) and after the dialyzer in the venous drip chamber. The ability to measure the pressure difference across the dialyzer (which would require monitoring at the dialyzer inlet and outlet) is not really needed, since improved technology in membranes and dialyzer fabrication has virtually eliminated the problem of major dialyzer obstruction due to clotting necessitating intradialytic replacement of the device.

The arterial pressure (prepump) monitor does not actually measure endogenous fistula pressure per se. It does provide several important pieces of information. One component measured is the resistance within the needle, which is a function of gauge size and length. It also provides an index of fistula supply relative to flow demand by the pump, and provides a guide to appropriateness of needle placement. In our experience, increasing negative arterial pressure over time has provided information on the adequacy of fistula blood flow. If one does not measure this segment of the circuit, the ability to monitor all these components is lost. Continued operation in the face of undetected high negative pressure can cause subclinical hemolysis with its undesirable effect on anemia or the introduction of air into the blood circuit with its attendant sequelae.

Routine monitoring of the venous pressure during dialysis (as measured in the venous drip chamber) also yields important information. It measures the resistance to flow through the needle as well as resistance to flow in the fistula. It will also detect needle placement problems. Over time, if needle placement is relatively constant, increasing venous pressure may indicate venous stenosis in grafts.

Therefore, the ability to routinely measure these pressures provides useful information to assess the integrity of the access as well as of the blood circuit.

With cannulas, the monitoring configuration will depend in part on the specific blood line that is used. Some blood lines with cannula connections place the arterial drip chamber between the blood pump segment and dialyzer, in other words, just before the dialyzer. This will allow monitoring of the pressure differential across the dialyzer, which can be used to assess clotting in the device. In this configuration both pressures will most likely be positive, with the arterial pressure always higher than the venous pressure. If the monitoring access points are the same as those used with fistulas, the same principles for interpretation will be used.

When using temporary access devices, such as double-lumen subclavian or femoral catheters or two femoral catheters, the monitoring configuration will be the same as with the usual fistula operation, and those principles will apply. The utilization of single-needle devices is described elsewhere in this chapter.

The important accessory function for the pressure monitors is that excursions outside the set limits activate the alarm sequence and stop the blood pump.

Whether the limits are preset or require operator selection, it is important to remember that limits should be placed so that they will guard against line separation. If separation occurs, the pressure will return to atmospheric pressure or zero. Therefore both limits on a pressure monitor should be set on the same side of zero so that pressure cannot cross to the opposite side of zero without alarming and stopping the blood pump.

Some individual delivery systems have preset limits incorporated into the software. Other systems require manual limit setting. These will vary, but should not exceed ± 50 mmHg. The most stringent limits that can be set will, in part, depend on the rhythmic fluctuations that occur with each blood pump revolution. The use of large-diameter monitor lines will result in larger swings in pressure readings. This will also be true if large-volume transducer protectors are used on the equipment.

There may be an additional safety factor in those monitors that do not allow manual manipulation of limits. In any case, excursion of pressures outside the defined limits should activate an audiovisual alarm and stop the blood pump. It is most helpful when attempting to troubleshoot the problem that the visual alarm lock in to indicate the source of the alarm condition. A mute and reset control are usually included in the pressure monitor.

Air detector. A serious complication of the dialysis procedure that is probably encountered more often than reported in the literature is iatrogenic air embolism. This event most often occurs when blood pumps are used for dialysis. It has been estimated that a major air embolism occurs in 1 per 2000 hemodialyses.

As noted earlier, the only segment of the blood circuit that experiences a negative pressure is that portion from the arterial fistula needle to the blood pump. Therefore this is the only area where air can be pulled into the system. Air can enter that system in several ways:

1. Air leaks around tubing joints, saline infusion sites, or heparin infusion lines placed before the blood pump

2. Excessive negative pressure related to inadequate fistula flow rate relative to pump demand or malposition of the arterial needle, which causes dissolved gases in blood to come out of solution

3. Unattended intravenous solution administration from a glass container attached to the prepump segment

4. If a prepump arterial drip chamber is used, a leak in the monitor line, drip chamber, transducer protector, or monitor diaphragm

If air is used to return the blood to the patient at the completion of dialysis, this is obviously another potential source.

The more common type of air embolism is due to foam rather than to a large bolus of air. Therefore, an air detector that is sensitive to foam should be incorporated into the blood circuit. The monitor should include the detector, a line clamp distal to the detector, and an independent circuit to stop the blood pump. The air detector is deployed on the venous drip chamber or on the venous blood line after the drip chamber.

The air detector should be sensitive to foam, but not saline, so that the dialyzer may be primed with saline and blood returned to the patient with saline while the detector is armed. Repetitive false nuisance alarms may result in the user disarming the system and forgetting to rearm it after completion of prime. If the detector can be disarmed or bypassed, there should be a persistent alarm that alerts the user to that condition.

Several types of air detectors have been used with varying success. One type is the level detector placed on the drip chamber and employing a photo-electric cell. When the level of air in the drip chamber reaches the cell, the alarm sequence is activated. This is the least reliable method since foam does not trigger the alarm. Also, a bright light will produce false positive alarms.

The type of air detector most commonly employed today is the ultrasonic foam detector, which uses ultrasonic waves to detect changes in the sound transmission between blood, saline, or foam. Activation of the alarm occurs only with the sensing of air or foam. These detectors have proven to be adequately sensitive to foam for patient protection. A sensitivity threshold of 0.2 ml/min of air is recommended in clinical operation.

The clamp device activated by the air detector should completely occlude the tubing and be competent in the face of high blood compartment pressure (+ 300 mmHg); occlusion should not damage the blood tubing. The time delay between detection and clamping should be in the microsecond range in order to assure air does not reach the patient.

The mechanisms used to stop the blood pump are triggered either by the detector itself or by pressure alarms resulting after the clamp activated by the detector has occluded the blood line. Either approach will work, although the pressure-triggered response again reinforces the need for appropriate limits on the venous pressure monitor.

Appropriate arming of the detector should be easily verified by visual inspection. Disarming of the air detector should be accompanied by a persistent audiovisual alarm that cannot be silenced without correction of the condition. Actual activation of the alarm during clinical operation should be followed immediately by the clamping operation and halt of the blood pump. This three-step sequence should be immediately followed by an audiovisual alarm that requires operator response.

Dialysate Circuit. As with the blood circuit, certain operating parameters of the dialysate circuit need to be monitored to adequately protect the patient. These parameters include conductivity, temperature, dialysate pressure, and blood leaks.

After the dialysate mixing point a conductivity probe measures conductivity and initiates a bypass mode if incoming dialysate is outside of specified limits. This is a crucial monitor, since patient exposure to hypertonic or hypotonic dialysate can result in cerebral damage and massive hemolysis; if it continues undetected, such exposure can be fatal. This probe is located before dialysate reaches the dialyzer and must result in fail-safe activation of the bypass mechanism to divert dialysate away from the dialyzer directly to the drain.

The types of proportioning methods were discussed earlier. In motor- or water-propelled fixed volume proportioning systems, usually only one conductivity probe is used to verify accuracy of dialysate concentration. In the conductivity feedback control delivery systems, two probes are used to ensure safe dialysate. As suggested by the guidelines for monitoring, the monitoring function and control function should be separate. Since the feedback control system uses one probe to properly adjust the concentrate pump, this is not considered an appropriate monitoring device. Therefore, another independent conductivity probe is included in the circuit to monitor the finished product before delivery to the dialyzer.

Temperature affects the conductivity measurement so that compensation for this effect is incorporated into all delivery systems. This separate circuit corrects the conductivity for temperature and therefore the meter reading or display.

There are important material constraints on conductivity probes. It is essential that they be noncorrosive, nontoxic, not easily fouled during use, and placed to minimize errors resulting from air bubbles in the dialysate. The conductivity meter or gauge should be accurate to $\pm 2\%$ and should be verified by an independent check frequently.

The placement of the probes must be at a point before the dialyzer and assure activation of the bypass valve immediately so that nonphysiologic dialysate does not reach the dialyzer. Activation of the monitor should produce an audiovisual alarm that alerts the operator to abnormal conditions. Limits for conductivity can be preset in the delivery system or manually set, which is considerably less desirable. Manual limits are subject to operator error and therefore do not provide sufficient safety for the patient. The manual system simplifies rinsing and sterilizing of the delivery system, since with preset limits, another operating mode is required for this step. It is essential that the system is designed so that it cannot operate in dialyze mode or with a dialyzer in place while in the rinse or sterilize mode.

As with conductivity, abnormal temperature can cause significant patient morbidity. In this instance, the greatest danger occurs with high temperature, in excess of 42°C. If blood is exposed to dialysate temperature in this range, hemolysis occurs. Dialysate temperature below 36°C can cause patient discomfort, but does not pose any substantial threat to patient safety. Therefore, the monitoring of dialysate temperature is most critical in avoidance of high temperature. This monitor is located before the dialyzer and activates the bypass mode when the upper limit is exceeded. Most delivery systems have incorporated a preset limit on the upper end of the temperature range, which cannot be manipulated by the operator. High temperature condition (>40°–42°C) should activate an audiovisual alarm and activate the bypass mechanism simultaneously. Some systems do not alarm with low temperature dialysate, while other systems produce an audiovisual alarm but no bypass. Whichever approach is used, the critical parameter is high-temperature dialysate with a fixed upper limit and bypass mode.

Another operating parameter of the dialysate circuit in single pass systems is the negative pressure used for ultrafiltration. Monitoring of this function with an upper limit avoids excessive levels (-500 mmHg) which could lead to rupture of the dialyzer. The other complication of continued dialysate pressure in excess of -500 mmHg is secondary degassing of dialysate, which causes air accumulation in the dialysate compartment, increased pressure drop across the dialysate compartment, and possible reduction in solute clearance due to air rather than dialysate contact with the membrane.

The dialysate pressure control systems have been discussed in some detail earlier. Negative or subatmospheric pressure in the dialysate is generated in modern delivery systems by a positive displacement effluent pump as shown in Figure 1-11.

The usual operating range for negative pressure is 0 to -500 mmHg. The pressure is optimally monitored on a gauge or meter with manually set limits, so that excursions outside the selected limits triggers an audiovisual alarm only. This does not interrupt any other operational system, but requires operator intervention to silence the alarm by returning the dialysate pressure to the desired level. In some delivery systems, monitoring is limited to a preset absolute upper limit that will alert the operator when pressure exceeds this value, with the objective of monitoring an upper limit where there is risk of dialyzer rupture and secondary degassing.

The actual monitor or gauge should be easily and frequently calibrated and should ideally be accurate to ± 10 mmHg. This goal is usually met with blood pressure monitors, but dialysate pressure gauges are often scaled in 25–50 mmHg increments. With high K_{UF} devices, this leads to considerable error in total fluid removed. With high K_{UF} devices dialysate pressure control to ± 20 mmHg would be the desired goal, but this is rarely achieved.

The regulation of dialysate flow is an important function of the delivery system in order to avoid compromising efficiency of the therapy, since clearance is dependent on Q_D. Usually, maintenance of the dialysate flow at the prescribed value ± 50 ml/min is the desired operating condition; the most commonly used flow rate is 500 ml/min. Some delivery systems use simple ball float flow meters that can be manually adjusted and monitored visually. Other delivery systems have no independent means of verifying flow, so that the operator must assume reliability and consistency in dialysate flow to the dialyzer. Independent verification of flow is desirable. At this time, there is no system that incorporates alarm limits for dialysate flow, which is reasonable, since clearance is relatively insensitive to Q_D in the range of 500 ml/min.

The last monitor function usually incorporated into modern single pass delivery systems is the blood leak detector, which guards against undetected blood loss during dialysis. With single pass dialysate flow of 500 ml/min, it is impossible to rely on visual inspection of the effluent stream. Therefore, ongoing sensitive detection for the presence of hemoglobin should be a part of every delivery system or bedside console. The critical objectives for this monitor are adequate sensitivity to hemoglobin and design of the measuring receptacle so as to avoid the interference of air bubbles in the outflow stream. The sensing apparatus should be cleaned frequently, since deposits from dialysate may render it incompetent.

There should be an upper maximum limit to hemoglobin present, on the order of 70 mg/L (corresponding to blood loss of about 0.4 ml/min), beyond which the blood pump is stopped to avoid excessive blood loss by the patient. Return of the blood contained in the dialyzer and lines to the patient in the event of a blood leak may require override of the monitor or removal of the dialysate lines from the monitor path before this can be accomplished.

Water Treatment. During dialysis the patient's bloodstream is typically exposed to approximately 120 L of dialysate across the dialysis membrane, which is highly permeable to low molecular weight solutes and has limited permeability up to mol wt ~10,000. Consequently, it is essential to remove any toxic contaminants that could diffuse into the bloodstream from tap water used to prepare dialysate. The quality of the tap water varies considerably, depending on the source, and can also vary as a function of the season in a given geographic location.

The contaminants of water may be grouped into sediments, ionized salts, un-ionized salts, organics, and microorganisms.

Visible contamination of water results from particulate sediments. Particulate materials would not cross dialysis membranes but may damage the equipment and must be removed, usually by passage through a 5-μm filter, as the first step in water treatment.

Ionized salts are most effectively removed by mixed bed cationic-anionic deionizers (DI), which will remove greater than 99% of ionic species. There are a number of ionized salts in city water, which may pose a hazard of toxicity to dialysis patients. These include salts of calcium, copper, fluoride, nitrates, sulfates, sodium, and zinc. These are most effectively removed by a deionizer.

Reverse osmosis (RO) membranes are required to remove most organics, microorganisms, and un-ionized salts. These are tight membranes with effective pore diameter of angstroms, which reject all solutes of mol wt >200. In addition, they operationally behave as uncharged salt rejection membranes and reject ~90% of all charged species irrespective of molecular weight. It is thus apparent that reverse osmosis has a broader range of water purification properties than deionization, but deionization is more effective for removal of charged species.

Aluminum is a very dangerous contaminant that can result in dialysis dementia and osteomalacia with multiple fractures. The proportion of ionic aluminum present is strongly pH-dependent, and in the common pH range of 6–7 only 30–50% of aluminum is ionized. Consequently, deionizers generally do not remove aluminum as effectively as reverse osmosis. If there is any question of toxic aluminum levels in the water supply, reverse osmosis is essential. The major source of aluminum is alum (aluminum sulfate) added to the water supply as a coagulant to purify the water for drinking.

The major organic contaminants of concern are pyrogens, which normally have mol wt ~1,000,000, but at times pyrogenic toxicity may be retained in pyrogen fragments with mol wt as low as 10,000. These organics will be completely removed by reverse osmosis membranes.

Chloramines are often added to municipal water supplies to reduce bacterial contamination. These are low molecular weight un-ionized compounds, which are not effectively removed by either deionization or reverse osmosis, but can be adsorbed on carbon filters. They can cause severe hemolytic anemia with denaturation of hemoglobin by both direct oxidation and inhibition of the hexose monophosphate shunt.

Bacterial colonization can readily occur in particulate filters, carbon adsorption filters, deionizers, and reverse osmosis units. It is not possible to sterilize particulate and carbon filters or deionizers, while sterilization of reverse osmosis units with formaldehyde is readily accomplished. These considerations dictate that, to assure that the purified water is free of pyrogens and bacterial contamination, the reverse osmosis unit should be located as the final step in water treatment with filters and deionizers deployed in the upstream flow path.

The optimal water treatment system consists of particulate filter, deionizer, and reverse osmosis units in series, and, if chloramines are known to be present, a carbon adsorption filter added between deionization and reverse osmosis units. Such a water treatment will readily meet the water standards proposed by the Association for the Advancement of Medical Instrumentation (AAMI). The product water of the carbon adsorption filter, deionizer, and reverse osmosis units must be regularly monitored to ensure that each component is operating properly. The filters and deionizers must be replaced relatively frequently, depending on the level of particulate and ionic contaminants, while the reverse osmosis membranes usually have a lifetime of 2–5 years.

The piping configuration of the water treatment system, subsequent dialysate preparation, and delivery system must be carefully designed to avoid stagnant and dead spaces where bacterial multiplication and formation of pyrogens can occur. All segments of the dialysate flow path, including the reverse osmosis unit, the final step of water treatment, must be regularly sterilized with formaldehyde.

Coagulation Monitoring. In order to maintain the patency of the extracorporeal circuit, anticoagulation is generally necessary. The anticoagulant nearly always used is heparin, although there have been some recent reports of trials with prostacycline used as a systemic anticoagulant. Regional anticoagulation of the dialyzer circuit by infusion of sodium citrate into the arterial blood line and calcium into the venous return line has also been reported. However, the only widely used anticoagulant for acute and chronic hemodialysis continues to be heparin.

Heparin is a particularly attractive anticoagulant for the relatively brief time span of dialysis because its anticoagulant effect is immediately and easily measured and can be almost immediately terminated if necessary by the administration of protamine. In addition, because of its relatively high molecular weight, it is not dialyzable and hence not lost across the dialyzer.

For the stable dialysis patient in whom heparin will not aggravate or precipitate bleeding, the goal is to prolong the patient's clotting time sufficiently to prevent clotting within the extracorporeal circuit and thus avoid compromising therapy. The amount of heparin required to accomplish this goal is usually prescribed in one of four ways:

1. An arbitrary dose administered to all patients
2. A dose based on an arbitrary number of units per kilogram of body weight
3. A prescribed dose based on the type of dialyzer used
4. Individual assessment of heparin activity in each patient and dose prescribed based on that information

There are two kinds of heparin administration: (1) an intravenous bolus dose at the start of dialysis and repeated intermittently during the course of therapy, and (2) a bolus dose just prior to the start of dialysis and then a slow constant infusion during all or part of the treatment. With the intermittent dose, the level of anticoagulation will oscillate over the course of dialysis, while with the infusion technique, a relatively constant level of anticoagulation will be maintained during the dialysis.

For the acute or chronic patient at risk of bleeding, there are two methods of heparin administration. The first method is called regional heparinization. The objective of this approach is to anticoagulate the blood circuit and not the patient, which requires simultaneous infusions of heparin and protamine (which neutralizes the heparin effect). Heparin is added to the blood after leaving the patient in the arterial blood line and protamine is administered after the dialyzer in the venous blood line before the blood returns to the patient.

The second method is called controlled or low-dose heparinization. This procedure aims to achieve and maintain a modest prolongation of clotting time during dialysis, using generally small doses of heparin by constant infusion. This method requires the manipulation of only one drug, therefore technically it is much simpler.

Regardless of the method of heparinization in either type of patient, for critical monitoring there must be a method for determining the level of anticoagulation through serial measurements of the clotting time. An early method used for this purpose was the Lee-White clotting time. A major problem with the use of this method for heparinized dialysis patients was the time required to obtain the results. Frequently values were in excess of 20 minutes and the test required constant attendance to obtain reliable results.

There are several requirements that should be addressed when selecting a clotting time method for the clinical setting: (1) the test should give rapid, reliable results; (2) the test must be done at the bedside; (3) the blood requirements must be minimal (<0.5 ml optimally); and (4) the test must be inexpensive. In the last 10 years, several tests have been introduced which meet some or all of these criteria.

The activated plasma partial thromboplastin time has been used in some instances to monitor anticoagulation in dialysis. This test requires separation of plasma from red cells, reconstitution of sample with calcium, addition of activating reagent, and automated measurement. The technique does not lend itself to bedside use and the time required to perform the necessary steps does not provide rapid feedback.

Another clotting time test used by many dialysis facilities is the activated clotting time (ACT) first described by Hattersley in 1966. The test can be done on whole blood and uses siliceous earth or ground glass as an activating agent.

The crucial parameters for accurate performance of the test consist of temperature control to 37°C, accurate measurement of the blood sample volume, timing, and consistent determination of the end point, which is described as the first evidence of clotting observed in the tube. This end point differs from other clotting time tests in that it is not a solid gel or typical "clot," which is easier to recognize.

The activated clotting time test involves the addition of 2 ml of whole blood to a prewarmed test tube (37°C) containing the reagent. The tube is incubated at constant temperature for generally 1 minute, then tilted at 5-second intervals until the initial formation of clot is observed, and the time is recorded to the nearest 5-second interval. The incubation, tilting, and timing processes have been incorporated into automated equipment, which can be used to obtain results comparable to the manual method. This automated test uses less blood, on the order of 0.5 ml per test. There is also equipment currently commercially available that uses ground glass as the activating agent.

The equipment requirements include the tubes containing the reagent, suitable syringes and needles for obtaining blood samples, and, if using the manual method, a constant temperature dry heat block and a stopwatch.

The normal activated clotting time values for baseline clotting times (measured before any heparin is given) are 90–120 seconds. Excursions above 120 seconds are considered to reflect inherent coagulation deficiencies. Target values during heparin administration will depend on the anticoagulation objective for a particular patient. For the stable patient an activated clotting time value of approximately 1.5 to 2 times the baseline value is often targeted. For the acute bleeding risk patient, a modest increase (e.g., 30 seconds) over baseline activated clotting time is usually selected as the target.

The major problem with the activated clotting time test is the lack of sensitivity encountered. In the presence of small doses of heparin, one may not be able to measure clotting time differences with this test. This is further complicated by the subjectivity of establishing the end point with the manual activated clotting time method. This latter problem may be diminished with the automated equipment.

Another test that has been used to monitor heparin administration in dialysis patients is the whole blood partial thromboplastin time (WBPTT), first described by Blakely in 1966. This test uses whole blood (0.4 ml) which is added to a test tube (12 × 75) containing an activating reagent (0.2 ml) and incubated at 37°C for 35 seconds followed by tilting at 5-second intervals measured by a stopwatch until a solid clot is achieved. The time is recorded to the nearest 5-second interval. To date, this test has not been automated so that the manual method is the only one employed in dialysis facilities. In our opinion, this test meets all the criteria for an optimal clotting time method as defined above.

Another factor influencing our preference for this particular test is the sensitivity of the method to modest increases in heparin doses. Unlike the activated clotting time test, the whole blood partial thromboplastin time test will track small changes in administered heparin doses, which is particularly useful in anticoagulation of the patient at risk for bleeding, where small amounts of heparin are used to maintain modest prolongation of clotting times. This test is also suitable for use with a heparin kinetic model to guide therapy. The equipment requirements are minimal and consist of tuberculin syringes, 20 G needles, a stopwatch and a constant temperature (37°C) heat block. The reagent is added to the tubes on site, using either a tuberculin syringe or constant volume sampler. The end point is easily determined and is thus more consistent and reproducible.

The normal baseline values for the whole blood partial thromboplastin time test, using Actin FS as the reagent, is 60–85 seconds. Excursions outside this range reflect either technical error or inherent coagulation defects. Target values for regular system heparinization in stable patients is 140 ± 10 seconds. The target for the bleeding risk patient will vary somewhat depending on the condition of the patient; our usual target range is 90–105 seconds, depending on the risk assessment.

Weight Monitoring.   One of the important goals to be achieved during dialysis is the removal of fluid (and hence weight change) that has accumulated between dialyses. Various configurations for scales exist to measure pre- and postdialysis weights. The one(s) selected will depend on the condition of the patient(s) and her or his ability or inability to stand or sit. The most important factor in selecting a scale should be accuracy, ± 0.1 kg, and linearity across the weights anticipated in an adult dialysis population. A standing scale should probably include some mechanism that will allow support of the patient who is unsteady without interfering with accurate weighing.

Patients who wear street clothes during their treatment should be weighed without shoes or heavy garments or objects frequently found in pockets. Whether street clothes or hospital garments are worn, the important object is consistency.

When determining total ultrafiltrate to be removed during dialysis, one should not neglect intake that may occur during the treatment. This should include all oral intake or saline the patient receives for the dialyzer prime and which is returned to the patient at the end of dialysis. Depending on the type of dialyzer used and the degree of red cell return desired, this can range from 100 to 250 ml for each treatment.

Ongoing weight measurement during dialysis may be desirable for acutely ill patients or if one is uncertain of the ultrafiltration coefficient of a dialyzer. If possible, the equipment should be versatile enough to allow use with chairs or beds. The patient's weight can then be obtained directly on the scale. The major requirement is that subsequent weights obtained during dialysis reflect the same conditions. In other words, attention should be paid to those items present when the initial patient weight is obtained, and these should be included with all subsequent weight measurements. Blood or other fluids received during dialysis should be included as intake when calculating the amount to be removed during the treatment so that the postdialysis weight will reflect the desired weight loss.

APPENDIX

Relative Importance of Diffusive and Convective Transport

Analogous to equation (1-13), dialysance (D) can be expressed as

$$D = Q_{Bi} \frac{C_{Bi} - C_{Bo}}{C_{Bi} - C_{Di}} + Q_F \frac{C_{Bo}}{C_{Bi} - C_{Di}} = Q_{Bi}(ER) + Q_F \frac{C_{Bo}}{C_{Bi} - C_{Di}} \quad (1\text{-}15)$$

Diffusive   Convective
dialysance   dialysance

The relative contributions of diffusion and convection to total dialysance are given by Equation (1-15). These relationships can be converted from dialysance to flux (the rate of solute removal rather than volume of blood cleared) by multiplying Equation (1-15) by $C_{Bi} - C_{Di}$, resulting in

$$\underset{\text{Total flux}}{(C_{Bi} - C_{Di})D} = \underset{\substack{\text{Diffusive} \\ \text{flux}}}{(C_{Bi} - C_{Bo})Q_{Bi}} + \underset{\substack{\text{Convective} \\ \text{flux}}}{Q_F C_{Bo}} \quad (1\text{-}16)$$

It is difficult to explore generally the relative importance of diffusive and convective flux using Equation (1-16) because it contains C_{Bo}. A more general relationship based on only inlet concentrations can be derived from consideration of mass balance across the device and is given by

$$J = (C_{Bi} - C_{Di})D + \left[C_{Bi} - \frac{D}{Q_{Bi}}(C_{Bi} - C_{Di}) \right] Q_F \quad (1\text{-}17)$$

Total   Diffusive   Convective
flux   flux   flux

Equation (1-17) provides a general definition of the relative contributions of diffusive and convective flux to total flux as a function of D, Q_{Bi}, C_{Bi}, C_{Di} and Q_F. It is instructive to vary these parameters in order to examine the effects Q_F may have on total flux of several important solutes.

In the case of urea, C_{Di} is usually zero and D/Q_{Bi} (equivalent to the extraction ratio in Equation (1-13) is quite high at usual blood flow rates of $\sim$200 ml/min. Typical values for urea transport parameters would be $C_{Bi} = 0.60$ mg/ml, $C_{Di} = 0$, $D = 170$ ml/min, $Q_{Bi} = 200$ ml/min, and $Q_F = 20$ ml/min. Substitution of these values in Equation (1-17) results in

$$J_{urea} = (0.60 - 0)(170) + \left[0.60 - \frac{170}{200}(0.60 - 0) \right] 20$$

$$= 102 \qquad\qquad + 1.80 \qquad\qquad = 103.80 \text{ mg/min}$$

It is apparent that high ultrafiltration rate contributes very little ($\sim$2%) to total urea removal because the diffusive flux is very high.

When D is low relative to Q_{Bi} or the difference between C_{Bi} and C_{Di} is small, the diffusive flux becomes smaller and variability in Q_F (and hence convective flux) can have a significant impact on total flux rate. This can be illustrated by consideration of HCO_3^- dialysis, where typical transport parameters would be $C_{Bi} = 0.026$ mEq/ml (26 mEq/L), $C_{Di} = 0.036$ mEq/ml, $D = 120$ ml/min, $Q_{Bi} = 200$ ml/min, and $Q_F = 0$ or 20 ml/min. Substitution of these values in Equation (1-17) with $Q_F = 0$ results in

$$J_{HCO_3^-} = (0.026 - 0.036)(120) + \left[0.026 - \frac{120}{200}(0.026 - 0.036) \right] 0$$

$$= -1.20 \qquad\qquad + (0.032)(0) \qquad\qquad = -1.20 \text{ mEq/min}$$

whereas, if $Q_F = 20$ ml/min,

$$J_{HCO_3^-} = -1.20 \qquad\qquad + 0.032(20) \qquad\qquad = -0.56 \text{ mEq/min}$$

Note that $J_{HCO_3^-}$ is a negative number because $C_{Bi} < C_{Di}$ and the sign convention used here for flux is positive for solute transfer from blood to dialysate (urea) and negative for transfer from dialysate to blood, as with HCO_3^-. A major effect of Q_F on $J_{HCO_3^-}$ can be seen above where flux is decreased by 33% from -1.20 to -0.56 when Q_F increases to 20 ml/min. The C_{Di} HCO_3^- required with $Q_F = 20$ ml to achieve $J_{HCO_3^-}$ equal to that at $Q_F = 0$ can also be calculated from the data above. These calculations show that C_{Di} HCO_3^- would have to be 42 mEq/L at the high Q_F to achieve net HCO_3^- flux equal to that with C_{Di} $HCO_3^- = 36$ mEq/L and $Q_F = 0$. The patient who routinely has high interdialytic weight gains and requires high Q_F will have substantially less alkalinization or buffer repletion during dialysis than the patient with minimal weight gain and low Q_F, even though dialysate HCO_3^- concentration is identical. Similar relationships apply to net acetate flux with acetate dialysis.

It is particularly instructive to examine the relative contributions of diffusive and convective flux to the Na concentration of ultrafiltrate removed. These relationships can be examined by dividing Equation (1-17) by Q_F, which, after rearrangement, results in

$$\frac{J}{Q_F} = C_{Bi} + (C_{Bi} - C_{Di}) \left(\frac{D}{Q_F} - \frac{D}{Q_{Bi}} \right) \qquad (1\text{-}18)$$

In the case of Na, the term J/Q_F is the rate of Na flux divided by the rate of H_2O flux, and therefore represents the net concentration of Na in the ultrafiltrate removed. It is apparent from inspection of Equation (1-18) that, when there is no diffusion gradient (i.e., $C_{Bi} = C_{Di}$ or $C_{Bi} - C_{Di} = 0$), $J/Q_F = C_{Bi}$ and the ultrafiltrate is isotonic to plasma. The concentration terms for charged solutes in blood such as Na^+ must be expressed for the aqueous phase of plasma and corrected for Donnan effects in order to determine the effective Na diffusion gradient between blood and dialysate. In the following discussion C_{Bi} values will be considered to represent aqueous, Donnan-corrected plasma Na concentration.

Typical Na transport parameters would consist of $D = 0.160$ L/min, $Q_{Bi} = 0.200$ L/min, $C_{Bi} = 140$ mEq/L, and $Q_F = 0.010$ L/min. If $C_{Di} = 130$ mEq/L, the Na$^+$ concentration of ultrafiltrate removed can be calculated using Equation (1-18) as follows:

$$\frac{J_{Na}}{Q_F} = 140 + (140 - 130) \left(\frac{0.160}{0.010} - \frac{0.160}{0.200} \right)$$

$$= 140 + \qquad 152 \qquad\qquad = 292 \text{ mEq/L}$$

If $C_{Di} = 150$ mEq/L, the value of $\dfrac{J_{Na}}{Q_F}$ would be

$$\frac{J_{Na}}{Q_F} = 140 + (140 - 150) \left(\frac{0.160}{0.010} - \frac{0.160}{0.200} \right)$$

$$= 140 \qquad\quad - 152 \qquad\qquad = -12 \text{ mEq/L}$$

The above examples show that if $C_{Bi} - C_{Di}$ varies from $+10$ to -10 mEq/L, the Na$^+$ content of ultrafiltrate can vary from 292 mEq/L to less than zero or -12 mEq/L. With a diffusive gradient of $+10$ mEq/L from blood to dialysate the ultrafiltrate removed is extremely hypertonic, while with a negative gradient of -10 mEq/L, Na$^+$ free water is removed with a small net infusion of Na$^+$ into the blood occurring simultaneously. Although fluid is removed at the same rate of 600 ml/h, hypertonic Na$^+$ and water removal would be far more likely to cause symptomatic hypotension than Na$^+$ free water removal. Thus Na$^+$ diffusion gradients may significantly relate to the morbidity of ultrafiltration and require individualized kinetic modeling of Na and water removal to minimize dialysis morbidity.

REFERENCES

Comty CM, Shapiro FL: Pretreatment and preparation of city water for hemodialysis. pp. 142–148. In Drukker W, Parsons FM, Maher JF (eds.): Replacement of Renal Function by Dialysis. Martinus Nijhoff, Boston, 1983

Drukker W: A historical review. In Drukker W, Parsons FM, Maher JF (eds): Replacement of Renal Function by Dialysis. pp. 3–44. Martinus Nijhoff, Boston, 1983

Gotch FA: Correlation of transport properties of new and reused hollow fiber dialyzers. In Multiple Use of Hemodialyzers. Final Report to the National Institute of Arthritis, Diabetes and Digestive and Kidney Disease. NIH, Contract No. N01-AM-9-2214, 1981

Gotch FA, Keen ML: Precise control of minimal heparinization for high bleeding risk hemodialysis. Trans Am Soc Artif Intern Organs 23:168, 1977

Gotch F, Lipps BJ, Weaver J, et al: Chronic hemodialysis with the hollow fiber kidney (HFAK). Trans Am Soc Artif Intern Organs 15:87, 1969

Grimsrud L, Cole JJ, Lehman GA, et al: A central system for the continuous preparation and distribution of hemodialysis fluid. Trans Am Soc Artif Intern Organs 10:107, 1964

Hemodialysis systems standard (proposed). Association for the Advancement of Medical Instrumentation, Arlington, VA, 1978

Henderson LW: Biophysics of ultrafiltration and hemofiltration. pp. 242–265. In Drukker, W, Parsons FM, Maher JF (eds): Replacement of Renal Function by Dialysis. Martinus Nijhoff, Boston, 1983

Hoenich NA, Kerr DNS: Dialyzers. pp. 106–137. In Drukker W, Parsons FM, Maher JF (eds): Replacement of Renal Function by Dialysis. Martinus Nijhoff, Boston, 1983

Keshaviah PR, Shaldon S: Hemodialysis monitors and monitoring. pp. 223–242. In Drukker W, Parsons FM, Maher JF (eds): Replacement of Renal Function by Dialysis. Martinus Nijhoff, Boston, 1983

Klein E, et al.: Evaluation of hemodialyzers and dialysis membranes. Report of a study group for the Artificial Kidney-Chronic Uremia Program of NIAMDD. DHEW Publ (NIH)77:1294, 1977

Lindsay RM: Practical use of anticoagulants. pp. 201–223. In Drukker W, Parsons FM, Maher JF (eds): Replacement of Renal Function by Dialysis. Martinus Nijhoff, Boston, 1983

Parsons FM, Stewart WK: The composition of dialysis fluid. pp. 148–171. In Drukker W, Parsons FM, Maher JF (eds): Replacement of Renal Function by Dialysis. Martinus Nijhoff, Boston, 1983

Sargent JA, Gotch FA: Principles and biophysics of dialysis. pp. 53–97. In Drukker W, Parsons FM, Maher JF (eds): Replacement of Renal Function by Dialysis. Martinus Nijhoff, Boston, 1983

2

ACCESS FOR DIALYSIS

William C. Krupski   Margaret Devney-Bruks
Ronald L. Webb   David J. Effeney

HISTORY

Gaining access to the circulation has been a major tour de force in the treatment of human disease. Sir Christopher Wren, most widely known and honored today for his achievements in architecture, in 1657 was the first to inject drugs into dogs, using a cannula fashioned from a quill. Sir Robert Boyle published Wren's experiments and in 1663 was first to successfully inject drugs intravenously into humans. As was often the case in early experiments, prison inmates were used as subjects.

Success in achieving chronic access to the circulation came to pass much later. In spite of Willem Kolff's invention of a usable artificial kidney machine in 1943, there was little enthusiasm for chronic hemodialysis. With each procedure a separate cutdown on artery and vein was required, quickly exhausting access sites. Thus, hemodialysis was used only in patients with acute renal failure.

In 1960, Scribner, Dillard, and Quinton made chronic hemodialysis practical by devising a Teflon-Silastic arteriovenous shunt. This external shunt, however, had some grave disadvantages—it was too often the source of infection, thrombosis, and restricted activity—which impelled scientists to further efforts at creating safer and more convenient access routes. In 1966, Brescia and Cimino developed the subcutaneous radial artery-to-cephalic vein arteriovenous fistula. Subsequently, a number of synthetic materials were introduced to create arteriovenous fistulas.

Peritoneal dialysis has been increasingly employed to treat patients with both acute and chronic renal failure. Continuous ambulatory peritoneal dialysis (CAPD), a relatively new technique with fast-growing clinical application, may be the therapy of choice for many patients with end-stage renal failure, as discussed in Chapter 4.

Access routes, either peritoneal or vascular, must be compatible with the individual patient's needs. The fact that access may be necessary for many years obliges attending physicians and nurses to preserve potential access sites at the onset of care of the patient with renal disease.

ACUTE DIALYSIS

External Arteriovenous Shunts

A number of external arteriovenous shunts are presently available. Some variety of the basic Scribner shunt introduced in 1960, is used most commonly in the United States, but the Thomas, Allen-Brown, and Buselmeier shunts are used in special circumstances. Unusual sites for shunt placement have been described by Hoeltzenbein, Belzer and Kountz, and Kauffman.

The basic components of the Scribner shunt are Teflon-beveled arterial and venous cannula tips, Silastic connecting tubing attached to each tip, and a Teflon shunt connection between arterial and venous tubing (Fig. 2-1). The curved connecting tubing introduced by Scribner and associates is still quite popular because the wrist or ankle joint is unencumbered. When these shunts thrombose, however, restoration of patency can be problematic because it is extremely dif-

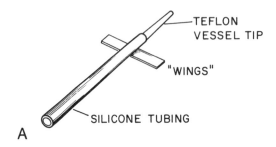

Fig. 2-1. (A) Straight and (B) curved Scribner shunts.

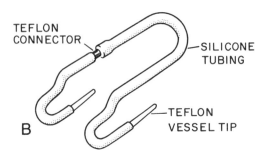

ficult to direct a Fogarty catheter around curves. In contrast, when straight connecting tubing is used, a thrombus can be removed easily with a Fogarty catheter. Accidental dislodgement, the major disadvantage of straight tubing, can be minimized by suturing the tubing to deep fascia and by attaching Silastic wings to the subcutaneous portion of the catheter. External splints, used as a contrivance to prevent dislodgement, are cumbersome and uncomfortable.

Certain basic principles apply to the placement of any external arteriovenous shunt. Most importantly, the patient's potential requirement for chronic hemodialysis must be considered so that choice vessels may be spared. The lower extremity should be used in most instances, employing either the posterior tibial artery or the dorsalis pedis artery and the greater saphenous vein. If vessels in the lower extremity are unsuitable because of peripheral vascular disease, phlebothrombosis, thrombophlebitis, or previous surgical use of the saphenous vein, the radial or ulnar artery and the cephalic or basilic vein may be used. Ingenuity and perseverance are occasionally necessary to find a suitable vein. A combination of a wrist artery and an upper arm vein should be avoided because of the thrombogenic long length of tubing required, the restriction of arm movement, and the propensity for dislodgement. When the easily accessible peripheral vessels have been used in all four extremities, a branch of the profunda femoris artery and saphenous vein in the thigh may be cannulated as described by Hoeltzenbein and later, independently, by Belzer and Kountz. Alternatively, the deep inferior epigastric artery and vein may be exposed and cannulated as described by Kauffman. We have also employed a branch of the external carotid artery and the external jugular vein.

Evaluation of the circulatory status is mandatory in choosing a site for shunt placement. If the patient describes symptoms of claudication or rest pain, arterial pulses in the lower extremity should be carefully palpated and assessed using the Doppler flow probe. In patients with compromised circulation, advanced ischemia may be precipitated by the ill-advised sacrifice of a pedal artery. The integrity of the collateral circulation in the hand cannot be predicted perfectly, but it can be evaluated best using the Allen test. This maneuver is performed by occluding both the radial and ulnar arteries while the patient induces blanching by repeatedly clenching the fist. One vessel is then released and the rapidity and distribution of color return is observed; the process is then repeated, releasing the other vessel. A normal test consists of equally rapid and full return of color upon release of either artery, implying that sacrifice of one vessel will be compensated by collateral flow from the other. Venous outflow must be adequate; it is unwise to employ diseased veins, since patency rate is markedly diminished.

Scrupulous attention to technical features is essential in the appropriate placement of external shunts. The arterial and venous tips must be large enough to maximize flow and to prevent leakage of blood around the cannula, yet not so large as to result in vessel injury. Tips are available in sizes ranging from 20 to 13 French, but tips smaller than 18 usually function poorly because of increased resistance. The arterial tip must not be larger than the venous tip in order to avoid high venous pressures and obligate ultrafiltration.

Local or regional anesthesia is preferable. When the artery and vein are in close approximation (as in radiocephalic shunts), a single longitudinal incision is used. Otherwise, separate incisions over artery and vein are required. Vessels are carefully dissected over a distance of 2–3 cm and are ligated distally. In placing the arterial cannula, care should be taken to avoid clamp trauma or the creation of an intimal flap. In order to avert the linear stress effect of traditional arterial dilators that can cause intimal disruption, several techniques may be useful: arterial inflow may be occluded by digital pressure; traction sutures may be placed on both sides of the arteriotomy; a small (3–4 French) Fogarty catheter may be placed through the shunt and into the arteriotomy to produce both inflow occlusion and gentle arterial dilation. The arterial inflow may also be compromised when the cannula rests against the vessel wall at a point of branching.

Both arterial and venous cannulas must be carefully secured by ligatures placed around the artery and then around the cannulas. Ligatures must be snug enough to prevent leakage of blood or accidental dislodgement, but not so tight as to deform the smooth inner lumen. Usually, ties are placed at the insertion site around the Teflon cannula and also around the subcutaneous portion of the Silastic connecting tubing. The connecting tubing is drawn out through separate subcutaneous tunnels and exits through small stab incisions. The tunnel must be wide enough to accommodate the wings of the tubing, which may be excessively large and may require trimming. The tip and connector should lie comfortably in the tunnel, which has been created in line with the vessel to prevent kinking (Fig. 2-2).

After completion of cannulation, the arterial line should exhibit brisk pulsation upon release of the shunt clamp. Heparinized saline should be easily injected into the arterial and venous lines. There should be little or no venous backflow from the cannula. Excessive venous return and high resistance upon irrigation suggest distal obstruction and stasis.

The arterial and venous lines are trimmed just before connecting them. The venous line should be cut shorter than the arterial line to facilitate thrombectomy, if necessary. The lines must be long enough to allow easy connection to the dialyzer, yet short enough to lie comfortably in the dressing.

After the arterial and venous lines have been connected, release of the arterial clamp should result in brisk migration of blood into the venous line. A small bubble of air left in the sterile connector aids in this assessment. Air should *not* be injected into the tubing, as it is not self-sealing and a leak will occur through the needle hole. A pulse should be palpable in the vein. The dressing should enclose most of the tubing, and thereby maintain alignment. A small portion of the tubing is left exposed to observe for clotting. It is important to stabilize the shunt firmly within the dressing, as excessive movement contributes to infection and thrombosis.

Special Shunts. The *Thomas shunt*, introduced in 1969, consists of Silastic tubing to which a "cobra head"-shaped patch of Dacron is attached (Fig. 2-3). Using vascular suturing technique, the dacron patch is affixed to the superficial

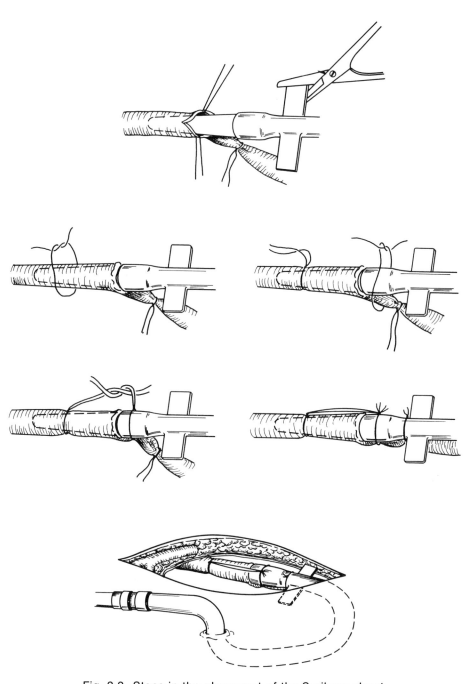

Fig. 2-2. Steps in the placement of the Scribner shunt.

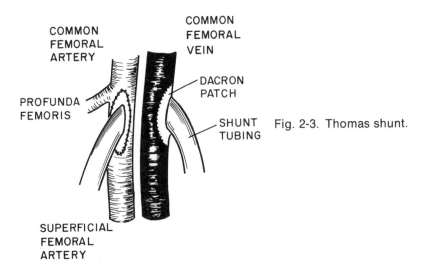

Fig. 2-3. Thomas shunt.

femoral artery, thereby creating a gentle angle of takeoff and a high rate of arterial inflow. The venous return may be through the greater saphenous vein using standard tubing or through the superficial femoral vein using Thomas shunt tubing with its Dacron patch. Normal flow is maintained by surgically established end-of-shunt to side-of-vessel anastamoses. Very high flow rates can be achieved using the Thomas shunt, which is especially useful when conventional shunt sites are unavailable.

The *Allen-Brown shunt* is similar in principle to the Thomas shunt, with Silastic tubing attached to a Dacron sleeve (Fig. 2-4). This shunt is designed for use with small arteries and veins. The Dacron sleeve is sewn in an end-to-end fashion to wrist or ankle arteries and veins or to a branch of the deep femoral

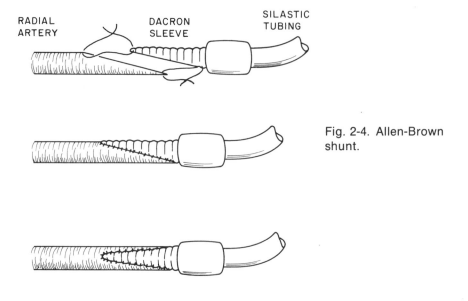

Fig. 2-4. Allen-Brown shunt.

artery in the groin. The distal artery and vein are ligated. Thrombectomy is especially easy in Allen-Brown shunts. These shunts are said to have greater longevity than Scribner shunts, although experience is limited.

The *Buselmeier shunt* consists of a short U shaped Silastic cannula with two side branches that are plugged with Silastic obturators (Fig. 2-5). Teflon tips identical to those used in the Scribner shunt are inserted into the artery and vein, and then into the Busselmeier shunt tubing. The U portion of this device is subcutaneous; only the side branches are external. When the patient undergoes dialysis, the obturators are removed.

Reported advantages of the Buselmeier shunt include low resistance to flow because of the short length of tubing; decreased vessel trauma and incidental dislodgement because of the stable subcutaneous location; and decreased incidence of suction-induced arterial spasm because of an inherent capacity for recirculation.

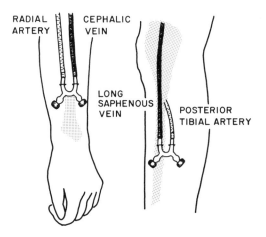

Fig. 2-5. Buselmeier shunt.

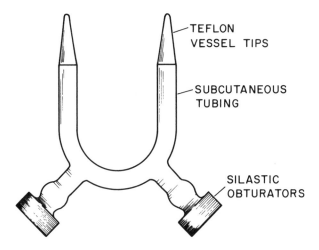

Care of External Arteriovenous Shunts. The extremity in which an external arteriovenous shunt has been placed should be elevated on pillows for 2–4 days to minimize edema. Since thrombosis often occurs shortly after operation, a pulse or bruit at the venous end of the shunt should be assessed hourly during the first 12 postoperative hours. Likewise, the amount of bleeding at insertion sites should be noted hourly. Usually, gentle direct pressure will control any bleeding; prolonged, excessive hemorrhage indicates a substantial problem that demands surgical correction.

If possible, dialysis should be delayed for 24 hours after shunt placement. Systemic heparinization tends to increase bleeding at exit sites. In children, however, immediate utilization of the shunt reduces venous spasm and helps to prevent thrombosis.

Long-term care of external arteriovenous shunts is based on commonsense principles. Cannulas are handled in a clean, rather than a sterile, mode. Dressings should be kept clean and dry. When patients bathe, the device should be protected by encircling the dressing in plastic. Shunts should be checked daily for thrombosis, which is manifested by fibrin layering, loss of warmth, or loss of pulse and bruit at the venous end. Watches, tight clothing, or other attire that potentially restrict blood flow in an extremity should be avoided. Blood pressure measurement or phlebotomy should not be performed in an extremity used for an external arteriovenous shunt. Above all, the patient should be advised to avoid activities that might result in shunt dislodgement, such as carrying heavy objects or repetitive movements of elbow, wrist, or fingers. Cannulas in legs should be elevated for 3–4 days following surgery. Patients should be instructed to stay off the leg completely during this time. For 5–10 days postoperatively, patients should ambulate using crutches to avoid weight bearing on the leg. At 2 weeks patients may begin light weight bearing. By 3 weeks most patients can fully bear weight and walk without the aid of crutches. Patients with leg shunts should be instructed to avoid crossing their legs and refrain from standing or sitting in one place for long periods of time. Footwear should accommodate the shunt body and dressing without constricting or pulling on the cannula limbs.

The procedures for using and cleaning arteriovenous shunt cannulas are outlined in Table 2-1.

The use of external arteriovenous shunts for routine blood drawing or administration of medications and solutions is strongly discouraged. Thrombosis and infection occur frequently when this is done.

Complications with External Arteriovenous Shunts. Thrombosis. A standard Scribner shunt provides a mean blood flow of 200–300 ml/min. Average patency rates range from several weeks to 8 months, but patency as long as 3 years has been reported. Thrombosis almost invariably occurs first in the venous end of the shunt.

When clotting occurs shortly after the placement of a shunt, a technical problem should be suspected. Diseased arteries or veins, indicated by poor inflow or outflow, are unfortunately common in the typical patient who requires acute

Table 2-1. Cannula Cleaning and Dressing

1. Remove old dressings and wash hands thoroughly.
2. Inspect incisions and exit sites for drainage, erythema, swelling, tenderness, and bleeding. Check cannula for evidence of clotting, twisting, or abnormal alignment. Check cannula connector and taping for kinks.
3. Open sterile applicators and soak in hydrogen peroxide.
4. Using separate applicators for each exit site, swab from exit site outward about 1–2 cm. Gently remove crusts around exit sites.
5. Dry each site.
6. Soak sterile applicator in povidone-iodine solution. Using a separate sterile applicator for each incision/exit site, gently wipe povidone-iodine solution outwardly 1–2 cm.
7. Dry each site.
8. Wipe the cannula body with an alcohol swab, using a separate swab for each limb.
9. Place a sterile gauze (4 × 4) under cannula limbs and over exit sites. Secure with tape. Tape should not be circumferential.
10. Wrap with gauze dressing, secure enough to stay in place, but not to constrict flow. Leave a small loop of cannula exposed so that patency can be assessed.
11. Place cannula clamps on dressing.

dialysis during severe illness. Kinking, misalignment, bending, and deformation of Teflon tips or Silastic tubing can result in early thrombosis.

Intimal fibrosis at the venous or arterial end of the shunt most commonly accounts for thrombosis that occurs after 2 or 3 weeks of dialysis. Additional complications at this site resulting in thrombosis are emboli that lodge in the outflow veins, causing a progressive increase in venous resistance, and thrombophlebitis.

Systemic factors that can lead to early or late thrombosis include hypotension and hypercoagulability. Less commonly, extrinsic compression by a dressing or flexed joint may be at fault.

Impending shunt thrombosis should be suspected when shunt flows decrease inexplicably during dialysis. Regular evaluation of the venous outflow network, using a Doppler flow probe, may be of some predictive value. Injection of 5–10 ml of radiopaque dye separately into the venous and arterial tubing will provide a satisfactory shunt angiogram. Specific problems can be identified and repaired before they lead to complete thrombosis.

Shunt thrombosis is obvious when separated clot and serum are visible in the tubing. Occasionally patients notice loss of a sense of pulsation. Attempts at reestablishment of flow should begin immediately, since propagation of the thrombus may result in an unsalvageable situation.

Arterial inflow can often be restored by simply disconnecting the venous and arterial tubing, allowing arterial pressure to flush out the clot. If this does not suffice, gentle suction should be applied, followed by a back and forth irrigation with warm heparinized saline. Cold saline should not be used because it may induce spasm. Above all, undue pressure should *not* be applied to the irrigant, since this may drive the thrombus proximally and even result in cerebral emboli. If these efforts are unsuccessful, a no. 3 Fogarty catheter may be advanced into the artery through the tubing. Straight tubing facilities passage of the catheter. The balloon tip should be gently inflated while withdrawing the catheter. An over-inflated balloon tip can cause arterial damage. Successful de-clotting should result in brisk arterial flow. If irrigation is unhindered but inflow is poor, an intimal flap should be suspected. Inadequate inflow requires appropriate surgical revisions.

The approach to thrombosis in the venous end of the shunt should be virtually identical to that applied at the arterial end. Because of the complexity of venous branching and the presence of valves, the Fogarty catheter is more difficult to use and less effective than in the arterial circulation. When using the Fogarty catheter in either the venous or arterial end of the shunt, care must be taken not to dislodge the entire apparatus by overinflation of the balloon as it emerges from the Teflon tip. In contrast to the risk of cerebral emboli as a consequence of flushing the arterial tubing, there is little risk of pulmonary emboli from flushing the venous end.

If mechanical efforts fail to restore patency, local infusion of the fibrinolytic agents streptokinase or urokinase may be effective. When streptokinase is infused locally, it rarely produces the hypersensitivity reactions, pyrexia, or bleeding complications reported with systemic therapy. Urokinase has less antigenicity than streptokinase, but is less readily available and much more expensive.

After reestablishment of flow, it is wise to begin a short course of continuous infusion of heparin through the shunt by way of a T-shaped sidearm connector. When heparin is administered at a dosage of 50–250 U/h for 24–48 hours, few bleeding complications occur, and the chance for immediate rethrombosis is lessened. Long-term patency of shunts reportedly has been prolonged by the use of anticoagulants and platelet-inhibiting agents.

Vessel exhaustion. Progressive loss of access sites is a major problem for patients on hemodialysis. With each placement of an external arteriovenous shunt a potential donor vessel may be destroyed. Internal fistulas provide superior long-term access routes.

Infection. Infection rates in Scribner shunts vary from 1 per 3.8 patient-months to 1 per 35 patient months, with an average rate of 1 per 6 patient-months. Staphylococci are the most common pathogens, causing over 90% of infections and motivating some investigators to recommend continuous prophylaxis using vancomycin. Conscientious attention to proper local care accounts for lower infection rates in most series.

Recognition of infection is not always easy. A slight redness around the exit sites of the Silastic tubing is common, but when erythema is extensive, or pus is present, or the patient experiences severe pain in the surgical site, antibiotics should be instituted promptly. Broad-spectrum systemic antibiotics, application of heat, rest, and elevation are generally adequate measures, but occasionally drainage of an abscess and removal of the shunt are necessary.

When infection occurs in a Thomas shunt, a more serious situation exists. The Dacron prosthesis must be removed entirely, and the artery repaired with a patch angioplasty of autogenous tissue. The same principle applies to infected Allen-Brown shunts, although the vessels involved are generally not as important.

Bleeding and dislodgement. A small amount of bleeding at the surgical site during dialysis is common in the immediate postoperative period, but excessive bleeding suggests some technical misadventure such as an unsatisfactory ligature around the vessel tip or disruption of the shunt connections. Late bleeding generally occurs because of accidental dislodgement and may be minimized by proper anchoring techniques and careful application of dressings to avoid accidents to the exposed portion of tubing.

Spontaneous dislodgement and bleeding are most commonly associated with infection. Infection may lead to necrosis of the vessel wall and lysis of the tissue holding the sutures in place, resulting in dislodgement. Alternatively, a pseudoaneurysm may form at the cannulation sites, usually presenting as a pulsatile mass associated with oozing or "herald" bleeding. Because of potential catastrophic hemorrhage from the superficial femoral artery, a false aneurysm or bleeding from a Thomas shunt requires immediate therapy. Emergency measures include discontinuation of dialysis and firm, direct pressure over the site until surgical intervention can be accomplished.

Skin erosion. Skin erosion occurs most often directly over the plastic tubing as it emerges from the skin over the sidearm wings. The incidence of this complication can be reduced by avoiding the use of a devascularized skin flap, creating a deep subcutaneous tunnel, and trimming the plastic wings. In most instances, it is not necessary to remove the shunt immediately. After removal of the shunt, the skin will ultimately heal.

Hemodynamic complications. Upper extremity digital ischemia is extremely unusual, even in patients who have had repeated cannulations of both radial and ulnar arteries. In the lower extremity, precipitation of ischemia is not infrequent. The best treatment, of course, is prevention by careful selection of access sites. Occasionally, arterial reconstruction is required.

High output cardiac failure is a very rare complication of external arteriovenous fistulas—with one exception. The Thomas shunt can provide flow rates as high as 1000 cc/min, resulting in cardiac decompensation.

Percutaneous Emergency Access

Percutaneous cannulation of the femoral or subclavian veins for acute hemodialysis has supplanted the use of external arteriovenous shunts in many medical centers. The original catheter developed for this procedure was introduced by Shaldon in 1961. The femoral artery, rather than vein, was first used for this technique, but presently venous access is favored because of lower complication rates.

The technique for placement of percutaneous catheters is similar for cannulation of either the femoral or subclavian vein. The patient is in the supine position for femoral cannulation, with the buttocks elevated on a pillow and the leg externally rotated. The femoral vein is located 2 cm below the inguinal

ligament and 1–2 cm medial to the femoral pulse. For subclavian vein cannulation, the patient is in the Trendelenberg position, with a pillow between
the shoulders and the head rotated away from the ipsilateral subclavian vein.
The subclavian vein should be punctured immediately beneath the clavicle at
the junction of its middle and lateral thirds.

A sterile field is prepared, and the skin over the cannulation site is injected
with local anesthesia. A small 18-gauge needle is inserted into the vessel, and
a Seldinger-type guide wire is threaded into either the inferior or superior vena
cava. The guide wire should never be advanced against resistance.

Once the guide wire is positioned properly, the femoral or subclavian catheter is advanced over it and the wire is removed. Blood return should be brisk.
This catheter is then attached to the dialyzer. Venous return may be accomplished in several ways. A peripheral vein may be cannulated, preferably one
that will not be needed for construction of a permanent arteriovenous fistula.
The contralateral femoral vein may be used, but this further impairs patient
mobility and increases the complication rate. When two ipsilateral femoral catheters are used, one catheter is positioned so that one extends farther up the vein
than the other (3–5 cm). To minimize recirculation, the lower catheter is used
as the arterial pull and the venous return is through the upper catheter. A coaxial
dual flow catheter may also be employed (Fig. 2-6). The dual catheter is very
stiff and should be placed under fluoroscopy to avoid perforation of the vena
cava.

If a solitary catheter is used, a single-needle device must be employed. This
device alternatively allows arterial pull and venous return to occur through the
same catheter. Blood flow (Q_B) should be 150–200 ml/min, with a stroke volume
(which is Q_B/cycles per minute) of 5–10 ml.

There are a number of advantages to percutaneous cannulation for hemodialysis. Most importantly, vessels that may be needed for permanent an-

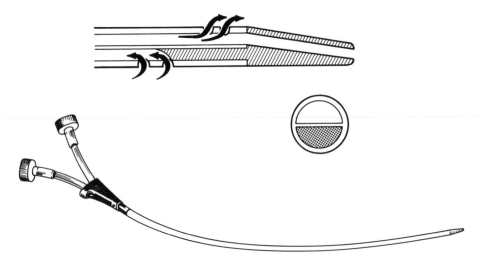

Fig. 2-6. Coaxial dual flow catheter.

gioaccess are spared. There is no need for an operating room, and dialysis may be instituted without delay. Incidence of infection is quite low, even when catheters remain in place for several days. Adequate flows are obtained with no additional cardiac workload, as occurs with shunts and fistulas.

Care of Percutaneous Catheters. Strict aseptic technique must be applied to femoral catheters placed for hemodialysis. Exit sites should be inspected daily for signs of infection. Dressings should be changed by the sterile technique, using procedures identical to those designed for hyperalimentation catheters. There should be minimal manipulation of the catheter in order to decrease the chances of accidental dislodgement or infection. Femoral catheters placed for hemodialysis should not be used for obtaining blood samples or administering medications or fluids.

The longevity of subclavian catheters is much greater than that of femoral catheters, which are usually left in place for only 24–72 hours. Furthermore, patients favor subclavian catheters over femoral because subclavian catheters allow greater mobility and require fewer reinsertions.

The subclavian catheter should be examined daily for evidence of infection at the exit site. Minimal handling of the subclavian catheter is strongly advocated, and then only by experienced personnel. Although not optimal, there are instances when the subclavian catheter is needed for administration of parenteral nutrition or blood. When parenteral solutions are administered, leur lock connections should be used to prevent accidental disconection leading to air embolus or blood loss. All connections should be scrubbed liberally with povidone-iodine for 3–5 minutes prior to disconnection. Indwelling heparin should be aspirated along with any clots.

Maintenance of femoral or subclavian catheter patency occasionally is difficult. Several techniques have been described to avoid thrombosis. Some authors suggest continuous heparin infusion of 500 U heparin/1000 ml saline given at a slow rate (<50 ml/h). Since this requires an automatic infusion system, limits patient mobility, and subjects the catheter to sepsis from the necessity of changing intravenous bottles, a preferable method of maintaining catheter patency is the instillation of 1000–5000 U of heparin into the catheter (which is then clamped) immediately following dialysis. Instillation of heparin should be repeated every 24–48 hours. The volume necessary to deliver the heparin depends on the size of the catheter, which should be determined before insertion to avoid administering systemic heparin to the patient.

Complications with Femoral or Subclavian Catheters. *Hemorrhage.* Minor hemorrhage may manifest as a small hematoma at the insertion site. This occurs quite commonly and is generally of little consequence. Major hemorrhage is secondary to arterial injury in most cases and may present as retroperitoneal bleeding when the femoral vein is used or hemothorax when the subclavian vein is used. The incidence of such major bleeding is less than 1%. Shock or a continually falling hematocrit are indications for urgent surgical exploration of the vessel.

Pneumothorax. Pneumothorax is a potential complication of all subclavian vein cannulations. This occurrence may be minimized by the proper positioning of patients, the use of small needles for insertion of the guide wire, and a thorough knowledge of the anatomy. A chest x-ray is mandatory after placement of any subclavian catheter.

Thrombosis. While thrombosis of indwelling catheters is not uncommon, occlusion of either the femoral or subclavian vein is rare. A swollen arm or leg is an indication for catheter removal and investigation of the venous anatomy. The Doppler flow probe may be used to assess lower extremity venous thrombosis, but this technique is unreliable in the upper extremity, for which phlebography is required. The patient with confirmed venous thrombosis should be treated with systemic heparinization, unless there is a contraindication to anticoagulation.

Infection. Careful attention to sterile technique in the placement and care of percutaneous catheters makes infection a very unusual complication. If the patient experiences unexplained fever or leukocytosis, or if redness or purulence appear at insertion sites, catheters should be removed and cultured.

Nerve injury. Rarely, the femoral nerve or brachial plexus may be injured during catheter insertion. Such injuries are due to improper technique in catheter placement. Most nerve injuries are transient.

Acute Peritoneal Dialysis

The technique of catheter placement for acute peritoneal dialysis is quite simple. The urinary bladder is decompressed and the skin is prepared with an iodinated antiseptic solution. Local anesthetic is injected at a point in the lower midline below the umbilicus approximately one third of the distance between that and the symphysis pubis. The skin is incised with a no. 11 scalpel, and a peritoneal dialysis catheter is inserted percutaneously. The trocar is advanced until it just penetrates the peritoneum. Once the peritoneum is penetrated, the trocar is removed and the dialysis catheter is advanced toward the pelvis. Alternatively, a small formal incision may be made to the peritoneum with direct inspection of the fascia and peritoneum. This is particularly applicable to those patients who have relative contraindiations to peritoneal dialysis, including previous abdominal surgery, pregnancy, and distended bowel.

Access to the peritoneal cavity may also be obtained by placing a "permanent" indwelling silicone rubber cannula modeled after Tenckhoff's original design. This requires an operating room environment, but may be done under local anesthesia. It offers the advantage of rapidly providing a means to begin long-term peritoneal dialysis.

Care of the Acute Peritoneal Dialysis Catheter. Since accidental dislodgement of the catheter placed for acute peritoneal dialysis is quite common, great care should be taken in securing the catheter in position once it is functioning properly. Generally, several sutures placed in the skin and then tied around the catheter ensure stability. Antibiotic ointment and bulky sterile dressings are applied to the exit site. Most acute catheters are left in place for the duration of the dialysis, usually 48–72 hours. Dressings should be observed for leakage or bloody drainage and changed in a sterile manner only if wet.

Complications with Peritoneal Dialysis. Peritonitis. Today, acute peritoneal dialysis rarely produces peritonitis. In the early experience, however, this was a common complication. Improvements in catheter design, the introduction of individual peritoneal dialysate bags, and the development of automatic equipment are responsible for the decline in peritonitis frequency with this modality.

Symptoms of peritonitis include abdominal pain, fever, nausea, vomiting, and diarrhea. The exit site of the catheter may show evidence of inflammation. Tenderness to abdominal palpation, including rebound tenderness, is often present. Bowel sounds are decreased. Abdominal x-rays generally reveal a pattern of diffuse ileus.

The diagnosis is confirmed by examination of the effluent, which is usually turbid. Fibrin or eosinophils can cause cloudiness, so a leukocyte count and differential should be performed on the effluent. Clear fluid contains <50–100 cells/mm^3. In peritonitis, the majority of the leukocytes in the dialysate will be neutrophils. In the absence of peritonitis, mononuclear leukocytes predominate. Gram stain is often, but not always, positive for organisms. About 75% of infections are due to gram-positive organisms and 25% to gram-negative organisms. Fungal infection is unusual.

Peritonitis in the patient undergoing acute peritoneal dialysis may be treated by lavage with antibiotics (cephalothin or vancomycin for gram-positive organisms and tobramycin for gram-negative organisms) and removal of the peritoneal catheter.

Most cases of peritonitis are the sequel to contamination at the catheter site. It must be remembered, however, that injury to the viscera can occur from catheter placement, and this complication should be suspected particularly if gram-negative organisms are present. Exploratory laparotomy is indicated if the patient remains ill after continuous peritoneal lavage and catheter removal.

The diagnosis and treatment of peritonitis is more fully discussed in Chapter 4.

Leakage. Leakage of dialysis fluid around the catheter can be minimized by using an acute angle when inserting the catheter so that it travels through a short tunnel of subcutaneous tissue before entering the peritoneal cavity. If an incision is made in fascia, meticulous closure of the wound will decrease the incidence of this complication. Patients who receive large volumes of dialysate and those who have poor abdominal musculature are most likely to sustain leakage. When it occurs, leakage may be decreased by placing the patient in a more upright position and by using smaller fluid volumes. If leakage persists, in spite of small inflow volumes, the catheter should be removed and another site selected. Dressings should be changed frequently to keep the exit site as dry as possible and to prevent the development of infection.

Catheter malfunction. Malposition and obstruction are the most common forms of catheter malfunction. A malpositioned catheter is usually the result of failure to direct the catheter caudally. There is little or no difficulty during inflow of dialysate, but effluent will not drain freely. Suction applied to the catheter produces pain. Treatment usually is replacement of the catheter, although repositioning is occasionally successful.

Obstruction of the catheter may be due to blood and fibrin or incarceration of omentum or bowel. When blood and fibrin clots are responsible for poor drainage, these elements generally appear in the effluent. Forceful irrigation of the catheter with heparinized saline solution usually restores patency. When soft tissue is incarcerated in the catheter, forceful irrigation will not relieve obstruction, and replacement of the catheter is necessary.

CHRONIC DIALYSIS

Autogenous Subcutaneous Arteriovenous Fistulas

Most of the complications of external devices for angioaccess were eliminated by the introduction of the internal arteriovenous fistula by Brescia and Cimino in 1966. The only disadvantages of an internal fistula are the necessity for repeated transcutaneous needle puncture, which some patients resist, and the delay required prior to use. These factors can be made to appear less objectionable to patients by soliciting their cooperation through clarification of the therapeutic process.

A logical and systematic approach to the creation of internal arteriovenous fistulas is essential in order to provide optimal access over a patient's lifetime. Periodic assessment of renal function should be performed in patients with progressive renal failure. An autogenous arteriovenous fistula should be created when creatinine clearance drops to about 15 ml/min or in anticipation of the institution of maintenance hemodialysis in 3–6 months, as discussed in Chapter 3. If emergency dialysis is required, peritoneal dialysis, percutaneous hemodialysis, or hemodialysis through an external shunt may be used while the internal fistula matures. When a Scribner shunt has been placed in the forearm, it is possible to convert this to an internal fistula.

The internal fistula of choice is the radiocephalic fistula, as illustrated in Figure 2-7. It provides adequate flow (300 ml/min), easy accessibility, a low incidence of thrombosis, and excellent longevity. The early failure rate is 5–10% (poor patient selection) and the average patency rate is 60–75% at 3 years.

Proper selection of a site for a radiocephalic fistula is essential. Preferably the nondominant extremity is used so that puncture by the patient is facilitiated. First consideration, however, must be given to the quality of artery and vein. An Allen test should be performed, as described previously. In an unconscious patient, a Doppler flow probe may be used to identify augmentation of flow in the ulnar artery upon compression of the radial artery. A weak radial pulse or inadequate collateral circulation precludes performance of a radiocephalic fis-

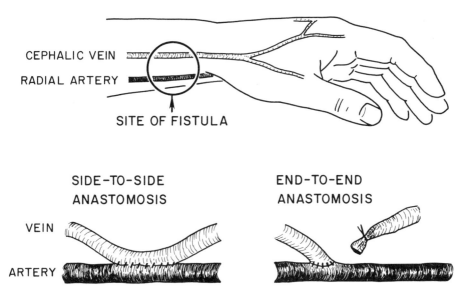

Fig. 2-7. Brescia-Cimino fistula.

tula. Venous outflow should be assessed by inspection and palpation of the cephalic vein and its tributaries after inflating a tourniquet on the upper arm. If veins are thrombosed, sparse, or particularly deep, an alternative site should be sought.

Local anesthesia is generally sufficient, but regional block is useful because it provides sympathetic blockade with vasodilation. Rarely, general anesthesia is required in a very apprehensive patient. A longitudinal incision is made between the radial artery and cephalic vein for a length of 3–5 cm. The artery and vein are dissected along the entire length of the incision, taking care to preserve all venous branches. It is particularly important to be gentle with the vein, since roughness and excessive stripping of adventitia may result in spasm and loss of endothelium.

Controversy exists as to the proper method of constructing the anastomosis. A side-to-side anastomosis generally has a better immediate patency rate, since outflow is both cephalad and caudad (Fig. 2-7). A side-to-side anastomosis also facilitates a relatively long anastomosis, extending 8–10 mm. However, venous hypertension in the hand occurs more frequently with this method of construction. An end-of-vein to side-of-artery anastomosis prevents venous hypertension, but care must be taken to avoid twisting the vein; to ensure an adequate anastomotic length it is necessary to spatulate the vein. End-of-artery to vein anastomoses have been described (Fig. 2-7) but should be avoided for two reasons: (1) forward arterial flow to the hand is permanently interrupted, and (2) one third of initial flow comes from the distal limb of the artery.

Several technical points are important in creating all internal fistulas. Gentle vascular clamps should be used to minimize clamp trauma that may lead to late fibrointimal hyperplasia. Wrapping vessels in gauze pledgets soaked with pa-

paverine directly relaxes smooth muscle. Excessive tension on the anastomosis should be avoided; it is better to dissect out a longer segment of cephalic vein and then perform an end-of-vein to side-of-artery anastomosis than to stretch the vein to the artery in an attempt to perform side-to-side anastomosis. Angles, abrupt changes in caliber, and intraluminal projections such as inverted adventitia or graft edges must be unobtrusive. Veins should be gently dilated with coronary artery dilators and irrigated with heparinized saline solution. Systemic heparinization is not essential, but it does eliminate the potential for in-situ thrombus formation during construction of the fistula.

At the completion of fistula construction a thrill should be palpable, and in nearly all cases a bruit is audible. Palpable venous pulsation and absence of a bruit indicates outflow obstruction and impending thrombosis, which will require revision of the anastomosis, thrombectomy, and dilation of venous outflow. Meticulous hemostasis is necessary before closing the wound to inhibit the development of a hematoma that would promote infection and early thrombosis. Postoperatively, the limb should be elevated 1–2 days to minimize swelling. Flow characteristics should be monitored at the arterial anastomosis and the proximal limb by auscultation of a bruit and palpation of a thrill. The limb should be evaluated consistently for changes in temperature, color, and sensation. Dressings should be loose and not circumferential to avoid possible constriction of flow. Skin sutures should not be removed for at least 2 weeks so as to accommodate the delayed healing of patients with end-stage renal disease. After the sutures are removed, patients may be encouraged to apply a tourniquet on the arm above the fistula for 2–3 minutes, 10–15 times a day, and to squeeze a rubber ball. These maneuvers promote venous dilation and fistula enlargement.

When a radiocephalic fistula cannot be constructed for some reason, alternative sites for an autogenous subcutaneous arm fistula are available. These include (1) ulnar artery to ulnar vein, (2) distal brachial artery to a branch of the antecubital vein, (3) middle brachial artery to the cephalic vein, and (4) middle brachial artery to the basilic vein.

Vascular Grafts for Hemodialysis

While a direct autogenous arteriovenous fistula is clearly the procedure of choice for angioaccess, there are many patients who require the interposition of a graft between an artery and a vein. The indications for a graft fistula include (1) severe obesity that makes repeated venipuncture difficult, (2) iatrogenic loss of superficial veins because of multiple cannulations, multiple cutdowns, or multiple external shunts, and (3) self-inflected loss of veins in drug addicts. Additionally, a graft fistula is generally easier to puncture than an autogenous fistula for patients performing home dialysis, but this is a very "soft" indication.

Graft fistulas are established by connecting the graft ends to the sides of an artery and vein. If the anastomotic sites are a distance apart, and most of the length of the graft is used in bridging this distance, the fistula is "straight." If the anastomotic sites to artery and vein are close together, the result is a "loop" or U fistula. These fistulas are illustrated in Figure 2-8. Proper selection of sites and avoidance of technical error are more important than graft configuration in determining patency rates.

Grafts may be placed in the upper extremity or thigh. While grafts in the leg between common femoral artery or superficial femoral artery and saphenous vein or common femoral vein provide high flows and leave the patient free to use the hands, such grafts are more prone to infection. In the upper extremity the preferred access is the straight graft between radial artery and antecubital vein below the flexion crease of the elbow. A loop fistula between the brachial artery and antecubital vein in the forearm is next best. Upper arm fistulas between the brachial artery at the elbow and the axillary vein are least desirable because of increased incidence of the steal syndrome, arm swelling, and nerve injuries, although they are of ultimate use in the long-term dialysis patient.

A variety of graft materials is available. Autogenous saphenous vein was used in the past, but this practice has been largely abandoned for the following reasons: (1) a separate incision is needed to harvest the vein, (2) future vascular procedures will be deprived of its availability, (3) patency rates are low, and (4) these grafts are difficult to puncture. Bovine carotid artery remains popular despite a greater risk of infection and false aneurysm; when infection does occur,

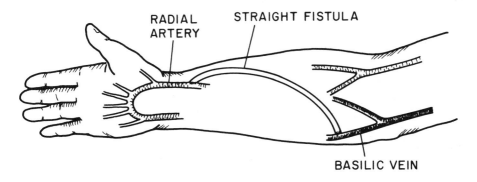

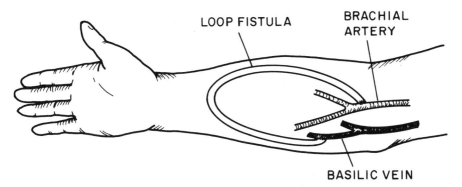

Fig. 2-8. Straight fistula and loop fistula.

it is extremely difficult to remove this graft. In comparison, polytetrafluoroe-thylene (PTFE) offers a slightly better patency rate, various diameters, better tolerance to infection, less propensity to form false aneurysms, and easy de-clotting. Its stiffness, however, makes it difficult to handle and prone to kink when used for loop fistulas. There has been a great deal of interest in the use of Dacron velour as graft material, but experience has been limited to date. Treated human umbilical veins are also available alternatives for graft fistulas.

Both diameter and length of the graft affect fistula flow. Grafts 6–8 mm in diameter usually provide good flows with few side effects. The longer the graft, the greater the internal diameter required to provide adequate flow because resistance increases. Grafts smaller than 5 mm have a high thrombosis rate, and those larger than 10 mm are associated with high output heart failure and distal extremity insufficiency.

Perioperative antibiotics are always administered. Local anesthesia may be used, but regional or general anesthesia is preferable because creation of a graft fistula demands much more dissection than a radiocephalic fistula. Vessels are exposed by standard techniques and the patient is given intravenous heparin. Just as in the radiocephalic fistula, the artery and vein must be of sufficient caliber and free of thrombus. Obliquely beveled anastamoses are performed in an end-of-graft to side-of-vessel fashion. Care must be taken to be certain the graft lies in a subdermal tunnel that is as superficial as possible to facilitate cannulation. Kinking occurs commonly in loop grafts; to prevent this compli-cation, some surgeons anastomose graft-to-graft in a V fashion at the apex of the loop. At the completion of the anastomosis to the vein a thrill should be palpable at both arterial and venous ends of the graft. In the presence of good venous outflow, prominent pulsations can be demonstrated only by digital compression.

Meticulous hemostasis must be obtained before closing the wound. Mild swelling of the arm and hand, frequently present in the early postoperative period, can be minimized by elevating the extremity. The grafts may be used for dialysis immediately, although most centers advocate waiting 10 days to 3 weeks if possible. Early cannulation may cause bleeding from the needle punc-ture site and dissection of blood throughout the subcutaneous tunnel. The re-sulting hematoma may compress the graft, and thus advance the development of thrombosis. Waiting to cannulate the graft allows for resolution of localized edema and results in better graft definition and cannulation and avoidance of perigraft hematomas and infection.

Meticulous preparation of the skin prior to cannulation is essential to pre-vent infection in the access. Povidone-iodine or hexachlorophene are the most widely used antimicrobial agents. After proper skin preparation, a local anes-thetic (usually 1–2% lidocaine) is injected intradermally where the needles are to be placed. A tourniquet can be applied above the fistula, if needed, to dilate and to stabilize the vessel. The needles are then inserted at a 45 degree angle, bevel up, directly into the lidocaine puncture sites. A more tangential approach may lacerate the graft and clot the needle. The needle should be advanced until a flush of blood is seen in the hub of the needle and tubing. The tourniquet is then released, and the needles are irrigated and examined for infiltration. Finally, the needles are taped securely and connected to dialysis lines.

Once fistula needles have been removed, hemostasis must be established before dressings are applied. Gentle pressure to puncture sites until bleeding stops prevents bleeding into the subcutaneous tunnel and prevents pseudo-aneurysms. A simple Band-Aid or dressing may be left in place for 4–6 hours or until the following day.

Care of Fistulas. Education of the patient in evaluating fistula function should begin in the preoperative period. Recognition of the presence or absence of a thrill should be done on a daily basis from the first postoperative day. The signs of infection should be familiar to the patients, as well as to dialysis personnel. Patients should not carry heavy objects or wear tight or circumferential clothes or jewelry that might compromise flow.

Brescia-Cimino fistulas generally take 2 or more months to "mature," although some patients with particularly large and good quality veins may undergo hemodialysis through their fistulas much sooner. Maturation of an autogenous fistula can be hastened by the temporary application of a tourniquet to the upper arm for a few minutes several times a day, or by having the patient repeatedly squeeze a rubber ball. Graft fistulas should not be cannulated for 2–3 weeks to allow tissue incorporation of the graft and diminish postdialysis perigraft hematoma formation.

In either autogenous or graft fistulas, cannulation sites should be carefully rotated to avoid repeated trauma to the same site that might result in late stricture or false aneurysm. The arterial needle should be the more distal of the two fistula needles. It may be placed pointing toward or away from the direction of flow. The venous needle is placed toward the heart in the direction of venous flow. The two needles should be at least 3–5 cm apart to avoid recirculation.

The ideal fistula needle for hemodialysis allows 200–300 ml/min blood flow with a minimal pressure drop across the needle. Most are available in metal or plastic with a gauge of 14–16. Needles with side holes near the tip have a decreased tendency to occlude against the vessel wall.

Complications with Fistulas. Thrombosis. With more than 60,000 patients on chronic hemodialysis worldwide, it is not surprising that thrombosis of angioaccess sites presents a challenging problem. The early failure rate of a Cimino fistula is 5–10%; once it is successfully constructed, a long-term patency rate of about 70% at 3 years can be expected. In contrast, the initial patency rate of graft fistulas is higher than that of radiocephalic fistulas, but long-term patency is much poorer. For these fistulas, 1-year patency rates ranging from 75% to 40%, and 2-year patency rates as low as 30%, have been reported.

Early thrombosis. Technical misadventures are usually responsible for early thrombosis.

The selection of an inadequate vein or an outflow obstruction will most often be the determinant of thrombosis of a Cimino fistula. In patients with atherosclerosis, particularly diabetics, the radial artery may not provide adequate inflow. A Doppler systolic pressure of 100 mmHg is mandatory, as is a normal Allen test.

Technical factors responsible for early thrombosis of a graft fistula include the following:

1. Improper selection of artery and vein
2. Narrowing of the lumen of the artery or vein
3. Incorporation of the back wall in the vascular suture
4. Entrapment of adventitia within the lumen of the anastomosis
5. Intimal dissection
6. Compression of the graft by hematoma due to inadequate hemostasis or premature puncture
7. Kinking or twisting of graft or vessel
8. Undue pressure over a needle puncture site or application of a tight compression dressing

If the selection of arteries and veins has been correct, early thrombosis of arteriovenous fistulas generally responds well to prompt operation, with thrombectomy and revision of anastomoses, if indicated.

Late thrombosis. Late thrombosis of a radiocephalic fistula is most often caused by repeated needle punctures leading to the formation of false aneurysm and/or fibrosis. Thrombectomy is rarely successful in this circumstance because the thrombus extends into multiple venous bifurcations, making it close to impossible to direct the Fogarty catheter into all potential outflow routes. Furthermore, the clot lodges behind venous valves and cannot be completely removed. Thus, a nidus for rethrombosis exists. Conversion of the radiocephalic fistula to a graft fistula is generally indicated.

Graft fistulas ultimately occlude in most cases because of stenosis at the venous anastomosis. The diagnosis can be suspected when the graft becomes increasingly pulsatile and increased venous pressure is noted on the dialysis machine. Angiography will confirm stenosis of the outflow tract. There are several causes of this anomaly. Mechanical factors such as angulation of the vein or repeated puncture in a confined area with extravasation of blood, fibrosis, and cellulitis can lead to stenosis. Endothelial damage may occur as a sequela to the shearing effect of turbulent blood flow and a marked difference in compliance between any graft material and vein. Intimal endothelial injury results in platelet aggregation and adherence to the subendothelium. Platelet degranulation is associated with the migration of injured smooth muscle cells to an intimal location and the transformation to fibroblasts. The result is neointimal fibrous hyperplasia.

Less common reasons for late thrombosis are poor arterial inflow and successful kidney transplantation. Poor arterial inflow is almost always due to hypovolemia rather than stenosis at the arterial anastomosis. Successful transplantation reverses the clotting abnormalities commonly associated with chronic renal failure and may lead to graft thrombosis. Fistulas placed for plasmapheresis or administration of chemotherapy have an increased thrombosis rate because of hypercoagulability.

Salvage of thrombosed fistulas. It is much easier to salvage an occluded graft fistula than an autogenous fistula. About 60% of established graft fistulas remain functional following thrombectomy and patch angioplasty. This can be accomplished even after a fistula has been occluded for several weeks. Unless there is some unusual reason for thrombosis, such as systemic hypotension, it should be assumed that venous outflow is responsible for late failure. The graft should be exposed at the venous end, and after systemic heparinization a Fogarty catheter should be directed through a graftotomy to retrieve the thrombus from the proximal graft and as many outflow veins as possible. Although pulmonary embolus is a theoretical consideration in performing this procedure, it is rarely observed.

Brisk arterial inflow and venous backflow should be apparent after successful thrombectomy. Intraoperative arteriography may disclose fibrous hyperplasia at the distal anastomosis, which should be repaired by widening the lumen with a patch angioplasty or graft interposition. If arterial inflow is diminished, revision of the arterial anastomosis is occasionally required.

Successful salvage of a fistula is indicated by return of a thrill along its course without a prominent pulse. Although implantation of a new graft fistula carries a greater chance of succeeding than does a declotted graft, it must be remembered that access sites are limited, and efforts to save established fistulas are worthwhile. Furthermore, the patient can be dialyzed the following day through the salvaged fistula, whereas a new fistula requires maturation.

Infection. Infection is second to cardiovascular disease as a cause of mortality in patients on chronic hemodialysis. Vascular access sites are common sources of bacteria in episodes of septicemia in dialysis patients. Deficient immune defense mechanisms and a particularly high rate of colonization with *Staphylococcus aureus* in the hemodialysis population are partially responsible for the high rate of infection of access sites. External shunts are most likely to become infected and Brescia-Cimino autogenous arteriovenous fistulas are least likely. Graft fistulas carry an intermediate risk. A recent review of the literature reported that there were 12 infections in 950 autogenous fistulas over 15,100 patient months. In contrast, there were 41 infections in 801 graft fistulas over 8606 patient months.

Infections that occur soon after the creation of angioaccess are a consequence of intraoperative contamination. The patient's skin organisms are responsible in most cases; this complication occurs more frequently when the graft is placed in the groin because of greater difficulty in preparing the sterile field. Inadequate hemostasis or premature puncture lead to hematoma formation, which predisposes to infection.

Late infections are usually due to direct inoculation of the graft by needle puncture of inadequately prepared skin. As many as 60% of patients on chronic hemodialysis are colonized with *Staphylococcus aureus,* compared with 10% of a control population. Septicemia from a distant infection may also lead to secondary infection of a fistula. This is most likely to occur shortly after access placement, since incorporation of a graft by surrounding soft tissue resists metastatic infection.

In order to minimize the risk of infection, a Brescia-Cimino fistula should be constructed whenever possible. Strict adherence to meticulous sterile technique and hemostasis must be maintained. Perioperative antibiotics should be given when prosthetic graft fistulas are employed. The type of graft material used cannot be conclusively correlated with graft infections, although there is suggestive evidence that bovine heterografts become infected more frequently than other materials. Prevention of late infection in any fistula is dependent on proper preparation of the skin prior to needle puncture.

Treatment of infected access sites depends on the type of access, the extent of infection, and the interval between operation and infection. When autogenous fistulas become infected, local drainage, dressing changes, and appropriate systemic antibiotics are often successful. Ligation of an autogenous fistula or complete removal of a graft fistula must be performed if infection occurs in the early postoperative period, if an anastomosis is involved, or if the entire graft is obviously involved. Local measures may be adequate if a short segment of graft becomes infected well after its placement.

Pseudoaneurysm. Pseudoaneurysms of arteriovenous fistulas will develop if inadequate hemostasis is obtained when dialysis needles are removed, and if one area of graft or vein is selectively weakened as a result of infrequent rotation of the needle puncture site. Rarely, a true aneurysm will occur in a graft or vein in patients with graft hypertension. The patient generally does not experience any symptoms from this complication unless the mass impinges upon contiguous nerves. Most aneurysms can be safely observed. Of course, alternative sites for needle puncture must be sought. When aneurysms cause pain or neurologic dysfunction, when they progressively enlarge, and when they are associated with marked thinning of overlying skin, repair should be performed. Usually this involves exploration and lateral repair of a small defect. Occasionally, patch angioplasty, resection and reanastomosis, or a short segment interposition graft, is required (Fig. 2-9). It is unusual for a consistently observed aneurysm to rupture. In the event of rupture the limb above with the aneurysm should have a tourniquet applied with direct pressure to the site. Immediate surgical intervention is imperative.

Vascular insufficiency. Steal syndromes due to anteriovenous fistulas manifest as pain of the small muscles of the hand on exercise. More severe ischemia results in nonhealing ulcers, pain at rest, and neurologic dysfunction. The involved hand or foot appears cold, clammy, and pale, with diminished Doppler digital pulsations. Vascular insufficiency occurs because of reversed flow from the artery distal to the anastomosis.

The incidence of vascular insufficiency due to arteriovenous fistulas is less than 1%. The occurrence of steal syndrome is more likely when large arteries (brachial or superficial femoral) are employed, or when patients have undergone

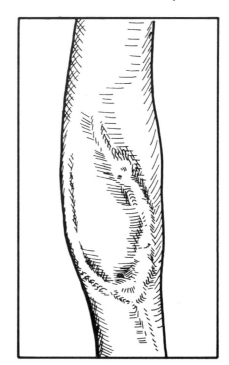

Fig. 2-9. Pseudoaneurysm of arteriovenous graft.

multiple operative procedures and arterial punctures previous to the fistula construction. Steal syndrome is particularly common in patients with peripheral vascular disease, vasculitis, or diabetes. Careful preoperative assessment of the circulation of the extremity aids in the prevention of vascular insufficiency. The diagnosis is made on clinical grounds, although arteriography assists in confirmation and therapy.

Operative intervention is required in patients with symptomatic vascular insufficiency from arteriovenous fistulas. Conversion of a side-to-side radiocephalic fistula to an end-to-side fistula is easily accomplished by ligation of the distal radial artery when steal phenomena occur in these fistulas. In fistulas arising from larger arteries, a banding technique may be used in which a Teflon tape progressively constricts the arterial end of the graft until flow rates decrease to 300 ml/min, as determined by an electromagnetic flowmeter. If banding is unsuccessful, it may be necessary to sacrifice the fistula. A tapered (5–7 mm) polytetrafluoroethylene graft is also available.

Venous hypertension. An uncommon complication of arteriovenous fistulas is venous hypertension, which occurs when arterial flow is possible both forward and backward in the recipient vein. This is particularly prevalent with venous outflow stenosis. Clinical features include swelling, bluish discoloration, hyperpigmentation, pain, and ulceration.

Intermittent elevation of the extremity and a light compression bandage are often effective in eliminating symptoms. If this is inadequate, ligation of the distal vein effectively converts the venous anastomosis to an end-type anastomosis, which usually alleviates the problem.

Congestive heart failure. When flow rates through arteriovenous fistulas are less than 20% of cardiac output, cardiac failure from this source does not occur. Since most Brescia-Cimino radiocephalic fistulas produce flows ranging from 200 to 400 ml/min, high output cardiac failure is extremely unusual. The incidence of congestive heart failure is positively correlated with the increased flow rates accompanying large donor arteries and large graft diameters. In many instances, inadequate dialysis with increased total body water is responsible for this complication. The fistula may be implicated, however, when temporary occlusion results in decreased heart rate (Branham's sign) and improved cardiac function, as determined by noninvasive measurements of cardiac contractility and ejection fraction.

Heart failure induced by arteriovenous fistulas can be avoided by using smaller arteries and grafts. When it occurs, operative correction involves banding of the fistula while measuring flow with the electromagnetic flow probe described above.

Carpal tunnel syndrome. In the general population, osteophytes, rheumatoid granulation tissue, benign tumors, and idiopathic thickening of the flexor retinaculum have been implicated in the development of the carpal tunnel syndrome. This syndrome is characterized by pain and numbness in the distribution of the median nerve, wasting of the muscles of the thenar eminence, and discomfort upon percussion of the median nerve at the wrist. There is an increased incidence of carpal tunnel syndrome in patients undergoing chronic hemodialysis that has been ascribed to edema of the hand during dialysis, venous compression of the median nerve, thickening of the carpal ligaments, and ischemia secondary to vascular insufficiency.

The diagnosis must be differentiated from uremic peripheral neuropathy. In general, uremic neuropathy is symmetrical and occurs in the upper extremity only after it is present in the lower. Nerve conduction velocity is uniformly slowed in patients with uremic neuropathy, while it is selectively slowed across the wrist in patients with carpal tunnel syndrome. Treatment consists of surgical decompression of the median nerve.

Vascular Access in Children
(Donald E. Potter)

A primary arteriovenous fistula in the forearm (Brescia-Cimino) is the preferred type of vascular access in children as well as adults. In children smaller than 20 kg, however, there is a higher incidence of thrombosis and primary failure of this type of fistula, although successful fistulas have been constructed in infants as small as 5 kg, using microvascular techniques. In very small children the optimum access is probably a primary fistula at the elbow, using the brachial artery. Alternatively, bovine or polytetraflouroethylene grafts can be implanted in the forearm or upper arm. Despite the needle insertions involved, children as well adults, prefer fistulas to arteriovenous shunts, which are still used occasionally in small children. In many pediatric centers single-needle devices are used exclusively.

Chronic Peritoneal Dialysis

Chronic peritoneal dialysis has become an alternative to hemodialysis because of two major technical advances made in the early 1970s: (1) a permanently implanted silicone rubber catheter providing safe, easy access to the peritoneal cavity, and (2) machines capable of delivering sterile dialysate at the patient's bedside. As discussed in Chapter 4, this allowed safe, unattended home dialysis with a reduced risk of peritonitis.

Chronic peritoneal dialysis requires placement of an indwelling catheter designed after that first described by Tenckhoff. Numerous models are commercially available. The catheters consist of teflon or silastic tubing, as shown in Figure 2-10. The external component of the tubing is separated from the intraabdominal tubing (with multiple holes) by a collar, flange, and Dacron cuff, which is "buried" in a subcutaneous tunnel. The flange and cuff allow for tissue ingrowth and protect against migration of bacteria along the tube track.

Strict adherence to sterile technique and standard surgical procedures are required for implantation of an indwelling peritoneal catheter. Prophylactic antibiotics to reduce skin flora are recommended in the perioperative period. After preparation of the skin with povidone-iodine, a vertical subumbilical midline incision is made and carried down to the midline fascia. The peritoneum is identified and opened. A pocket for the flange is prepared subcutaneously to one side of the incision. The pocket should be made as close as possible to the

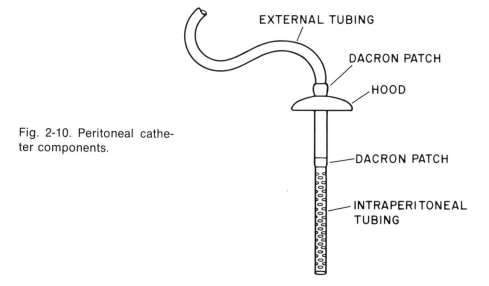

EXTERNAL TUBING

DACRON PATCH

HOOD

DACRON PATCH

INTRAPERITONEAL TUBING

Fig. 2-10. Peritoneal catheter components.

skin surface without destroying the dermal blood supply. This will prevent catheter retraction as well as encourage prompt fibroblastic migration into the upper surface of the flange.

A tunnel is created through the full thickness of the abdominal wall centered under the skin flap. A trocar may be attached to the tubing to facilitate guiding the catheter through the peritoneum. Proper tunneling is important in preventing extraperitoneal estravasation of dialysis fluid.

The distal end of the catheter is then drawn through the tunnel, and the insertion trocar is removed. The undersurface of the flange rests on the posterior surface of the dissected skin pocket and the edges of the flange should be anchored to underlying tissue with absorbable sutures. The catheter is directed into the pelvis, taking care to avoid malposition or entanglement of omentum or bowel. Irrigation of the catheter confirms unobstructed flow.

The skin exit site is directly above the subcutaneous flange and collar. A small circle of skin is excised so that snug skin apposition is present. The collar should protrude completely through the skin. If the skin around the collar appears to be too loose, it may be secured with a suture. If the skin opening is too tight, necrosis may occur. If it is too loose, infection is increased and retraction of the device may occur. After a final irrigation as a check for patency, the wound is meticulously closed in layers (Fig. 2-11).

Care of the Chronic Peritoneal Dialysis Catheter. Proper care of the peritoneal dialysis catheter is imperative for its long-term survival. Dialysis should begin immediately after placement to maintain patency. Small volumes of dialysate (e.g., ≤1000 ml) are used initially with gradual increase in the volume of exchange. If exit site leakage is observed, volumes are adjusted downward.

Sterile dressings should be used on exit sites for a week to 10 days post-

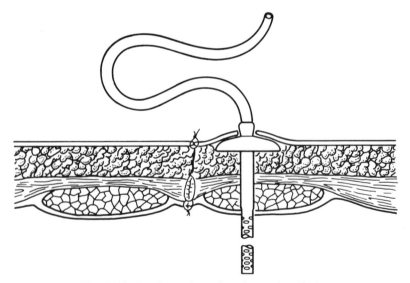

Fig. 2-11. Implantation of peritoneal catheter.

operatively. After healing has occurred and sutures have been removed, patients should be instructed to wash the exit site and surrounding skin once or twice a day. Hydrogen peroxide may be used to remove crusting around the catheter. Patients and dialysis center staff must check the exit site and subcutaneous tunnel routinely for any evidence of infection. Additionally, the catheter itself should be regularly inspected for cracks or tears or debris in the adaptor. Initial line attachments are performed in a sterile manner following catheter insertion. Subsequently the changes are performed at 4- to 8-week intervals, according to unit policy.

Complications with Chronic Peritoneal Catheters. Peritonitis. The development of peritonitis in patients undergoing chronic peritoneal dialysis is much more frequent than in patients undergoing acute peritoneal dialysis. Improper technique in performing home dialysis is the most common cause. Despite newer infection-resistant materials, an indwelling catheter remains a foreign body that increases the risk of infection.

The diagnosis of peritonitis in the chronic situation is based upon the same criteria established for acute peritoneal dialysis. Since chronic peritoneal dialysis does not require hospitalization, the responsibility for making the diagnosis rests with the patient. Abdominal symptoms or turbidity of the dialysate effluent should signal the patient to obtain a dialysate leukocyte count and culture and to advise the physician promptly. The approach to the diagnosis and treatment of peritonitis is discussed in Chapter 4.

Removal of the catheter must be undertaken in cases refractory to conservative management. Some investigators have recommended that a new catheter be implanted immediately after the old one is removed, but this carries a high incidence of a recontamination. In most cases the patient should be maintained on hemodialysis for 2–3 weeks, following which a new abdominal catheter may be placed if the patient is free of symptoms.

Catheter malfunction. Malposition of indwelling peritoneal catheters usually occurs shortly after placement and rarely occurs when catheters have been functional for 10–14 days. Failure to direct the catheter into the pelvis or improper tunneling technique are the commonest causes. The clinical criteria for diagnosis are identical with those of acute peritoneal dialysis. If the catheters are not radiopaque, instillation of a small amount of contrast material aids in demonstrating catheter position on x-ray examination of the abdomen. Catheter repositioning or replacement is the treatment.

In addition to obstruction by blood and fibrin in the immediate postoperative period, chronic indwelling catheters are subject to encasement by a fibrous sheath that may result from recurrent bouts of symptomatic or asymptomatic peritonitis. Inability to drain the dialysate freely is the primary clinical finding. Contrast material injected into the catheter reveals tracking along the catheter sheath and poor diffusion into the peritoneal space. While forced irrigation is often successful in flushing blood or fibrin from indwelling catheters, catheter replacement is necessary when obstruction is due to encasement.

Exit site infection. Exit site infection may result from poor catheter care, poor personal hygiene, traction on the catheter, or improper technique in catheter placement. *Staphylococcus aureus* or *S. epidermidis* are commonly the infecting organisms, although gram-negative organisms such as *Pseudomonas* and *Serratia* are encountered with increasing frequency. Clinical manifestations include erythema, tenderness, edema, and purulent drainage at the exit site. Increased local care of the exit site and a 3- to 4-week course of appropriate antibiotics is generally effective therapy. If signs of infection persist beyond a month, replacement of the indwelling peritoneal catheter is recommended. See Chapter 4 for further discussion.

Sinus tract infections. Sinus tract infections develop secondary to infections of the exit site or of the catheter cuff. If sinus tract infection is not recognized and treated, peritonitis will recur. The chief clinical manifestation is a persistently cloudy dialysis effluent that does not clear with antibiotic treatment. Occasionally drainage at the exit site is noted. In contrast to exit site infections, therapy with local care and antibiotics is ineffective. Removal of the indwelling catheter is essential. A new catheter may be placed later at another site after the sinus tract infection has subdsided. See Chapter 4 for further discussion.

Catheter cuff erosion. Catheter cuff erosion occurs because the subcutaneous tunnel was not made long enough. Pressure necrosis at the catheter exit site results in skin breakdown and exposure of the cuff. Infection invariably results, and a new catheter is mandatory. Many newer catheters have double cuffs, and there have been reports of successful treatment of this problem by trimming the superficial cuff.

REFERENCES

Appel GB: Vascular access infections with long term hemodialysis. Arch Int Med 138:1610, 1976

Bell PRF, Calman KC: Surgical aspects of hemodialysis. Churchill Livingstone, London, 1974

Bergman H: The double lumen subclavian cannula. Dial Transplant 11:73, 1982

Bone GE, Pomajzl MJ: Management of dialysis fistula thrombosis. Am J Surg 138:901, 1979

Bone GE, Pomajzl MJ: Prospective comparison of polytetrafluoroethylene and bovine grafts for dialysis. J Surg Res 29:223, 1980

Brescia MJ, Cimino JE, Appel K: Chronic hemodialysis using venipuncture and a surgically created arteriovenous fistula. N Engl J Med 275:1089, 1966

Butt KMH, Friedman EA, Kountz SL: Angioaccess. Curr Probl Surg 13:1976

DeCubber A, DeWolt L, Lameire N: Single needle hemodialysis with the double head pump via the subclavian vein. Dial Transplant 7:1261, 1978

Geis WP, Giacchino J: A game plan for vascular access for hemodialysis: systematic approach for 10 to 20 year access survival. Surg Rounds 12:92, 1980

Giacchino JL, Gesi WP, Buckingham JM, Vertuno LL, Bansal VK: Vascular access: Long term results, new techniques. Arch Surg 114:403, 1979

Gloor H: Peritoneal access and related complications in CAPD. Am J Med 74:560, 1983

Hammill FS, Johnston GG, Collins GM, et al: A critical appraisal of the changing approaches to vascular access for chronic hemodialysis. Dial Transplant 9:325, 1980

Henderson IS: Peritoneal dialysis. J Med Eng Technol 5:229, 1981

Humphries AL, Nesbit RR, Caruana RJ, et al: Thirty-six recommendations for vascular access operations. Am Surg 47:145, 1981

Johnson G, Blythe W: Hemodynamic effects of arteriovenous shunts used for hemodialysis. Am Surg 171:715, 1970

Larson E, Lindbloom L, Davis K: Development of the clinical nephrology practitioner. Mosby, St. Louis, 1982

Light JL: A review of vascular access management. Dial Transplant 4:20, 1975

Mandel SR, Martin RL, Blumoff RL, et al: Vascular access in a university transplant and dialysis program. Arch Surg 112:1375, 1977

Moncrief JW, Popovich RP: CAPD Update. Masson, New York, 1981

Oblath RW, Buckley FO, Green RM, et al: Prevention of platelet aggregation and adherence to prosthetic vascular grafts by aspirin and dipyridamole. Surgery 89:37, 1978

Palmer R, Newell J, Gray E, Quinton W: Treatment of chronic renal failure by prolonged peritoneal dialysis. N Engl J Med 274:248, 1966

Schmidt RW, Blumenkrantz MJ: IPD, CAPD, CCPD, CRPD: Peritoneal dialysis: Past present and future. Int J Artif Organs 4:124, 1981

Shaldon S, Chiandussi L, Higgs B: Hemodialysis by percutaneous catheterization of the femoral artery and vein with regional heparinization. Lancet 1:857, 1961

Wedall R: Subclavian cannulation for hemodialysis: The present state of the art. Artif Organ 6:73, 1980

Wilson SE, Owens ML: Vascular Access Surgery. Year Book Medical Publishers, Chicago, 1980

3

CARE OF THE PATIENT ON HEMODIALYSIS

Frank A. Gotch   Marcia L. Keen

INDICATIONS FOR DIALYSIS IN CHRONIC RENAL FAILURE

In principle, it would seem that the decision to initiate dialysis therapy should be based on the development and identification of dialysis-responsive clinical abnormalities in patients with slowly progressive renal insufficiency. Unfortunately, it is not a simple decision because the clinical response to dialysis therapy is quite variable. Ideally, the patient should not start dialysis until clearly necessary because it is a complex therapy with side effects, requires a major patient time commitment, and is very costly. On the other hand, it is equally important that dialysis be started before severe clinical abnormalities develop and result in major disability.

The uremic syndrome is a complex entity with multisystem manifestations. Manifestations of advanced uremia that constitute unequivocal indications to initiate dialysis are uremic malnutrition, symptomatic peripheral neuropathy, pericarditis, uncontrollable severe hypertension or congestive heart failure due to sodium overload, and uremic coma. The symptoms typically preceding these catastrophic manifestations are fatigue with progressive restriction of physical activity, decreased mental concentration, nausea, and intermittent vomiting (and occasionally diarrhea) with reduced intake of protein and calories resulting in weight loss. These are unfortunately nonspecific symptoms characteristic of many illnesses, including the depression commonly accompanying a major illness such as progressive renal failure. Consequently, it is important also to correlate clinical symptoms with more objective measures of renal function and nutritional status in patients with slowly progressing renal failure.

73

Urea Clearance and Protein Catabolic Rate

Protein is the major dietary constituent contributing to the uremic syndrome in chronic renal failure. The major protein catabolites are renally excreted and consist of urea, phosphorous, mineral acids, and potassium. Nearly all of the nitrogen content of protein is excreted as urea, and, although urea per se is not highly toxic, it can serve as a useful marker solute to monitor dietary protein intake relative to the level of renal function in progressive chronic renal failure. The rate at which renal function is lost varies widely in chronic renal disease, but is generally slow enough to consider that the patient is in a steady state at any given time. The term "steady state" in this context means that the renal excretion rates of substances such as urea and creatinine equal their generation or production rates, and hence the body content is neither increasing nor decreasing. Although renal excretion of urea and creatinine is not mechanistically analogous to dialyzer function, it is a first-order process and can be described as clearance that is fully analogous to dialyzer clearance (see Chapter 1). The rate of excretion of these solutes by the kidney is therefore given by the product of the clearance and blood concentration, and in steady state can be defined mathematically as

$$G = K_r \cdot C \tag{3-1}$$

where G is the solute generation rate, K_r is renal clearance, and C is the blood concentration, and all units are consistent. In the case of urea,

$$G_U = K_{rU} \cdot \text{BUN} \tag{3-2}$$

where G_U is the net urea nitrogen generation rate, K_{rU} is residual renal urea nitrogen clearance, and BUN is the blood urea nitrogen concentration.

In order to determine the level of residual renal urea clearance, K_{rU}, we need to measure G_U and BUN, and then calculate K_{rU} by rearranging Equation (3-2) to give

$$K_{rU} = \frac{G_U}{\text{BUN}} \tag{3-3}$$

The net generation rate of urea nitrogen can be determined by measuring the total urea nitrogen content of a timed urine collection, since in the steady state all of the urea nitrogen generated during the collection period will be excreted in the urine. The total urea nitrogen content of the urine is given by the product (urine volume, V_u) (urine urea nitrogen concentration, U_u), and the minute rate of urea nitrogen generation (G_U) is found by dividing the total amount excreted by the collection time (t). Thus, since

$$G_U = \frac{V_u \cdot U_u}{t} \tag{3-4}$$

the urea clearance (K_{rU}) is then calculated from Equation (3-3) as

$$K_{rU} = \frac{(V_u \cdot U_u)/t}{BUN} \tag{3-5}$$

A note of caution is in order regarding consistency of units. The U_u and BUN are usually reported as mg/dl and must be changed to mg/ml by multiplying by 0.01 or simply moving the decimal point 2 places to the left.

The length of the urine collection should be at least 12–24 hours, or 720–1440 minutes, to minimize the effect of collection errors. Typical data reported for a chronic renal failure patient might be as follows: collection time = 20 h (1200 min); V_u = 2100 ml; U_u = 250 mg/dl (2.5 mg/ml); BUN = 70 mg/dl (0.70 mg/ml). Using Equations (3-4 and 3-5), we can calculate

$$G_U = \frac{V_u \cdot U_u}{t} = \frac{2100(2.5)}{1200} = 4.4 \text{ mg/min}$$

$$K_{rU} = \frac{G_U}{BUN} = \frac{2100(2.5)/1200}{0.70} = \frac{4.4}{0.7} = 6.3 \text{ ml/min}$$

The calculations show that G_U is 4.4 mg/min and K_{rU} is 6.3 ml/min. These values provide objective measurements of the level of renal function and dietary protein intake for correlation with the clinical manifestations of uremia. There is a predictable relationship between the net protein catabolic rate (PCR, g/day) and G_U, which is given by

$$PCR = 9.35(G_U) + 11 \tag{3-6}$$

Equation (3-6) can be used to compute the PCR for the patient example above where G_U is 4.4 mg/min. The calculation shows

$$PCR = 9.35(4.4) + 11 = 52 \text{ g/day}$$

The PCR calculation provides a measurement of the number of grams of protein catabolized daily to waste products. It can be used to assess compliance with the prescribed dietary protein intake and/or nitrogen or protein balance. If the patient's weight is stable or increasing (and there is no evidence of water and salt retention), it would be expected that the body content of protein is stable; therefore, the PCR must be equal to the dietary protein intake. If the diet records indicate a substantial discrepancy between dietary protein intake and PCR, it is very likely that there are errors in the patient's estimation of protein intake, and hence willful or inadvertant poor compliance with the prescribed diet. If PCR exceeds reported dietary protein intake, and there is associated weight loss, negative body protein balance is probable, due to inadequate protein and caloric intake. Such malnutrition is possibly in consequence of uremic toxicity, which would be a clear indication to initiate dialysis therapy.

The PCR provides a valuable objective method to assess nutritional therapy. However, it would be cumbersome and somewhat expensive to routinely measure G_U in accordance with Equation (3-4) by urine collection. If K_{rU} is known, it is apparent from Equation (3-2) that G_U can be calculated simply by measuring the BUN and multiplying this value by K_{rU}. Since K_{rU} is usually slowly decreasing, it cannot be assumed to be constant over several months. Consequently, if the BUN changes, it may not be clear whether K_{rU}, G_U, or both have changed.

In the steady state Equation (3-1) can also be applied to creatinine generation (G_{Cr}, mg/min), clearance (K_{rCr}, ml/min), and blood level (Cr, mg/ml) in accordance with

$$G_{Cr} = K_{rCr} \cdot Cr \quad \text{or} \quad K_{rCr} = \frac{G_{Cr}}{Cr} \tag{3-7}$$

from which can be derived

$$K_{rCr} = \frac{G_{Cr}}{Cr} = \frac{(V_u \cdot Cr_u)/t}{Cr} \tag{3-8}$$

Unlike G_U, which will vary from day to day directly with PCR (and hence dietary protein intake), G_{Cr} remains quite stable over long intervals if the skeletal muscle mass remains constant, since G_{Cr} is directly proportional to the amount of skeletal muscle. Consequently, if G_{Cr} has been previously measured, K_{rCr} can be computed simply by measurement of the blood creatinine (Cr) (Equation 3-8) if there has been no substantial change in muscle mass or body weight. The K_{rU} is always substantially lower than K_{rCr}, but there will tend to be a fairly constant ratio (R_{K_r}) of K_{rU}/K_{rCr} in the absence of acute fluid and electrolyte disturbances or drastic change in K_{rCr}. Thus it follows that

$$K_{rU} = R_{K_r}(K_{rCr}) \tag{3-9}$$

Since K_{rU} is now calculated and BUN is measured, G_U can be calculated from Equations (3-2) and (3-9):

$$G_U = R_{K_r} \cdot K_{rCr} \cdot BUN$$

In this way creatinine clearance, urea clearance, and net urea generation rate (from which PCR is calculated) can all be determined simply by measuring the serum creatinine and BUN.

If the patient has very slowly declining renal function, G_{Cr} and R_{K_r} may be stable for many months. However, periodically these parameters should be remeasured, particularly if serum creatinine increases substantially, because this is associated with increasing degradation of creatinine in the gut and reduction in the net generation appearing in blood.

There is generally somewhat more variability in R_{K_r} than in G_{Cr}. If G_{Cr} is believed to be stable, R_{K_r} can be determined from the plasma creatinine and

BUN and the urine urea (U_u) and creatinine (Cr_u) measured in a spot urine sample. Appropriate combination of Equations (3-5), (3-8), and (3-9) results in

$$R_{K_r} = \frac{Cr}{BUN} \cdot \frac{U_u}{Cr_u} \tag{3-10}$$

The use of Equation (3-10) with blood concentrations and concentrations in a spot urine is easier for the patient in that only a single spot urine sample is required, and it may be more accurate, since it eliminates collection time errors. These relationships can be illustrated by further consideration of the patient example given above. Assume that, in addition to the urea measurements listed, the following creatinine measurements were made: Cr_u = 39 mg/dl (0.39 mg/ml) and blood creatinine = 5.4 mg/dl (0.054 mg/ml). Using Equations (3-7) and (3-8) it can be calculated that

$$G_{Cr} = \frac{2100(0.39)}{1200} = 0.68 \text{ mg/min}$$

$$K_{rCr} = \frac{2100(0.39)/1200}{0.054} = 12.6 \text{ ml/min}$$

It is thus established that G_{Cr} = 0.68 mg/min, K_{rCr} = 12.6 ml/min, and R_{K_r} = 6.3/12.6 = 0.50. Assume that 4 months later the following measurements are made: Cr = 6.0 mg/dl (0.06 mg/ml); BUN = 120 mg/dl (1.20 mg/ml); U_u = 355 mg/dl (3.55 mg/ml), and Cr_u = 33 mg/dl (0.33 mg/ml) measured in a spot urine.

We can assume that G_{Cr} is unchanged, so that K_{rCr} can be calculated as 0.68/0.060 = 11.3 ml/min. Next, using Equation (3-10), we compute R_{K_r} as

$$R_{K_r} = \frac{0.060}{1.20} \cdot \frac{3.55}{0.33} = 0.54$$

Using Equation (3-9) we can compute K_{rU} = 0.54(11.3) = 6.1 ml/min, and from Equation (3-2) compute that G_U = 1.20(6.1) = 7.3 mg/min. Finally, using Equation (3-6), PCR is computed as

$$PCR = 9.35(7.3) + 11 = 79 \text{ g/day}$$

These calculations indicate that there has been a minimal decrease in K_{rCr} from 12.5 to 11.3 ml/min and negligible change in K_{rU}. The sharp increase in BUN from 70 to 120 mg/dl was due entirely to an increase in PCR from 52 to 79 g/day. If the patient was not losing weight, the conclusion must be reached that dietary protein intake increased to 79 g/day; dietary counseling is indicated to return the dietary protein intake to ~50 g/day, which will result in BUN ~65 mg/dl. These calculations provide a definitive analysis of the clinical data, showing that renal function has not changed but that protein ingestion has increased by 27 g/day. The quantified increase in dietary protein intake permits the renal dietitian to approach the patient with precise knowledge of how large the error is in dietary protein intake, which facilitates a more quantitative discussion of protein sources and serving sizes. Other blood chemistry changes would likely be found in association with the increase in BUN in such a patient. Since phosphate intake and metabolic hydrogen ion generation are strongly dependent on PCR, the rise in BUN would likely be associated with a rise in serum phosphorus and a fall in bicarbonate concentration, both of which would return toward normal when PCR is reduced.

Clinical Correlates of K_{rU}, BUN, and PCR in Chronic Renal Failure

As discussed in the preceding section, the major uremic symptoms that actually result in initiation of dialysis therapy are often rather nonspecific. The most objective and commonest dialysis responsive clinical manifestation is impaired nutrition and weight loss and negative nitrogen balance due to uremic gastrointestinal toxicity with anorexia, nausea, and intermittent vomiting. When impaired nutrition due to uremic toxicity is established, dialysis is clearly indicated. However, both excessive and inadequate protein intake relative to the degree of renal failure may occur and complicate the clinical picture. Consequently, it is very helpful to examine K_{rU}, BUN, and PCR together as shown in Figure 3-1, which is derived from the steady-state relationships discussed above.

Figure 3-1 shows the relationship of BUN to K_{rU} at constant levels of PCR ranging from 20 to 130 g/day. The lettered domains indicate approximate regions in which dialysis or dietary management are indicated.

Domain A is the region in which dialysis usually becomes indicated, the indications increased as the patient moves to the left in this domain. It is apparent that the BUN will vary widely when dialysis is initiated, depending heavily on PCR. For example, if K_{rU} is 2 ml/min and PCR is very low at 20 g/day due to nutritional failure, the BUN will be only 48 mg/dl. In contrast, if at this level of K_{rU} PCR is 40 g/day, the BUN will be 150 mg/dl. The BUN alone provides no insight into either nutrition or the level of renal function.

Domains B, C, and D are regions in which dialysis is usually not yet clinically required for optimal management of the uremic syndrome. Domain B is a region of optimal matching of PCR (or dietary protein intake) to the level of K_{rU}, with BUN ranging from 50 to 80 mg/dl. As K_{rU} falls from 10 to 4.5 ml/min, it is necessary to progressively restrict dietary protein to prevent sharp increases in BUN. For example, to maintain BUN at 70 mg/dl, protein intake and PCR would have to decrease from ~75 to 40 g/day as K_{rU} falls from 10 to 4.5 ml/min.

Domain C is a region of excessive protein intake relative to K_{rU}. The change in PCR and dietary protein intake required to produce a desired change in BUN at a specific level of K_{rU} can be read directly from the figure. For example, if K_{rU} is 8 ml/min and the BUN is 120 mg/dl, the PCR is 100 g/day. To reduce the BUN

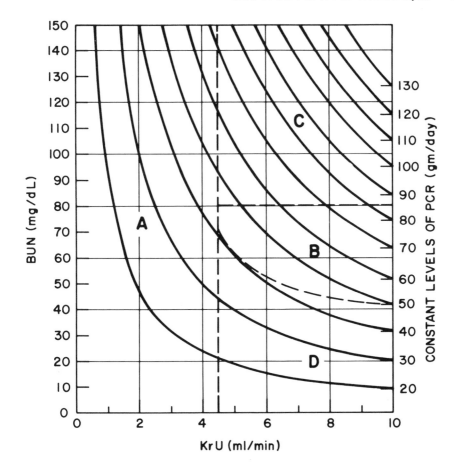

A . Increasing clinical indications for dialysis as KrU falls below 4.5 ml/min.

B . Optimal dietary protein intake relative to KrU.

C . Excessive dietary protein intake relative to KrU.

D . Excessive restriction of dietary protein intake relative to KrU or anorexia not likely due primarily to uremic toxicity.

Fig. 3-1. Clinical correlations of residual renal urea clearance (K_{ru}), blood urea nitrogen concentration (BUN), and protein catabolic rate (PCR) for patients with chronic renal failure. See text for discussion, including explanation of lettered domains.

to 70 mg/dl the PCR (actually dietary protein ingestion) would have to be reduced to ~65 g/day.

The relationships shown in Figure 3-1 do not relate PCR to body size, which should also be considered in both large and small patients. In large patients it is probably not wise to restrict protein intake to less than 0.8 g/kg/day where weight is ideal body weight. In very small patients it is difficult to construct palatable diets with less than 40 g protein intake per day. Thus, in a 40-kg patient restriction of protein intake below 1.0 g/kg/day is often not realistic.

Domain D is a region of either excessive protein restriction or anorexia which is not likely to be due primarily to uremic toxicity. For example, if K_{rU} is 8 ml/min and the BUN is only 25 mg/dl, the PCR is very low at 30 g/day. Although the patient clearly has chronic renal failure, it is quite unlikely that the nutritional impairment is due to uremic toxicity that will be corrected by dialysis. Other clinical explanations for anorexia must be sought.

It must be pointed out that the dialysis and nutritional therapy relationships depicted in Figure 3-1 refer to conventional therapy of chronic renal failure with whole food diets containing adequate amounts of high biologic quality protein. There are currently experimental protocols for management of chronic renal failure with synthetic diets containing essential amino acids and/or their keto-acid analogs. If these therapies prove to be clinically successful and realistic, the relationships in Figure 3-1 could change, so that the clinical indications to initiate dialysis would move to the left and down in domain A by virtue of maintaining nitrogen balance with reduced clinical uremia at very low levels of nitrogen intake and urea clearance.

CLINICAL GUIDELINES FOR AN ADEQUATE DIALYSIS PRESCRIPTION

When dialysis is clinically indicated, the hemodialysis prescription must provide therapy adequate to control fluid, electrolyte and acid-base balance, and the clinical syndrome of uremia. Furthermore, this therapy must result in minimal intradialytic morbidity. Adequate dialysis only partly controls the clinical uremic syndrome, so there is usually variable residual morbidity in these patients. Ongoing abnormalities include variable levels of anemia, impaired immunocompetence, hyperparathyroidism, hypertension, cardiomyopathy, and nutritional impairment, as discussed more fully in Chapter 5. Precise relationships between many of the clinical manifestations of uremia and dialyzable toxic solutes remain unknown and continue, in part, to confound a comprehensive quantified approach to the dialysis prescription.

Middle Molecules

In an attempt to approach this dilemma conceptually, correlations between dialyzer solute transport properties and residual morbidity in the dialyzed patient have been studied in a search for clues to the molecular size of toxic materials that must be removed. As discussed in Chapter 1 (see Figure 1-6), the mechanism underlying dialyzer solute removal is diffusion; consequently, clearance is inversely proportional to molecular size. For a number of years it was argued that poorly cleared "middle molecules," mol wt 1000–1500, were responsible for much of the residual morbidity in dialysis patients. There has been little success in proving this hypothesis either from clinical studies or measurement of endogenous peptide materials in this molecular weight range. Although some controversy remains, the current consensus is that middle molecule transport is not a significant consideration in the dialysis prescription.

Creatinine

Creatinine continues to be used to some extent as a marker solute to define adequate dialysis. Net generation of creatinine is relatively constant and proportional to the size of the skeletal muscle mass and serves as an extremely useful solute to measure the glomerular filtration rate and to follow the course of renal disease. In the dialysis patient predialysis serum creatinine reflects the ratio of creatinine generation (magnitude of skeletal muscle) to the amount of dialysis prescribed. If uremic toxicity were proportional to the skeletal muscle mass, the predialysis serum creatinine would be a useful marker to assure that the level of dialysis was adequate relative to the skeletal muscle mass. However, there is no evidence that uremic toxicity is proportional to the mass of skeletal muscle; consequently, the predialysis serum creatinine may range from 6 to 25 mg/dl in adequately dialyzed patients. In male patients who come to dialysis with marked wasting and then undergo nutritional recovery with restoration of skeletal muscle, it is not uncommon to see predialysis creatinine increase from 8 to 25 mg/dl over the first 1 to 2 years of dialysis therapy. There is no need to increase dialysis in such patients to maintain some arbitrary lower level of predialysis creatinine when the prescribed dialysis therapy has been adequate for nutritional recovery and restoration of skeletal muscle.

Protein Nutrition: BUN

The protein catabolic rate, which equals dietary protein intake in the steady state, has a major influence on the level of uremic toxicity and nutritional status. Inadequate levels of protein intake can result in protein malnutrition, while excessive levels of intake are associated with high phosphorus intake and with high rates of mineral acid production and urea generation. Since nearly all of the nitrogen content of protein is excreted as urea nitrogen, the rate of urea nitrogen generation can be used to measure the protein catabolic rate, and the BUN can be used to assess the level of protein catabolism relative to the amount of dialysis prescribed. These relationships in dialysis are analogous to the steady-state relationships in Equation (3-1) and can be described in a word equation as

$$BUN = \frac{\text{Protein catabolic rate}}{\text{Amount of dialysis}} \qquad (3\text{-}11)$$

It is important to note in Equation (3-11) that BUN represents the ratio of protein catabolic rate to the amount of dialysis prescribed and that, if the amount of dialysis is held constant, the BUN will increase linearly as the protein catabolic rate increases. A quantitative discussion of these relationships will be provided later.

A National Cooperative Dialysis Study (NCDS) of the relationships among morbidity and BUN, protein catabolic rate, and the amount of dialysis has recently been reported. The results of mechanistic analysis of the study are depicted in Figure 3-2. For this analysis protein catabolic rate is expressed as pcr (g/kg

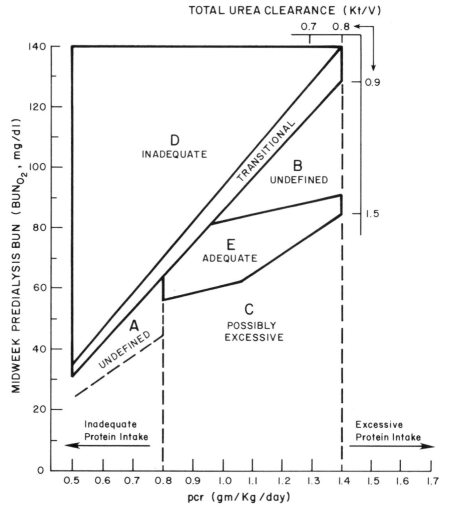

Fig. 3-2. Clinical outcome of hemodialysis treatment as a function of protein catabolic rate (pcr), midweek predialysis BUN, and total urea clearance, as defined by the National Cooperative Dialysis Study.

of normalized body weight/day). Note that that PCR discussed earlier is now transformed to pcr by dividing by ideal body weight. All patients were dialyzed thrice weekly, and BUN is expressed as the midweek predialysis level (BUN_{o_2}, mg/dl). The level of dialysis is expressed as the product of dialyzer urea clearance (K, L/min) and treatment time (t, min) divided by the body urea distribution volume (V) or as Kt/V, which is a dimensionless parameter describing the fractional body water urea clearance prescribed. These interrelationships between pcr, BUN_{o_2} and Kt/V will be treated more quantitatively in discussion of the dialysis prescription. In the NCDS patients K_{rU} was near zero.

In the NCDS, patients were followed for 6 months at various levels of dialysis. Appearance of uremic manifestations or medical indications for hospitalization was carefully noted and used to define treatment failure expressed as the fraction of patients failing due to uremic manifestations and/or hospitalization. The uremic manifestations resulting in failure were gastrointestinal toxicity with anorexia, nausea, vomiting, or gastrointestinal bleeding; cardiac toxicity with pericarditis, pleuritis, congestive heart failure, or sudden death; and hematologic toxicity with increased anemia or transfusion requirements. The results are shown in Figure 3-2, where five lettered domains are depicted.

Domain D was shown to be clearly inadequate therapy with high and constant probability of failure of 0.57, indicating that 57% of patients in this domain of therapy developed uremic manifestations or required hospitalization during the 6 months of the study. All of these patients were treated with Kt/V less than 0.8. It can be noted that this domain of failure encompasses a wide range of BUN_{o_2} values (40–140 mg/dl), depending on the pcr.

Domain E in Figure 3-2 represents the patient group for whom Kt/V was prescribed ranging from 0.9 to 1.5 and increasing with pcr, so that BUN_{o_2} values were less than 90 mg/dl at maximum pcr of 1.4 g/kg/day. Clinical outcome was excellent with constant 13% failure over this treatment domain.

The transitional zone depicted in Figure 3-2, where $0.8 < Kt/V < 0.9$, represents the region of abrupt decrease in the probability of failure from 57% to 13%, which appeared as a discontinuity in the outcome data. The exact relationship between clinical outcome and Kt/V was not defined by the study, hence the label "transitional."

Since clinical outcome appeared to be constant in domain E as Kt/V increased from 0.9 to 1.5, it can be tentatively concluded that higher levels of dialysis will not further reduce morbidity. Therefore, domain C is considered to be a region of possibly excessive dialysis.

Because of the design of the NCDS, no patients with pcr < 0.80 were treated with $Kt/V > 0.90$; consequently, clinical outcome of patients in domain A must be considered to be undefined. For similar reasons, domain B is undefined. As pcr increased from 0.8 to 1.4, Kt/V was increased in proportion to pcr in this study and, therefore, BUN_{o_2} was constrained to levels less than $\sim$90 mg/dl as shown by domain E.

The data in Figure 3-2 provide a comprehensive definition of both adequate and inadequate dialysis as well as indicating undefined and possibly excessive domains of dialysis. This figure portrays the only data base describing clinical outcome as a function of both protein nutrition and the level of dialysis.

KINETICS OF THE DIALYSIS PRESCRIPTION

Clear guidelines for an adequate dialysis prescription were identified by the National Cooperative Dialysis Study and are defined by BUN, pcr, and the amount of dialysis. However, in order to prescribe optimal therapy, it is necessary to consider the kinetics of urea nitrogen generation and removal, which determine the relationships among BUN, pcr, and the amount of dialytic urea removal in the patient requiring dialysis therapy. Rigorous mathematical solution of the urea kinetic model for each patient is complex and realistically requires computer assistance. Computer services for this purpose are now available through time share or with an in-house microcomputer using purchased software. These systems provide the most efficient means of managing long-term data for a sizable population of patients. However, it is possible to develop relatively simple yet rigorous graphic and algebraic relationships among these parameters without dependence on a computer. In addition, this approach can provide greater understanding of the kinetics underlying the prescription.

In the following sections, an overview of the relationship of optimal predialysis BUN to pcr and total fractional urea clearance (K_T, the sum of dialyzer and effective residual renal clearances divided by V) can be explained. Finally, when dialyzer clearance is chosen, the dialysis prescription (for dialyzer, blood flow, and dialysis duration) can be defined.

The BUN Concentration Profile

The BUN oscillates in a sawtooth pattern with intermittent dialysis therapy, as shown in Figure 3-3 for a typical asymmetric thrice-weekly dialysis schedule. The profile is depicted here beginning with the end-dialysis BUN on Friday for reasons which will become clear later. The predialysis BUN's are designated as BUN_o and postdialysis values as BUN_t. These respective values are designated for the first, second, and third dialyses of the week with subscripts 1, 2, and 3, so the midweek values would be BUN_{o_2}, BUN_{t_2}.

The decrease in BUN during each dialysis is determined by the amount of dialysis prescribed, which is Kt/V, where K is the urea clearance on dialysis of duration t, and V is the volume of distribution of urea in the patient. The basis

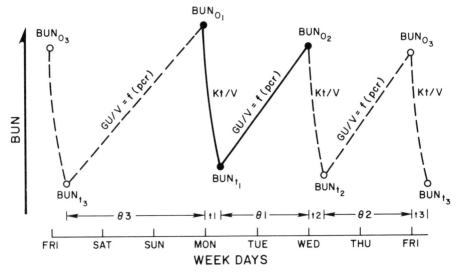

Fig. 3-3. Typical BUN profile with thrice-weekly dialysis.

of the definition can best be seen from a simplified version of the urea kinetic modeling equation

$$BUN_t = BUN_o e^{-Kt/V} \tag{3-12}$$

or

$$\frac{BUN_t}{BUN_o} = e^{-Kt/V} \tag{3-12}$$

It can be seen in Equation (3-12) that Kt/V is the exponent relating BUN_t to BUN_o and determines the fractional decrease in BUN during dialysis.

Although the dialyzer removes urea only from the bloodstream flowing through it, urea is distributed throughout body water and rapidly diffuses out of the intracellular volume and extracellular volume into the blood volume across cell and capillary membranes as the blood concentration falls during dialysis. Although only a small fraction of the blood volume passes through the dialyzer each minute, the concentration of urea in whole blood volume falls uniformly because the blood volume is well mixed. The cardiac output is 6–8 L/min, while the total blood volume is only 3–5 L; thus the entire blood volume is recirculated through the vascular system 2 to 3 times per minute. Urea rapidly diffuses across cell membranes so that minimal concentration differences (i.e., diffusion gradients) result between intracellular and extracellular compartments. Somewhat larger concentration gradients across cell membranes may occur in specialized tissue, particularly the brain, and may contribute in part to cerebral edema in patients with very high BUN and a rapid rate of dialysis.

The rise in BUN between dialyses in the patient with no residual renal function is determined entirely by the amount of urea generated over the interdialytic interval (θ) divided by its volume of distribution. This is depicted in Figure 3-3 as $(G_u \cdot \theta)/V$.

Earlier in the discussion of steady-state chronic renal failure, urea generation (G_U) was related to protein catabolic rate (PCR) or total grams of protein catabolized per day. In the dialysis patient in whom K_{rU} often is near zero, virtually all urea generated accumulates in the body water. In order to establish generalized relationships using BUN, it is essential to consider urea generation divided by V which relates directly to concentration change. A new term is needed, called pcr, which is a function of the urea generation rate factored by body weight. Thus, pcr is defined as PCR/normalized body weight. Normalized body weight is defined as $V/0.58$ or 1.72 (V), which considers the normalized body mass to be 58% water. Thus,

$$pcr = \frac{PCR}{V/0.58} = 0.58\frac{PCR}{V} = \frac{PCR}{1.72V} \tag{3-13}$$

This definition of pcr expresses PCR relative to V and hence directly relates to G_U/V and change in BUN. Furthermore, it preserves the important nutritional concept that the requirement for protein intake is related to body size with average normal intake of 1 g/kg/day. This corresponds to 70 g in a 70-kg individual, for instance. Since the average body water content is ~58%, the normalized body weight used above will generally correspond quite closely to actual body weight. In the obese patient the normalized body weight will be substantially less than actual body weight and provides a measure of body weight corrected for excess fat.

The Impact of Residual Renal Urea Clearance (K_{rU})

In the patient with some residual renal urea clearance (K_{rU}) there is continuous urea excretion between dialyses, which reduces the stable midweek, predialysis BUN (BUN_{o_2}) relative to pcr and Kt/V. This effect is shown in Figure 3-4, where the stable BUN profile from Monday to Wednesday is calculated for BUN_{o_2} target of 75 mg/dl with pcr = 1.0 g/kg/day, and variable K_{rU}.

Examination of Figure 3-4 shows that as K_{rU} increases, the interdialytic rise in BUN becomes smaller. In fact the slope of the BUN buildup curve is precisely determined by K_{rU} for any specified values of BUN_{o_2} and pcr. It is apparent in this example with pcr = 1.0 that the amount of dialysis required (the decrease in BUN during dialysis determined by Kt/V) in order to achieve BUN_{o_2} of 75 mg/dl is determined by the K_{rU}, since it fixes the slope of the buildup curve. Inspection of the curves shows that when $K_{rU} = 0$, postdialysis BUN (BUN_{t_1}) must be 36. When $K_{rU} = 3.0$ ml/min, the BUN_{t_1} is 55 mg/dl. Calculation of the corresponding Kt/V values shows that for $K_{rU} = 0$, the amount of dialysis needed (Kt/V) = 1.0, whereas when $K_{rU} = 3.0$ ml/min, $Kt/V = 0.51$.

The graphic relationships seen in Figure 3-4 suggest that it should be possible to transform K_{rU} to a parameter, the effective renal urea clearance (K_{rE},

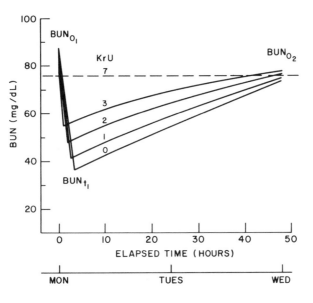

Fig. 3-4. Impact of residual renal function (K_{rU}) on the BUN profile.

L), which is equivalent to an amount of dialysis. This transformation of K_{rU} could then be used to estimate the decrease in Kt/V required for any specified midweek predialysis BUN target at a given level of pcr. The coefficient required is dependent on the dialysis schedule or number of dialyses per week and, since it transforms K_{rU} (ml/min) into K_{rE}, which provides equivalent units of Kt (L), the coefficient will have units of L/ml/min. The value for the coefficient for twice-weekly dialysis is 10.1 L/ml/min, and for thrice-weekly dialysis is 5.9 L/ml/min.

For instance, the equivalent urea clearance on dialysis for a K_{rU} of 1 ml/min for thrice-weekly dialysis is 5.9 L/ml/min. This is the amount of urea clearance by dialysis saved by the residual renal function, compared with that necessary in an anephric individual. Total urea clearance (K_T) is the liters of urea clearance provided by dialysis plus that provided by residual renal function, expressed as K_{rE}.

Therapy Assessment

Now that the interrelationships of BUN, pcr, and total fractional urea clearance (K_T, urea clearance by dialysis added to the effective clearance by residual renal function (K_{rE}) and divided by V) have been explained, the optimal values for these three parameters can be given. In Figures 3-5 and 3-6, therapy assessment plots relating midweek predialysis BUN (BUN_{o_2}) to pcr at variable levels of K_T are shown for twice weekly (Figure 3-5) or thrice-weekly dialysis (Figure 3-6).

These figures are three variable plots which show the pcr, midweek predialysis BUN lines for constant values of K_T ranging from 0.8 to 3.0 in the case of Figure 3-5 for dialysis twice a week, and from 0.2 to 1.8 in Figure 3-6 for dialysis three times per week. In addition, the clinical outcome domains from the National Cooperative Dialysis Study are depicted so that on a single plot the risk of clinical morbidity can be correlated to pcr, BUN_{o_2} values, as well as to the magnitude of K_T (clearance by dialysis as well as by residual renal function) that is required to achieve the pcr and BUN_{o_2} values. It is apparent that total fractional urea clearance must be substantially higher for twice-weekly dialysis than for thrice-weekly dialysis to achieve the same pcr and BUN_{o_2} values. This, of course, reflects the need to achieve lower postdialysis BUN values with only two dialyses per week.

The dotted modeling lines in Figures 3-5 and 3-6 describe the target pcr, BUN_{o_2}, and K_T values that must be achieved for an adequate dialysis prescription as defined by the NCDS. In the case of thrice-weekly dialysis, the modeling line provides a K_T of 1.0 over a pcr range 0.50 to 1.1 g/kg/day. This will assure that K_T is 25% greater than 0.8, the level at which discontinuity was seen with a sharp morbidity increase in the NCDS. Although domain A in Figure 3-2 is undefined, it is clearly undesirable to reduce dialysis in patients with low pcr and treat these patients in either the transitional zone or domain D where morbidity was shown to be high. The BUN_{o_2} will increase from 30 to 85 as pcr increases from 0.5 to 1.1 with constant $K_T = 1.0$, a result that points up the unsuitability of BUN alone as a criterion for an adequate dialysis prescription.

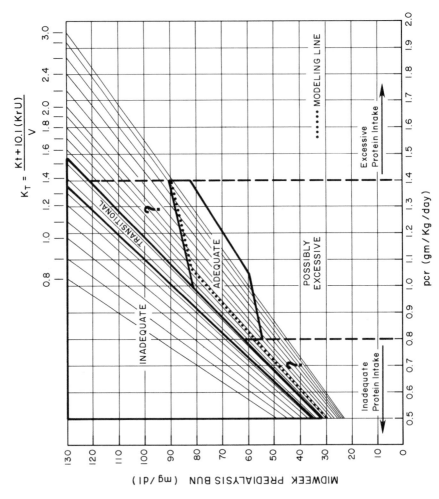

Fig. 3-5. Therapy assessment plot for twice-weekly dialysis.

88

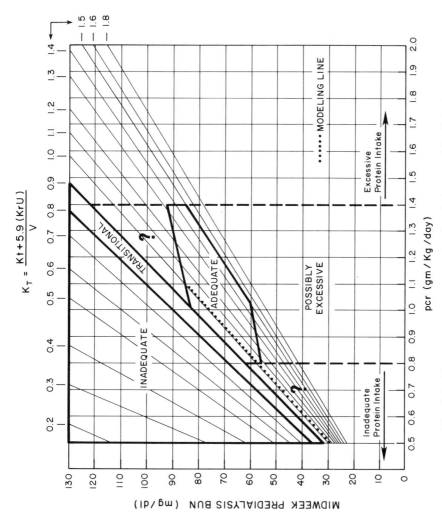

$$K_T = \frac{Kt + 5.9\,(KrU)}{V}$$

Fig. 3-6. Therapy assessment plot for thrice-weekly dialysis.

89

The modeling line in Figure 3-6 follows the upper bound BUN level of region E in Figure 3-2, the domain of adequate dialysis over the pcr range 1.1 to 1.4. There was no increase in morbidity in domain E with either vertical or horizontal movement of pcr, BUN_{o_2} points in this domain. Since clinical morbidity was constant across domain E, the modeling line follows the upper bound of the domain for $1.1 < pcr < 1.4$. However, it can also be pointed out that, although domain B is undefined by the NCDS, a recent report suggests it may also be adequate therapy.

There are no guidelines for recommending an adequate dialysis prescription for high levels of pcr greater than 1.4 g/kg/day. Dietary counseling for both low (<0.8) and high (>1.4) pcr would be a major therapeutic approach. If pcr remains high, the level of dialysis probably should be increased to maintain BUN_{o_2} at a level the medical team feels is reasonable. Fortunately, less than 5% of patients persistently maintain average pcr > 1.4 except during a catabolic response to acute intervening illness.

The therapy modeling line for twice-weekly dialysis in Figure 3-5 describes the same family of pcr, CO_2 values as for thrice-weekly dialysis, but K_T values required are much higher because of less frequent dialysis.

CALCULATION OF THE DIALYSIS PRESCRIPTION

The clinical correlates of an adequate dialysis prescription and the kinetics underlying the prescription have now been discussed. The prescription calculation is somewhat complex conceptually because all of the prescription parameters are interrelated. Consequently, it is highly desirable to calculate the prescription in a systematic way with a clear separation and understanding of the prescription variables. The following is a logical sequence of calculation steps (Table 3-1).

1. Calculate the urea volume of distribution, V.
2. Calculate the renal urea clearance, K_{rU}, and effective renal clearance, K_{rE}.
3. Determine the protein catabolic rate, pcr.
4. Determine total fractional urea clearance, K_T, from Figures 3-5 and 3-6.
5. Calculate dialyzer fractional clearance, Kt/V.
6. Select rate of dialysis, K/V, and calculate dialyzer urea clearance, K.
7. Select most appropriate dialyzer and blood flow.
8. Calculate treatment time, t.
9. Evaluate ultrafiltration, Q_F, requirements and determine the transmembrane pressure, TMP.
10. Determine dialysate sodium and potassium.

In order to calculate a prescription it is necessary to have values for V, K_{rU}, and pcr (Steps 1–3). In the new patient, V and pcr will not be known. The initial prescription is based on an estimated V and usually assumes pcr = 1.0. If K_{rU}

Table 3-1. The Dialysis Prescription

Step	Calculation	Method	Use Figure	Prescribe
1	V	a) Initially assume 0.58 body weight, and subsequently b) Measure from intradialytic ΔBUN and Kt	3-7	
2	K_{rU}	Urine urea cleared in specified interval: a) $K_{rU} = \dfrac{V_u \cdot U_u}{t(0.25\ BUN_{t_1} + 0.75\ BUN_{o_2})}$ (3×/week dialysis) b) $K_{rU} = \dfrac{V_u \cdot U_u}{t(0.16\ BUN_{t_1} + 0.84\ BUN_{o_2})}$ (2×/week dialysis)		
3	pcr	a) Initially assume 1.0 g/kg/day, and subsequently b) Measure from pcr $= 0.22 + 0.036\ \Delta$BUN $+ \dfrac{0.054\ (K_{rU})(\overline{BUN})}{V}$		
4	Total fractional urea clearance (K_T)	Use target predialysis midweek BUN and known pcr	3-5, 3-6	
5	Kt/V	a) $Kt/V = K_T - \dfrac{5.9\ K_{rU}}{V}$ (3×/week dialysis) b) $Kt/V = K_T - \dfrac{10.1\ K_{rU}}{V}$ (2×/week dialysis)		
6	K	Select $K/V \simeq 0.0060$ and calculate K	3-9	Dialyzer, Q_B
7	Evaluate dialyzer choices	Use available dialyzer function curves to achieve desired K	3-10	t
8	Length of treatment (t)	Kt/V divided by K/V	3-11	TMP
9	Q_F	(Weight − estimated dry weight) $= t \cdot K_{UF} \cdot$ TMP		
10	Evaluate dialysate Na^+ and K^+ requirement	Measure predialysis Na^+, K^+ and assign target postdialysis Na^+, K^+	3-12, 3-13	Dialysate Na^+, K^+

and pcr have been followed prior to initiation of dialysis, which should be the case, the most recent value can be used to calculate the initial prescription. During the course of the first four dialyses pre- and post-BUN measurements and two interdialytic urine collections should be made to determine V, pcr, and K_{rU}. These values can then be used to refine the initial prescription.

The 10 steps in prescription calculation can now be considered in more detail.

Step 1. Determination of V

As shown in Equation (3-12), the drop in BUN on dialysis is directly related to Kt/V. Therefore, if Kt is known, and BUN_t/BUN_o are measured, V can be determined. Figure 3-7 shows V as a function of BUN_t and BUN_o for constant Kt values ranging from 20 to 60 L. For example, if $Kt = 30$ L, predialysis BUN $= 80$ mg/dl, and postdialysis BUN $= 32$ mg/dl, $V = 28$ L. The curves in Figure 3-7 were derived from the rigorous variable volume urea model assuming an average fluid removal of 2 L and pcr of 1 g/kg/day.

If Kt is overestimated, erroneously large V's will be calculated. This is a common error and may happen with faulty blood pump calibration, recirculation in the fistula, or clotting in the dialyzer. Likewise, if BUN_t/BUN_o is erroneously high due to laboratory measurement errors, erroneously high volumes will be estimated. With good control of Kt and BUN measurement, the V should be reproducible to better than $\pm 10\%$. Because of the possibility of this significant measurement error, an average V representing the last four to six measurements should be used for prescription calculations.

It is very useful to evaluate V as a fraction of body weight and habitus. In lean patients it would be expected to be in the range of 58 to 65% of body weight, while in obese patients it may be as low as 35% of body weight. If V is 80 to 100% of body weight, it can be concluded with certainty that Kt is overestimated (commonest error) or that BUN_t/BUN_o is erroneously high due to measurement error. In the new patient prior to the first dialysis V must be estimated. A value of 58% of body weight is assumed for lean patients (e.g., 40.6 L in a 70-kg patient).

Step 2. Determination of K_{rU}

In patients with residual K_{rU} factored into treatment, it is essential to periodically measure K_{rU}, since in all patients K_{rU} eventually declines to near zero but at widely varying rates. Although it is somewhat inconvenient for the patient to periodically do urine collections to measure K_{rU}, it is well worth the effort. The dialysis treatment time can be decreased ~30 minutes per 1.0 ml K_{rU} for the average-sized patient, and with $K_{rU} \geq 2.5$ ml/min the average patient can often be treated with twice-weekly dialysis.

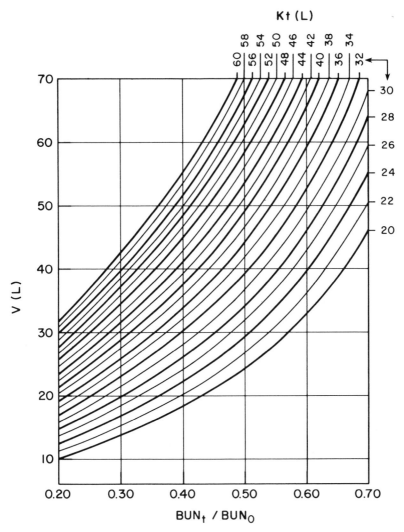

Fig. 3-7. Plot for determination of urea distribution volume (*V*) from the ratio of end-dialysis BUN/predialysis BUN (BUN$_t$/BUN$_o$) and the product of urea clearance and dialysis time (*K*t).

The measurement of K_{rU} in patients on dialysis is more complex than measurement in steady state (see Equation 3-5) because the BUN is not constant. The most rigorous method to determine K_{rU} is to collect urine through the total interdialytic interval and determine the average BUN over the interval. A simpler, yet adequate, technique is to collect for ~24 hours prior to dialysis and estimate the mean BUN during the interval. It is most convenient to measure K_{rU} between the first and second dialyses of the week. The mean BUN during the collection interval on twice-weekly dialysis will be defined as a function of BUN$_{t_1}$ +

BUN_{o_2}, and the formula for calculating K_{rU} is

$$K_{rU} = \frac{(V_u \cdot U_u)/t}{0.16\ BUN_{t_1} + 0.84\ BUN_{o_2}} = \frac{V_u \cdot U_u}{t(0.16\ BUN_{t_1} + 0.84\ BUN_{o_2})} \quad (3\text{-}14)$$

with units as in Equation (3-5).

In the case of thrice-weekly dialysis, the formula for K_{rU} is

$$K_{rU} = \frac{(V_u \cdot U_u)/t}{0.25\ BUN_{t_1} + 0.75\ BUN_{o_2}} = \frac{V_u \cdot U_u}{t(0.25\ BUN_{t_1} + 0.75\ BUN_{o_2})} \quad (3\text{-}15)$$

Nearly all patients with chronic renal failure start dialysis with significant K_{rU}, and in our experience ~30–50% of these patients can initially be treated with twice-weekly dialysis if K_{rU} is ≥2.5 ml/min and is factored into the prescription calculation. The rate of decline in K_{rU} during the first year of dialysis is fairly rapid in the majority of patients; at the end of 1 year, ~75% of patients starting twice-weekly therapy will have to be converted to thrice-weekly treatment, although a small number of patients may be able to continue twice-weekly dialysis for 2–3 years. It is desirable to measure K_{rU} monthly during the first 6 months to clearly define the rate of loss of renal function and hence changes required in the dialysis prescription. If K_{rU} is found to be fairly stable after several determinations, measurement every 2 months is adequate. In the average patient a K_{rU} of 0.5 ml/min results in treatment time reduction of ~15 minutes, so that when K_{rU} clearly falls below 0.5 ml/min, further measurement is unnecessary, and K_{rU} can be considered to be zero with respect to the dialysis prescription. Equations (3-14) and (3-15) are used to calculate renal urea clearance for twice- and thrice-weekly dialysis. As described below, these values will then be converted into equivalent amounts of dialysis. For instance, for thrice-weekly dialysis, K_{rU} is multiplied by 5.9 and divided by V to obtain the equivalent fractional urea clearance provided by residual renal function. It is probably not appropriate to prescribe twice-weekly dialysis if t > 4.5 hours is required, which reflects very low K_{rU}. Depending on patient size, the K_{rU} must usually be at least 2 ml/min for twice-weekly therapy to be suitable.

Step 3. Calculation of Protein Catabolic Rate, pcr

The pcr is calculated directly from the rate of urea nitrogen generation between dialyses, which is determined from the rate of accumulation of urea nitrogen in body water plus, in patients with some residual K_{rU}, the rate of excretion in the urine. Solution of the urea nitrogen mass balance equations, assuming an average fluid gain of 0.75 kg/day between dialyses, provides reasonably simple algebraic expressions to calculate pcr. The expression to calculate pcr (normalized to body weight, g/kg/day) is

$$\text{pcr} = 0.22 + 0.036(\Delta \text{BUN}) + \frac{0.054(K_{rU})(\overline{\text{BUN}})}{V} \quad (3\text{-}16)$$

where ΔBUN = the increase in BUN, mg/dl/24 hr; $\overline{\text{BUN}}$ = mean BUN, mg/dl, over any specified interval, usually 24–72 hours; K_{rU} = residual renal urea clearance, ml/min; V = urea distribution volume, L.

It can be noted in Equation (3-6) that, when $K_{rU} = 0$, the pcr is calculated from ΔBUN alone. This is the case, of course, in the majority of dialysis patients. The pcr can be calculated over any interval with Equation (3-6) as long as BUN values are measured at the beginning and end of the interval in order to calculate ΔBUN and $\overline{\text{BUN}}$ for the interval. In the stable patient, in whom BUN_{o_1}, BUN_{t_1}, and BUN_{o_2} are measured monthly, Equation (3-16) would be used to calculate pcr from postdialysis Monday to predialysis Wednesday (or Tuesday to Thursday) for the typical thrice-weekly schedule.

It is also possible to estimate reasonably accurately the average pcr over the 3-day weekend preceding the BUN_{o_1} measurement. If it is assumed that pcr between BUN_{t_2} and BUN_{o_3} is the same as that calculated between BUN_{t_1} and BUN_{o_2} and that Kt/V has remained constant, BUN_{t_3} can be estimated and assumed to be equal to BUN_{t_3} at the end of the preceding week. An approximate expression for BUN_{t_3} is $0.94\ \text{BUN}_{t_1}(\text{BUN}_{o_3})$, and from this approximated BUN_{o_3} and measured BUN_{o_1} the weekend pcr can be estimated in accordance with

$$\text{Weekend pcr} = 0.22$$

$$+ 0.036\ \frac{\text{BUN}_{o_1} - 0.94\ (\text{BUN}_{t_1}/\text{BUN}_{o_1})(\text{BUN}_{o_2})}{\theta_1} \quad (3\text{-}17)$$

$$+ \frac{0.0542(K_{rU})(\overline{\text{BUN}})}{V}$$

where the units are the same as for Equation (3-16).

The use of Equations (3-16) and (3-17) with monthly measurement of BUN_{o_1}, BUN_{t_1}, and BUN_{o_2} permits calculation of pcr for 5 days of each month, or 17% of the time, which provides an excellent sampling of protein nutrition in the patient.

Determination of PCR. The PCR represents the total grams of protein catabolized per day and equals the product of pcr times normalized body weight. Since the mean normalized body weight ($\overline{\text{NBW}}$) is defined as 1.72 ($\overline{V}$) and is known since $\overline{V}$ has been determined, calculation of PCR is simply

$$\text{PCR} = \text{pcr}(1.72\overline{V}) \quad \text{or} \quad \text{pcr}(\overline{\text{NBW}}) \quad (3\text{-}18)$$

The pcr is required to calculate the dialysis prescription in accordance with Figures 3-5 and 3-6 and also provides a valuable nutritional index to the appropriateness of dietary protein intake relative to body size. The PCR yields a precise determination of the total dietary protein intake when the patient is in zero nitrogen balance, the usual case in stable patients. It also provides an invaluable measurement for the renal dietician counselling the patient with respect to dietary protein intake. The PCR serves as a quantified measure of protein intake to be compared to the reported dietary protein intake and thus determine errors in diet records due to some combination of patient misconception of diet instruction and/or noncompliance. In the patient with an associated acute illness or acute renal failure and receiving parenteral nutritional support, the difference between PCR and protein intake permits assessment of nitrogen balance.

Step 4. Determination of Total Fractional Urea Clearance (K_T)

The K_T required is determined from the modeling lines in Figures 3-5 and 3-6 for twice- and thrice-weekly therapy, respectively. In the new patient, if pcr is assumed to be 1.0 g/kg/day, the K_T's for twice- and thrice-weekly therapy will be 1.8 and 1.0, respectively.

Step 5. Calculation of Kt/V

The fractional dialyzer urea clearance required, Kt/V, is calculated from the value determined for K_T, subtracting the contribution of residual renal clearance.

$$\frac{Kt}{V} = K_T - \frac{10.1 K_{rU}}{V} \quad \text{(for twice-weekly dialysis)} \quad (3\text{-}19)$$

$$\frac{Kt}{V} = K_T - \frac{5.9 K_{rU}}{V} \quad \text{(for thrice-weekly dialysis)} \quad (3\text{-}20)$$

Step 6. Designation of K/V and Calculation of K

The rate of dialysis can be described by the normalized dialyzer urea clearance, which is defined as K (L/min) divided by V (L) and thus has units of min^{-1}. K/V is a rate constant describing the rate at which BUN decreases during dialysis and therefore provides an index to how rapidly the patient is dialyzed. Since the clearance (dialysance) values for sodium, potassium, acetate, and other low molecular weight solutes are all proportional to urea clearance, the K/V also provides an index to the rate of concentration change of these solutes. Intradialytic morbidity is believed to be in part a function of the rate of dialysis, although precise correlations have not been established, particularly for individual patients.

Acetate is widely speculated to contribute to intradialytic morbidity, with morbidity increasing as some function of acetate flux rate. Consequently, the blood acetate concentration as a function of K/V are shown in Figure 3-8. The end-dialysis plasma acetate concentrations are calculated at three levels of dialysate acetate concentration.

There are several studies that have shown a relationship between morbidity and rate of dialysis, which in turn can be correlated with blood acetate levels. Whether acetate is really the factor responsible for morbidity in these studies is unknown. Furthermore, absolute levels of K/V or acetate have not consistently been found to be deleterious. Morbidity is undoubtedly multifactorial in etiology, as is considered more fully under Complications of Dialysis. It is our empirical policy generally to limit K/V to ≈ 0.0060 in stable chronic patients, which will minimize plasma acetate accumulation, but a forceful recommendation cannot be made in this regard. Some patients may have less morbidity with $K/V <$ 0.0060, while some patients may tolerate K/V levels substantially higher than 0.0060.

After K/V is determined, the dialyzer urea clearance can either be computed from the product of prescribed K/V in accordance with

$$K = \frac{K}{V} \cdot V \qquad (3\text{-}21)$$

or read off the plot in Figure 3-9, which shows K as a function of K/V with constant values of V ranging from 20 to 60 L. Figure 3-9 is useful because it permits one to "go shopping" over the total range of K and K/V values for an individual patient with known V. For example, with a V of 44 L and maximum K of 0.220 L/min, it is immediately apparent that the maximum K/V that can be prescribed is 0.0050. At the other extreme, with $V = 20$ L, K will only be 0.120 L/min, with $K/V = 0.0060$.

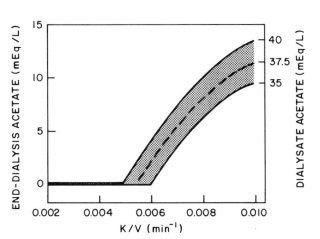

Fig. 3-8. End-dialysis acetate concentration as a function of the rate of dialysis (K/V) and dialysate acetate concentration.

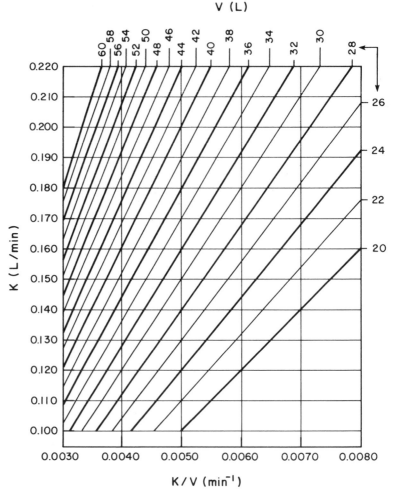

Fig. 3-9. Plot for determination of urea clearance (K) as a function K/V at constant values of V.

Step 7. Selection of Dialyzer and Q_B

Once K is determined, it is necessary to select a dialyzer and Q_B that will deliver that K. It is very helpful to have a plot available that shows K as a function of Q_B for each type of dialyzer used in the facility, such as illustrated in Figure 3-10, which shows two prototypical dialyzers used commonly. Many considerations are involved in the choice of dialyzer and Q_B but some general guidelines can be given. With conventional transmembrane pressure control systems the device with the lowest K_{UF} (but adequate to meet the patient's ultrafiltration requirements) should be used, since this will maximize the precision of ultrafiltration control (see Chapter 1). The maximum Q_B, without inducing recirculation and excessive pressures, is usually in the range of 300–350 ml/min, with an excellent blood access. In some instances it will not be possible to reach this level without recirculation or excessive negative arterial pressure and/or positive venous pressure. Operating at very low arterial pressure (exceeding − 250 mmHg) may induce hemolysis, while high venous pressure may result in obligatory excessive ultrafiltration in patients with minimal weight gain and require saline replacement during dialysis. Thus there may be a constraint on maximal Q_B in some patients.

Some examples can be given to illustrate selection of dialyzer and Q_B. If the patient has a low V and an average ultrafiltration requirement, and K of 0.150 L/min is prescribed, it is clear from Figure 3-10 that dialyzer B would be the best choice. The Q_B required is only 0.180 L/min and lower K_{UF} will give better precision for ultrafiltration control. If the patient has a large V and a high or low ultrafiltration requirement, and K of 0.220 L/min is prescribed, dialyzer A must be prescribed, since this K cannot be reached with dialyzer B. If this patient had a marginal blood access, and the maximal Q_B feasible is 200 ml/min, the difference in K between dialyzers A and B decreases but may still be highly significant with respect to the treatment time required. The effect on treatment time must be weighed against the importance of maximizing precision of ultrafiltration control.

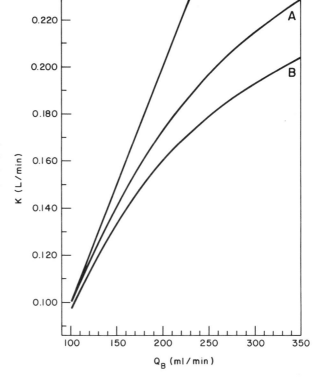

Fig. 3-10. Urea clearances (K) as a function of blood flow rate (Q_B) for two typical hollow fiber dialyzers, A and B.

Step 8. Definition of Treatment Time (t)

The treatment time is calculated by dividing the prescribed dialyzer fractional urea clearance, Kt/V, by the rate of dialysis prescribed, K/V, in accordance with

$$t = \frac{Kt/V}{60(K/V)} \tag{3-22}$$

where the coefficient 60 converts t from minutes to hours.

The treatment time can be calculated from Equation (3-22) or determined from Figure 3-11, which is a three-variable plot showing t as a function of K/V for constant Kt/V values ranging from 0.6 to 1.6. For example, if Kt/V of 1.0 and K/V of 0.0060 are prescribed, t will be 2.8 hours. However, if K/V of 0.0040 is prescribed, t must increase to 4.2 hours to achieve a Kt/V value of 1.0.

Step 9. Calculation of TMP

The clinical procedure to prescribe precise levels of ultrafiltration during dialysis has been discussed in Chapter 1. Assessment of the ultrafiltration requirement is also important, since the prescription calculated in Steps 1–8 may not be realistic if the patient either does not comply with dietary sodium and fluid restriction and has excessive weight gains or tolerates ultrafiltration poorly.

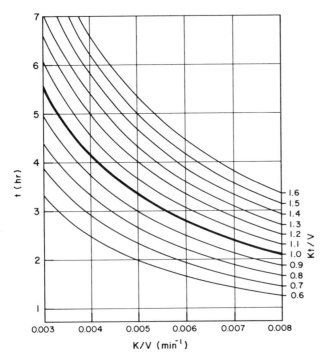

Fig. 3-11. Plot for determination of t as a function of K/V and Kt/V.

It is therefore useful to determine the mean total ultrafiltrate removed over the past four to six dialyses and compute the rate of ultrafiltration (Q_F, ml/hr) which will be required with the frequency of dialysis and t calculated in Step 8. Interpretation of these values is difficult, however, since ultrafiltration morbidity is still poorly understood, multifactorial in etiology, and difficult to predict as a function of Q_F in individual patients. This will be considered in more detail later under Complications of Dialysis.

The average fluid gain in most patients is about 1.0 L/day and on a thrice-weekly schedule average total ultrafiltration will be 3.0 L during the first dialysis of the week and 2.0 L for the other two dialyses. If t is 2.8 hours, the average Q_F on the first dialysis will be 1070 ml/hr and on the other dialyses 714 ml/hr. These Q_F rates can often be tolerated without undue morbidity, particularly if patients are regularly surveyed for reversible clinical causes of ultrafiltration morbidity as discussed below. Increasing t will reduce Q_F moderately. In the average patient on thrice-weekly dialysis described above, increasing t to 3.5 hours would reduce Q_F during the first dialysis of the week to 857 ml/hr and to 571 ml/hr during the other two dialyses or result in absolute decrease of 150–200 ml/hr. Although in individual patients this may empirically be found to reduce morbidity significantly, there is not an adequate data base in the literature to predict the effect of Q_F changes in this range on ultrafiltration morbidity.

When twice-weekly dialysis is considered, it is particularly important to evaluate total ultrafiltration needs because of the less frequent dialyses. Since there must be significant residual renal function present to consider twice-weekly dialysis, the urine volume is usually at least 500 ml/day and results in interdialytic weight gains that do not greatly exceed the average values for patients with negligible renal function on thrice-weekly therapy. If this is not the case due to poor compliance with dietary sodium and fluid restriction, twice-weekly therapy may not be realistic.

Step 10. Determination of Dialysate Sodium and Potassium

In the typical stable chronic dialysis patient, the optimal average dialysate Na^+ and K^+ values are 140 and 2 mEq/L, respectively, which will result in end-dialysis plasma Na^+ and K^+ values of 138 and 3.5–4.0 mEq/L, respectively. However, as discussed in Chapter 1, the net concentration of Na^+ in the ultrafiltrate removed can vary widely if the predialysis plasma Na^+ deviates as little as 5–10 mEq/L from dialysate Na^+ and may contribute to variable morbidity with ultrafiltration.

A graphic portrayal of Na^+ kinetics is contained in Figure 3-12, where end-dialysis plasma Na^+ is shown as a function of predialysis Na^+, dialysate Na^+ and constant Kt/V. Four plots of constant urea Kt/V ranging from 0.80 to 1.40 are shown, which should cover the usual range of Kt/V prescribed. The end-dialysis aqueous concentration of Na^+ in plasma will be quite accurately predicted by these graphs but the flame photometer Na^+ value measured in plasma

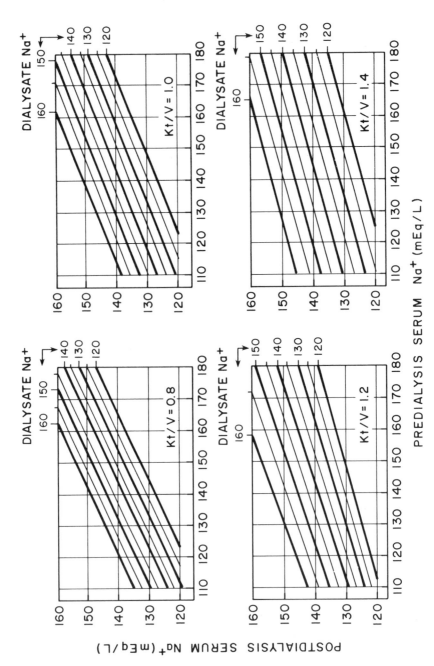

Fig. 3-12. Plots for determination of dialysate Na$^+$ concentration as a function of the predialysis serum Na$^+$ concentration and targeted postdialysis serum Na$^+$ concentration at different levels of prescribed Kt/V.

may vary somewhat depending on changes in plasma protein concentration due to ultrafiltration or fluid administration during dialysis.

The graphs in Figure 3-12 are most useful for patients with acute renal failure or chronic renal failure with an acute intervening illness. In these circumstances markedly abnormal predialysis Na$^+$ values may be seen as a result of either the coexisting illness or intravenous fluid therapy.

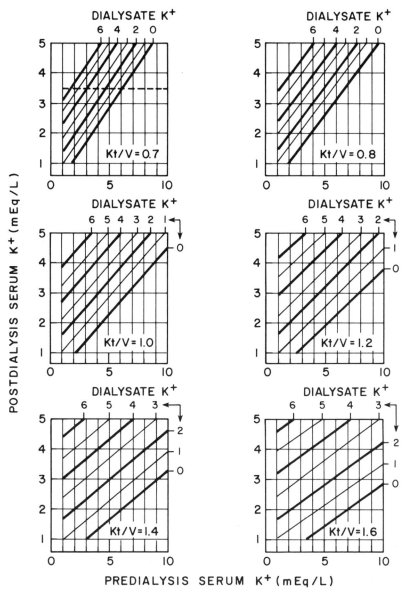

Fig. 3-13. Plots for determination of dialysate K$^+$ concentration as a function of the predialysis serum K$^+$ concentration and targeted postdialysis serum K$^+$ concentration at different levels of prescribed Kt/V.

In the chronic dialysis patient intradialytic morbidity is clearly reduced as dialysate Na^+ increases. Arbitrarily increasing dialysate Na^+ for all patients without modeling Na^+ balance carries a risk of substantially increasing body Na^+ content with possible consequences of increasing hypertension or congestive heart failure. However, a reasonable guideline would be to generally avoid hypertonic ultrafiltration in the stable patient: that is, do not prescribe dialysate Na^+ below the maximal predialysis plasma Na^+ values measured in the stable patient. The interdialytic Na^+ and water loading ratio varies between patients and in the same patient from time to time, resulting in variability in predialysis Na^+. Some patients regularly come to dialysis with Na^+ values of 145 mEq/L so that, assuming $Kt/V = 1.0$, in order to avoid hypertonic ultrafiltration (which results in decreased postdialysis Na^+) the plot in Figure 3-12 would indicate a dialysate Na^+ of 145–150 mEq/L should be used. The average predialysis Na^+ is ~138 mEq/L in our experience, and the plot for $Kt/V = 1.0$ shows that dialysate Na^+ of 140 mEq/L will result in end dialysis plasma Na^+ of 138 mEq/L.

The graphs in Figure 3-13 can be used to select dialysate K^+ required to achieve a specified end-dialysis K^+ as a function of predialysis K^+ and the urea Kt/V prescribed. In the average patient treated with $Kt/V = 1.0$, the predialysis K^+ is usually 5–6 mEq/L and, as can be seen in Figure 3-13, a dialysate K^+ of 2.0 mEq/L will result in end-dialysis plasma K^+ of 3.5–3.8 mEq/L. This demonstrates the basis for choosing an average dialysate K^+ of 2.0 mEq/L. If a much larger Kt/V of 1.6 is prescribed, the end-dialysis K^+ for this patient would be ~3.0 mEq/L.

Although the commonest predialysis K^+ is 5–6 mEq/L, some patients, particularly if there is some residual renal function, have predialysis K^+ levels of ~4 mEq/L, while other patients tend to have values between 6 and 7 mEq/L due to excessive intake. In these instances Figure 3-13 can be used to select the optimal dialysate K^+ to achieve the desired end-dialysis serum K^+. Both hyperkalemia and hypokalemia must be avoided as far as possible because of the life-threatening risk of cardiac arrhythmias.

The use of Figure 3-13 to target end-dialysis serum K^+ is particularly useful for the acutely ill chronic dialysis patient and the patient with acute renal failure. In these circumstances, particularly with gastrointestinal losses and parenteral nutrition therapy, predialysis serum K^+ can vary from high to low values over short intervals; it must be measured frequently and Figure 3-12 used to prescribe an appropriate dialysate K^+.

MONITORING THE DIALYSIS PRESCRIPTION

The 10 steps outlined above provide a rigorously calculated prescription, which will assure low-level morbidity as defined by the NCDS data. It should be monitored by monthly measurement of BUN_{o_1}, BUN_{t_1}, and BUN_{o_2}, which provides for independent calculation of pcr from BUN_{t_1} and BUN_{o_2} and verification of Kt/V from BUN_{o_1} and BUN_{t_1} by determination if the calculated V is reproducible and realistic. Thus it provides ongoing quality control of the dialysis parameters and protein nutrition. Unless there is careful regular attention to technical details (e.g., calibration of blood pumps), dialysis treatment parameter (Kt/V) can vary markedly. It is not uncommon to find improperly occluded blood pumps in a facility with Q_B errors of 50–100 ml/min. Consequently, the rigorous prescription calculation with monthly monitoring by measurement of BUN_{o_1}, BUN_{t_1} and BUN_{o_2} and calculation of V and pcr are recommended as the best way to provide adequate, quality-controlled therapy.

It is possible to progressively reduce the number of measurements and use the concepts presented above, although each decrement in data collection reduces the level of quality control. It can be noted in Figures 3-5 and 3-6 that, if K_T and BUN_{o_2} are measured, the pcr can be calculated directly from the graph, since these are three-variable plots relating BUN_{o_2} to both pcr and K_T. If only BUN_{o_2}, BUN_{t_2} are measured and used to calculate V and thus verify that the prescribed K_T has been in fact delivered, pcr can be determined from the K_T, BUN_{o_2} coordinants using Figure 3-5 or 3-6, depending on the treatment schedule.

This simplification might be reasonably valid for monthly monitoring of the established chronic dialysis patient. This technique cannot be used to determine pcr at the start of dialysis therapy, since the relationships in Figures 3-5 and 3-6 are based on a stable treatment schedule and are valid only for BUN_{o_2} and after 2 to 3 weeks on the fixed schedule with relatively stable pcr. There will be more "noise" in this type of pcr calculation, since it reflects only midweek pcr with no consideration of weekend pcr. When K_{rU} is measured, a BUN_{t_1} is required to calculate the mean BUN for the collection interval. However, subject to these considerations, it may be a reasonably valid simplification to monitor stable therapy.

A further simplification for consideration would be to measure BUN_{o_2} only, assume that the prescribed Kt/V has been accurately delivered and calculate pcr from Figures 3-5 and 3-6. This ultimate simplification provides no quality control checks on Kt/V and pcr and is not recommended as a method to provide quantified and quality-controlled nutritional/dialysis therapy.

The basic dialysis prescription is complex and comprised of five variables: frequency of dialysis, selection of dialyzer, Q_B and t, and the dietary protein prescription. In the absence of clear-cut criteria for targeting adequate treatment, these variables are often not quantitatively considered, and frequently all patients are treated relatively similarly in a given facility.

The treatment time and frequency of dialysis are particularly strongly rooted in clinical empiricism. Many patients are routinely started on thrice-weekly dialysis empirically and highly significant levels of residual renal function ignored. This stems to a considerable extent from the experience 20 years ago when a major improvement in clinical outcome was seen when routine therapy was increased from twice to thrice weekly. The criteria for initiation of dialysis were much stricter then and patients with K_{rU} of 3–4 ml/min were not started on dialysis as they are today.

The concept of middle molecule uremic toxicity which is treatment time dependent led to consideration of treatment time as an independent, primary treatment variable. As discussed earlier, there is little evidence to support this concept, but there are still some strong empirical feelings about an optimal "treatment time." Dialysis is still categorized as "short time" and "long time" without consideration of total fractional clearance, normalized clearance, and ultrafiltration rate.

The treatment time is strongly controlling on the cost of in-facility dialysis and also has a major impact on the time available to patients for activities other than dialysis. Treatment time has empirically decreased enormously over the past 20 years as dialyzer small molecule clearances have increased. The increasing impact of cost containment on therapy must inevitably produce still greater pressure to reduce treatment time, which is the single most costly component of therapy. Consequently, we believe it is now particularly important to quantify therapy and target it in domain E of Figure 3-2. This was less important when nearly all patients received high levels of therapy, but as t decreases below 4–5 hours, avoidance of domain D can only be assured by quantification of therapy.

OTHER ASPECTS OF THE DIALYSIS PRESCRIPTION

Isolated Ultrafiltration

A few years ago Bergstrom made a remarkable observation: if ultrafiltration was entirely separated from dialysis (isolated ultrafiltration), it was better tolerated in a patient who had a high incidence of hypotension during simultaneous ultrafiltration and dialysis. This interesting phenomenon was initially thought to reflect the osmotic effect of rapid urea removal during dialysis with shift of fluid from the plasma and extracellular compartments to the intracellular compartment. This would appear to be an unlikely explanation because urea equilibration is extremely rapid and unlikely to result in any substantial intracellular shift of water other than in very specialized tissue such as brain. Subsequent studies by Bergstrom showed that equivalent tolerance to ultrafiltration could be achieved by using a dialysate sodium of 145 mEq/L.

It was also initially thought that ultrafiltration to remove all the fluid immediately before or after the dialysis might improve the tolerance to ultrafiltration in patients particularly susceptible to hypotension. Clinical studies of this technique have shown it is not very useful, since hypotension often occurs during dialysis after or during isolated ultrafiltration when it is preceded by dialysis. This procedure increases treatment time, since the ultrafiltration phase must be added to dialysis time.

When ultrafiltration is done on a separate day and thus is completely isolated from dialysis, it can be an extremely useful technique to manage large fluid overloads and correct acute heart failure with reduced risk of hypotension. However, it should be reserved for unusual circumstances such as this because it is not realistic to manage sodium and water balance by isolated ultrafiltration on a regular basis, which would double treatment frequency.

Large quantities of fluid (3–4 L) can be removed in 2 or 3 hours with isolated ultrafiltration. Because of the Donnan effect of negatively charged plasma proteins, the concentration of Na^+ and K^+ in ultrafiltrate will be lower than plasma concentration, and chloride and bicarbonate ion concentrations will be higher in ultrafiltrate. If the plasma potassium is at the upper bound of normal or slightly elevated, it may rise 1 or 2 mEq/L during isolated ultrafiltration and become significantly abnormal. This effect should be anticipated and may require a short period of dialysis with zero dialysate potassium or the administration of an exchange resin.

Acetate and Bicarbonate Dialysis

For technical reasons (discussed in Chapter 1), dialysate containing acetate has been routinely used over the past 15 years to correct metabolic acidosis. In recent years there has been growing concern regarding the suitability of acetate for a variety of reasons. There was concern that dialysate acetate might increase cholesterol production, but this has not been shown to occur. As dialyzer clearances have increased, acetate flux rates may substantially exceed the rate of acetate metabolism and result in high acetate blood levels, which have been inconsistently implicated as causative in dialysis morbidity, as discussed earlier. It has been shown in both animals and human subjects that acetate at very low blood levels can induce significant vasodilation, and is thus suspected to contribute to hypotensive episodes during dialysis. There are some data suggesting that acetate dialysis may be inadequate to fully correct metabolic acidosis and may lead to slow progressive dissolution of bone buffer salts. Despite all of these considerations, acetate continues to be widely used, and properly so, until more definitive evidence of adverse effects is obtained. The concentration of dialysate acetate prescribed varies usually from 35 to 40 mEq/L. A consideration of bicarbonate and acetate flux rates with efficient dialyzers suggests that for optimal correction of acidosis the dialysate acetate should not be less than 40 mEq/L.

Bicarbonate dialysate has been strongly recommended recently to reduce dialysis morbidity, particularly hypotension, muscle cramps, nausea, and fatigue by some investigators but not by others. The general advantages of bicarbonate over acetate have not been clearly shown to date, although there is a growing feeling that in selected patients bicarbonate dialysis may reduce morbidity. It is possible that bicarbonate dialysis would increase the K/V tolerated without undue morbidity, but carefully controlled studies of this have not been reported to date.

Calcium and Magnesium

Impaired calcium absorption and low dietary intake have been implicated in the hypocalcemic stimulus to secondary hyperparathyroidism. Calcium flux studies have indicated that to assure a positive net calcium flux into the patient during dialysis a dialysate calcium of 3–3.5 mEq/L is required. Consequently, this level of dialysate calcium is widely employed, although in many patients it does result in mild end-dialysis hypercalcemia in the range of 12 mg/dl.

The use of dialysate containing 0.5 mEq/L of magnesium results in near-normal predialysis serum magnesium levels, and skeletal magnesium may fall with improved chemical composition of bone. A magnesium concentration of 1.5 mEq/L in dialysate, still fairly widely used, results in substantially elevated predialysis magnesium levels and may contribute to renal osteodystrophy.

HEPARIN ADMINISTRATION

It is necessary to administer an anticoagulant during hemodialysis to prevent clotting in the extracorporeal circuit; intravenously administered heparin is used almost universally for this purpose. If the level of anticoagulation is too low, clotting of the circuit can occur, while with excessive anticoagulation there is increased risk of patient bleeding during or after dialysis. The goal of heparinization is to achieve a uniform, adequate level of anticoagulation. The dose of heparin required may vary considerably between patients because of variability in sensitivity of the clotting mechanism to heparin and variability in the rate at which heparin is eliminated from the blood.

In view of the above considerations it is apparent that the optimal heparin dose for an individual patient must be based on a test that reliably measures the level of anticoagulation resulting from a quantified heparin dose. In the following sections, methods of calculating the heparin prescription for an individual patient based on measurement of heparin anticoagulant activity, sensitivity of the clotting mechanism to heparin and heparin elimination rate will be discussed.

Measurement of Heparin Anticoagulant Effect

A number of clotting time tests are used to measure heparin anticoagulant effect. The requirements for an ideal test in dialysis are considered in Chapter 1 and are summarized here as follows: (1) Prolongation of the test clotting time must increase linearly with heparin dose over the therapeutic dosage range (linear dose-response); (2) clotting should be abrupt and complete in order to give a sharp easily determined end point; (3) the sensitivity of the test to heparin (prolongation of clotting time) must be adequate to reliably measure heparin effect with both low-dose and regular-dose prescriptions; (4) the dialysis nurse or technician should be able to reliably perform the test at the bedside because rapid feedback of test results is essential.

Unfortunately there is no clotting time test that perfectly satisfies all of these criteria. The whole blood partial thromboplastin time (WBPTT) best fulfills these criteria in our experience. The technical details of performing this test must be carefully followed for reliable results. This test provides a linear dose-response, has a sharp end point, and can readily be performed at the bedside. The sensitivity of the test can vary considerably depending on the reagent used. Actin FS appears to be the most suitable reagent currently available. It gives a baseline clotting time without heparin of ~70 seconds, which increases to ~105 and ~140 seconds with low-dose and regular-dose prescriptions, respectively. The sensitivity can vary somewhat with different batches of this reagent. One disadvantage of the WBPTT is that the end point cannot be determined closer than ±5 seconds; this can be a problem, particularly with low-dose prescriptions, as will be discussed below.

There are several other important technical considerations in assessing the anticoagulant response to the heparin dose. It is essential that the dose be accurately delivered, which is facilitated by using larger volumes of heparin diluted to 200, 250, or 500 U/ml. The solution used to prime the circuit and fistula needles must not contain any heparin. Reliable and well-calibrated infusion pumps delivering at least 1.5 to 2.0 ml/hr of dilute heparin must be used for constant heparin infusion.

Heparin Kinetics

The target anticoagulation profiles for regular- and low-dose heparin are depicted in Figure 3-14. In the case of regular-dose heparinization, full-level anticoagulation is induced with a heparin loading dose [D_L, units (U)] predialysis. During dialysis a constant heparin infusion rate (I_r, U/hr) is administered to maintain a constant level of anticoagulation. The heparin infusion is discontinued at a time calculated to allow the level of anticoagulation to decay to a specified lower value so that bleeding risk, when the needles are removed and postdialysis, is negligible. The low-dose profile is similar, except the target level is much lower and equal to the end-dialysis level targeted with regular-dose

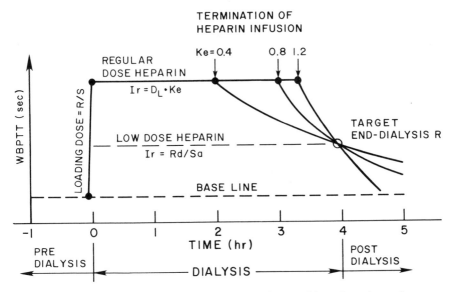

Fig. 3-14. Anticoagulation profiles for regular- and low-dose heparin.

heparinization. In order to develop heparin prescriptions that will result in these profiles it is necessary to utilize a heparin pharmacokinetic model.

An intravenous dose of heparin is uniformly distributed in the plasma volume within 3 minutes. It is taken up by the reticuloendothelial system and eliminated from plasma by a first-order mechanism analogous to dialyzer urea clearance. There is no significant removal of heparin by the dialyzer because of its high molecular weight. Thus heparin is distributed in a single compartment, the plasma volume, and is eliminated by a first-order process, as depicted in Figure 3-15.

The amount of heparin in the plasma at any time is the difference between input and elimination (Fig. 3-15). The anticoagulant response, prolongation of WBPTT, is linearly related to the amount of heparin in plasma, and this measured value can therefore be used to determine plasma content of heparin at any time.

Heparin Sensitivity. The anticoagulant response (R, sec) to heparin is determined from the measured prolongation of WBPTT, which increases linearly with plasma heparin content. The slope or rate of increase in WBPTT with increasing plasma heparin is called sensitivity (S) and has units of seconds prolongation WBPTT per unit of heparin, or sec/U. It defines the sensitivity of the clotting mechanism to heparin and can vary markedly between patients. Each individual patient has a characteristic S; since our purpose is to achieve a similar R for all patients, S must be known for a patient in order to determine the appropriate loading dose of heparin required just prior to initiation of dialysis.

Sensitivity is determined from the anticoagulant response to an intravenous bolus dose (D) of heparin. The baseline WBPTT ($WBPTT_{BL}$) is measured just prior to the dose and remeasured 3 minutes after the dose ($WBPTT_{3\,min}$). Over this short interval it can be assumed that a negligible quantity of heparin has been eliminated and the administered dose is well mixed in plasma. The R is calculated from

$$R = WBPTT_{3\,min} - WBPTT_{BL} \qquad (3\text{-}23)$$

Since R is linearly related to D with slope S, it follows that

$$R = S \cdot D \qquad (3\text{-}24)$$

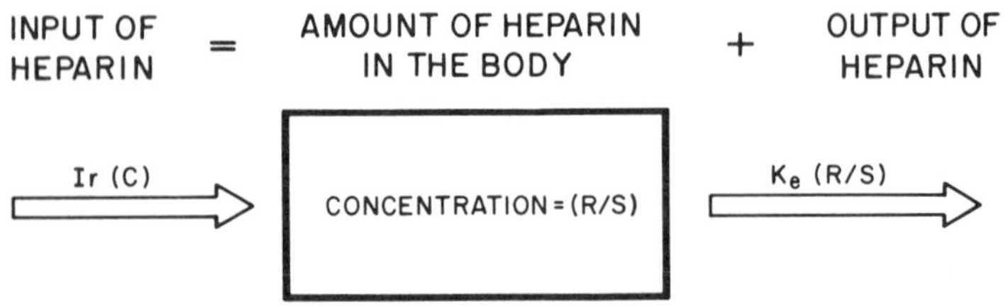

Fig. 3-15. Heparin kinetic model.

and S can be determined by rearrangement of Equation (3-24), giving

$$S = \frac{R}{D} = \frac{\text{WBPTT}_{3\,\text{min}} - \text{WBPTT}_{\text{BL}}}{D} \qquad (3\text{-}25)$$

After the mean S has been determined for a patient, the relationship between R and D is established and can be used to calculate the D required to achieve any desired value of R (R_d) in accordance with a rearrangement of Equation (3-25)

$$D = \frac{R_d}{S} \qquad (3\text{-}26)$$

Equation 3-26 is the operational expression used to calculate the loading dose (D_L) of heparin required to achieve any desired level of anticoagulation. Its use can be illustrated by consideration of some typical patient parameters and desired levels of anticoagulation. Assume a patient for whom WBPTT_{BL} = 70 sec and S = 0.040 sec/U. The WBPTT desired for low-dose heparinization would be 105 sec and R_d = 105 − 70 = 35 sec. The loading dose of heparin required is calculated from Equation (3-26) as 35/0.040 = 875 U heparin. If regular-dose heparinization were planned with WBPTT targeted at 140 sec, the R_d would be 140 − 70 = 70 sec, and required D_L = 70/0.040 = 1750 U.

In contrast, patients with substantially increased and decreased heparin sensitivity can be considered. If S = 0.080 the required loading doses for R_d 35 and 70 sec would be 35/0.080 = 440 U and 70/0.080 = 875 U, respectively. In the case of a low S = 0.030, the loading doses for R_d 35 and 70 sec would be 35/0.030 = 1165 U and 70/0.030 = 2335 U, respectively. Thus, the loading doses for similar, low-level anticoagulation could range from 440 to 1165 U, and for regular anticoagulation the loading doses would range from 875 to 2335 U. These examples illustrate the need to measure S in order to determine the loading dose required for an individual patient.

Equation (3-26) is also used to calculate a bolus dose of heparin during dialysis when the WBPTT is found to be low and it is desirable to increase it abruptly. In this case, the R_d is determined by subtracting the current low WBPTT from the desired higher WBPTT and dividing by S to calculate the bolus dose.

Heparin Elimination Constant. Heparin is quite rapidly eliminated from plasma with an average half-life of ~50 minutes. This means that, on the average, one half of the loading dose must be infused every 50 minutes to maintain a constant WBPTT. In some patients the half-life is as short as 30 minutes, while in others it may be as long as 2 hours. Since the heparin infusion rate must equal the elimination rate to maintain a constant anticoagulation level, it is clearly important to measure the elimination rate in order to prescribe the proper infusion.

As discussed earlier, heparin elimination is first-order, and the elimination mechanism is quantitatively described by an elimination rate constant (K_e), which is analogous to the dialyzer urea clearance, K. The units for K_e are hr^{-1}. The K_e can be measured after a bolus dose of heparin, after a constant infusion is turned off or during a constant heparin infusion. In each case, the K_e is determined from serial measurements of R, which is directly proportional to the plasma content of heparin.

The mathematics describing the decrease in R measured after a single bolus dose or after termination of a constant infusion are similar to those describing the decrease in BUN during dialysis [see Eq. (3-12)] and are given by

$$R_t = R_o e^{-K_e t} \qquad (3\text{-}27)$$

where t is an interval of time (hour) and R_o and R_t are the R values at the beginning and end of t, respectively.

Equation (3-27) when solved for K_e yields

$$K_e = \frac{\ln(R_o/R_t)}{t} \qquad (3\text{-}28)$$

The K_e can be determined using Equation (3-28) or graphically using Figure 3-16 where Equation (3-27) has been solved or R_t/R_o and t over a range of K_e from 0.20 to 1.60. The average heparin K_e is ~0.80 in dialysis patients but can range from ~0.40 to ~1.40. Since the WBPTT cannot be measured to accuracy greater than ±5 seconds, the accuracy of K_e determination will generally be higher with high values of R_t and R_o which will have smaller fractional measurement errors. As R_o and R_t approach baseline, it becomes more difficult to measure them because the measurement error (±5 sec) becomes large relative to R_o and R_t.

For optimal determination of K_e, measure R_o and then measure R_t at 20 and 30 minutes. Each of these R_t values can be used to calculate K_e values for 20 and 30 minutes using the R_o value at $t = 0$ for each calculation with Equation (3-28) or Figure 3-16. The mean of the two determinations is then taken to be the average K_e. It is convenient to measure K_e during the last half hour of dialysis with the heparin infusion turned off. In this way the K_e data can be taken during dialysis, and extra patient and nursing time is not required.

The use of Figure 3-16 can be illustrated by example. Assume the WBPTT$_{BL}$ = 70 sec. When the Ir is terminated 0.5 hour prior to end of dialysis, the WBPTT is 150 seconds. At 20 and 30 minutes later WBPTT values of 130 and 120 seconds, respectively, are measured. The R_o = 150 − 70 = 80 sec; the R_t at 20 min is 130 − 70 = 60 sec and R_t at 30 min is 120 − 70 = 50 sec. Thus at 20 min, R_t/R_o = 60/80 = 0.75 and K_e in Figure 3-16 is 0.88 hr^{-1}. At 30 min R_t/R_o = 50/80 = 0.63 and K_e is found to be 0.98 hr^{-1}. The average K_e found with these measurements is 0.93 hr^{-1}.

If the above data were analyzed with Equation (3-28), the K_e at 20 minutes would be [ln (80/60)]/(20/60) = 0.288/0.33 = 0.87 hr^{-1} and at 30 min would

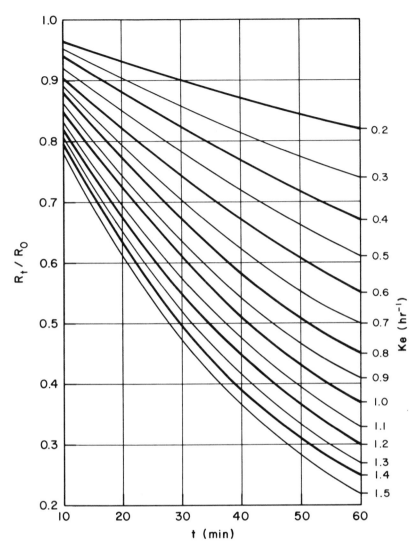

Fig. 3-16. Plot for determination of heparin elimination constant (K_e) from ratio of anticoagulation responses (R_t/R_o) and time (t) after heparin bolus dose or cessation of heparin infusion.

be $[\ln (80/50)]/(30/60) = 0.470/0.50 = 0.94$ hr^{-1}. The values determined by visual interpolation on Figure 3-16 agree closely with those calculated from Equation (3-28).

The K_e can also be determined during a constant heparin infusion, although the mathematical relationships are more complex and involve interaction of Ir, S, K_e, R_o, and R_t. However, these mathematical relationships can be graphically portrayed as in Figure 3-17, which can be used to determine K_e during a constant heparin infusion. Figure 3-17 is a three-variable plot in which constant K_e values are shown as a function of $Ir \cdot S/R_o$ and R_t/R_o when R_t is measured exactly 1.0

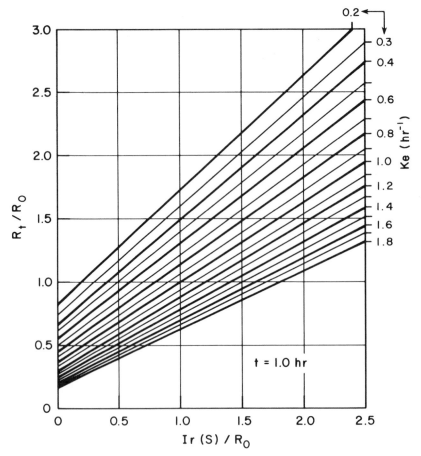

Fig. 3-17. Plot for determination of heparin elimination constant (K_e) from ratio of anticoagulation responses (R_t/R_o) at an interval of 1 hour as a function of the expression: heparin infusion rate (Ir) multiplied by the heparin sensitivity (S) divided by the initial anticoagulation response (R_o).

hour after R_o is measured. Although the relationships in Figure 3-17 are solved for exactly 1.0 hour between R_o and R_t, an error of up to 10 minutes in the time between R_o and R_t measurements will not result in significant error in the K_e determined from the graph. It is essential that the Ir be held constant during the interval.

Figure 3-17 can be used to calculate K_e during a constant heparin infusion over any 1.0-hour interval of dialysis. However, it should be used only for regular dose heparinization because with low-dose heparinization, the R values are too low relative to the WBPTT measurement error to permit calculation of reliable K_e values. In order to calculate K_e from Figure 3-17 it is necessary to know S, which must be measured predialysis when the heparin loading dose is given.

The use of Figure 3-17 is illustrated by the following example. Assume that $S = 0.040$ sec/U, $Ir = 1500$ U/h, $R_o = 60$ sec, and 1.0 hour later R_t is 75 seconds.

The calculation of $Ir \cdot S/R_o$ is $1500(0.040)/60 = 1.0$ and $R_t/R_o = 75/60 = 1.25$. The point with these coordinates on Figure 3-17 shows that K_e is ~0.65 hr^{-1}. If R_t were found to be 50 sec, and all other data in the example were the same, then $R_t/R_o = 0.83$ and K_e would be 1.30 hr^{-1}. The average K_e in dialysis patients is ~0.80 but can be as low as 0.40 and as high as 1.40 hr^{-1} in individual patients. The importance of accurate measurement of R is also illustrated in this example, which shows calculated K_e increasing from 0.65 to 1.30 hr^{-1} as measured R_t decreases from 75 to 50 sec.

In the above examples the patient was not at steady state (where the Ir is equal to the rate of heparin elimination). Instead, the plasma content of heparin was increasing or decreasing toward the steady-state value, where R is constant and the rates of heparin infusion and elimination are equal. This will be discussed more fully below.

The relationships in Equation (3-28) are also used to calculate the time at which the Ir should be terminated to allow the R value to decay to the targeted end-dialysis level (see Fig. 3-14). Solution of Equation (3-28) for t yields

$$t_{dc} = \frac{\ln[R_o/R_t]}{K_e} \tag{3-29}$$

The term R_o in this expression refers to the R value when the Ir is terminated, R_t is the targeted end-dialysis R value and t_{dc} (hour) is the time interval between R_o and R_t. The value of t_{dc} will depend primarily on K_e, since R_o and R_t are targeted at the same level for most patients.

The calculation of t_{dc} can be illustrated from an example where R_o and R_t are 70 and 35 seconds, respectively. If the K_e were quite low, 0.50 hr^{-1}, t_{dc} would be $[\ln (70/35)]/0.50 = 0.693/0.50 = 1.4$ hr, and for a 4-hour dialysis, the infusion would be terminated at 2.6 hr, or 1.4 hr before the end of dialysis. If the K_e were 1.2 hr^{-1}, t_{dc} would be $[\ln (70/35)]/1.2 = 0.693/1.2 = 0.6$ hr, and for a 4-hour dialysis the infusion would be terminated at 3.4 hours.

Figure 3-18 can also be used to calculate t_{dc}. For this purpose, R_o is assumed to be in a steady state (R_s). Figure 3-18 is a three-variable plot where Equation (3-29) is solved for constant values of K_e as a function of R_t/R_s and t_{dc}. Thus, from a known value for K_e and targeted value for R_t/R_s, t_{dc} can be determined from the plot.

Steady-State Heparin Kinetics. During constant heparin infusion the amount of heparin in plasma (and its linear correlate, R) will reach a constant, steady-state value. The steady state will be reached when the rate of heparin infusion is equal to the rate of elimination. Recalling that the amount of heparin in plasma can be expressed as the anticoagulant response R, the steady state (R_s) can be expressed as

$$Ir \cdot S = R_s \cdot K_e \tag{3-30}$$

The left-hand side of Equation (3-30) is the product of Ir (U/hr) and S (sec/U), which describes the rate at which anticoagulant effect or prolongation

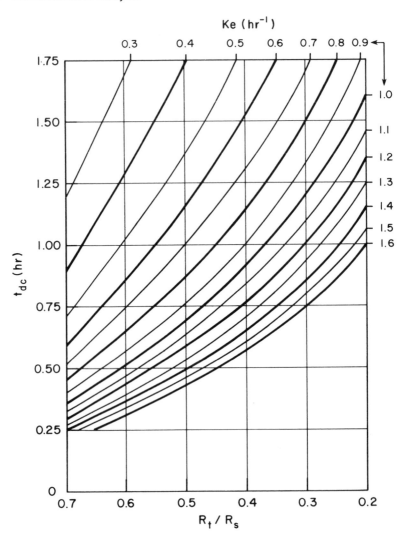

Fig. 3-18. Plot for determination of the time before dialysis that the heparin infusion should be terminated (t_{dc}) as a function of the heparin elimination constant (K_e) and of the heparin response desired at the end of dialysis (R_t) divided by response in the steady state (R_s).

of WBPTT is infused, expressed as sec/hr. The right-hand side of Equation (3-30) is the product of the steady state R (R_s, sec) and K_e (hr^{-1}), which describes the first-order rate at which anticoagulant effect is eliminated, expressed as sec/hr. The time required to reach steady state during constant heparin infusion is 2 to 3 half-lives and can be estimated as $\simeq 1.7/K_e$ so that with an average K_e of 0.80 the time required to reach steady state is $\simeq 1.7/0.8 \simeq 2.1$ hr after an infusion is started. However, in dialysis the loading dose administered is calculated to result in R equal to the steady-state value so that steady state is present virtually from the beginning of the Ir in a stable patient with a properly calculated prescription.

Equation (3-30) provides the basis for calculating the Ir required to maintain the constant level of R targeted during dialysis. Solution of the expression for Ir gives

$$Ir = \frac{R_s}{S} \cdot K_e \qquad (3\text{-}31)$$

Recall that the heparin loading dose (D_L) administered 3 minutes prior to start of dialysis is calculated from R_d/S [see Equation (3-26)] and that R_d equals the desired R_s. It follows that, since $D_L = R_d/S = R_s/S$, the Ir can also be simply calculated as

$$Ir = D_L \cdot K_e \qquad (3\text{-}32)$$

Equation (3-32) depicts quite clearly the meaning of K_e with respect to the heparin prescription. In order to maintain the level of anticoagulation achieved with the loading dose, the Ir must be equal to the hourly elimination of the loading dose which is equal to the product of K_e and D_L. Thus if $K_e = 0.50$, one half of D_L must be administered each hour by constant infusion, whereas if $K_e = 1.2$, the Ir must deliver 1.2 times the loading dose each hour.

Regular Dose Heparin Prescription

The three primary components of the prescription have been discussed, consisting of loading dose, constant infusion rate and time at which the infusion is terminated. There are five steps in development of the prescription.

Step 1. Select Target WBPTT Profile. The shape of the profile is shown in Figure 3-14, but the absolute values of clotting times will depend on the clotting time test used, the reagent used and the level of anticoagulation considered optimal by the staff. As discussed earlier, we believe the WBPTT is the best test for monitoring heparin in dialysis and currently use the Actin FS reagent, which gives $WBPTT_{BL} \sim 70$ seconds. We target the WBPTT at 140 seconds during dialysis ($R = 70$ sec) and 105 seconds end-dialysis ($R = 35$ sec) with this reagent.

Step 2. Measure S. A loading dose (D_L) of heparin is prepared in a dilution of 200 to 500 U/ml. The D_L is calculated from R_d/S [see Equation (3-26)]. For a new patient an average S (0.040 with Actin FS) is assumed. Subsequently, the measured S is used in the patient to calculate D_L.

One of the fistula needle sets is then cleared withdrawing 10 ml blood. A 0.4-ml blood sample is put in a tube to measure $WBPTT_{BL}$. Finally, the 10 ml blood drawn to clear the line is returned.

After clearing the line as above, the D_L is injected and the blood drawn to clear the line is returned. A stopwatch is started immediately after D_L is injected and exactly 3 minutes later, a 0.4-ml sample is taken to measure $WBPTT_{3\ min}$, following the technique used to draw the $WBPTT_{BL}$ sample. If the $WBPTT_{3\ min}$ is too low, another bolus should be administered and S remeasured. Remember that the solutions used to prime the circuit must not contain heparin when S and/or K_e measurements are made.

Step 3. Measure K_e. Immediately after the $WBPTT_{3\ min}$ measurement is found to be adequate, dialysis is begun simultaneously with the prescribed Ir. The infusion rate is calculated from Equations (3-31) or (3-32). For a new patient Equation (3-31) is used with the R_s targeted, the S measured in the patient, and an assumed K_e of 1.0. Subsequently the average S and K_e values measured in the patient will be used to calculate both D_L and Ir.

During dialysis R_o and R_t are measured over two consecutive 1-hour intervals (requires two consecutive WBPTT measurements) to calculate two consecutive K_e values using Figure 3-17.

About 35 minutes prior to the end of dialysis the Ir is terminated, and WBPTT measured to calculate R_o. If $R_o \geq 50$ sec, the Ir is left off and WBPTT is measured exactly 20 and 30 minutes later in order to calculate R_t values 20 and 30 minutes after the infusion is discontinued. The K_e values are then calculated from either Equation (3-28) and Figure 3-16.

The procedures followed in Steps 1–3 are called a heparin modeling study, which is designed to determine the heparin kinetic model parameters S and K_e for an individual patient. During each such modeling study, eight WBPTT measurements are made with a total blood sample requirement of $\sim 3\frac{1}{2}$ ml. All measurements and calculations can be done at the bedside. Because there is significant unavoidable measurement error as well as biologic variability in these parameters, it is recommended that these modeling studies be done on three consecutive dialyses and the mean S and K_e values used to write the final regular-dose heparin prescription for the patient.

Step 4. Writing the Prescription. After the three modeling studies are completed, the mean values for S and K_e are determined to calculate D_L from Equation (3-26), Ir from Equation (3-32) and time to terminate the Ir (t_{dc}) from Equation (3-29) or Figure 3-18. This prescription is then routinely administered each dialysis.

Step 5. Follow-up Studies. The kinetically derived heparin prescription will result in the anticoagulation profile depicted in Figure 3-14 and generally results in the targeted WBPTT values ± 20 sec. In some patients there is more day to day variability in S and K_e, and the confidence limits on the prescribed profile are correspondingly greater.

If the initial modeling studies are done during severe uremia and/or associated acute illness, the S and K_e values may change substantially after the patient is stabilized. Consequently, under these circumstances it is strongly recommended that random WBPTT measurement be made during several subsequent dialyses to evaluate continued suitability of the prescription. Acute severe uremia is at times associated with a greatly prolonged $WBPTT_{BL}$ and increased S, both of which decrease substantially during a single dialysis, resulting in difficult if not impossible modeling. Coumadin typically increases $WBPTT_{BL}$ and can occasionally result in $WBPTT_{BL} = 140$ sec, so that heparin may not even be required during a dialysis.

We routinely reevaluate the heparin prescription twice a year or whenever there is evidence of increased dialyzer clotting or excessive bleeding. Acute intercurrent illness and febrile episodes often result in decreased S and increased K_e with increased heparin requirements.

Low-Dose Heparin Prescription

The most demanding situation in which heparin is administered is dialysis of the uremic patient with high risk of bleeding. This population includes those with a recent major surgical procedure, pericarditis, gastrointestinal bleeding, and eye surgery, to name a few. As discussed in Chapter 1, one approach to this problem is so-called regional heparinization. This is based on a complex technique of regulating heparin and protamine infusions whose interaction is often not stable. Another approach is kinetic guidance of heparin infusion at a low dose calculated to produce minimal prolongation of WBPTT as depicted in Figure 3-14. In our experience over the past 10 years, this has been an extremely successful approach and we feel fully confident using this technique in any patient at high risk of bleeding. The R targeted throughout dialysis with low-dose heparinization is equal to the end-dialysis R targeted for regular dose heparinization (see Fig. 3-14).

The techniques described for measuring K_e during regular-dose heparinization cannot be reliably used with low-dose heparin because the ± 5 second measurement error is excessive with very low R values. Consequently, a different approach is used based on the value of S/K_e and assuming steady-state kinetics.

The steady state relationships in Equation (3-30) can be rearranged to give

$$\frac{S}{K_e} = \frac{R}{Ir} \quad \text{or} \quad S_a = \frac{R}{Ir} \qquad (3\text{-}33)$$

and

$$Ir = \frac{R_d}{S/K_e} \quad \text{or} \quad Ir = \frac{R_d}{S_a} \qquad (3\text{-}34)$$

A new term, the apparent sensitivity or S_a, has been introduced in Equations (3-33) and (3-34). The S_a is defined as the ratio S/K_e with units of sec · hr/U. It can be considered to be the steady-state analog of S measured 3 minutes after a bolus dose of heparin. In the latter case R is measured 3 minutes after the bolus, during which time the amount of heparin eliminated is considered to be zero. In Equation (3-33) at steady state with no net gain or loss of heparin from plasma, the Ir is an analog of the bolus dose and S_a is calculated from R/Ir. In similar analogy, D_L is calculated from R_d/S, while in Equation (3-34), the Ir is calculated from R_d/S_a.

The assumption of steady state underlying the use of S_a to control the Ir during low-dose heparinization is not rigorously correct but is sufficiently valid to use S_a to guide therapy. However, as will be discussed below, if the S_a calculation indicates need for a very large increase or decrease in the Ir during dialysis, clinical judgment may take precedence to select an intermediate level change in the Ir.

Low-dose heparinization must be closely monitored by the nurse with WBPTT measurement every half hour. It is necessary to tightly control the heparinization in order to prevent either too little anticoagulation and circuit clotting, or excessive anticoagulation resulting in increased risk of patient bleeding.

A nursing procedure flow diagram describing the feedback control algorithm used to tightly control low-dose heparinization is shown in Figure 3-19. The left-hand column shows the timing of procedures, the central blocks describe the procedures done, and the right-hand column blocks depict the parameters measured (S and S_a) or adjusted (Ir). The five discrete procedural steps can now be considered.

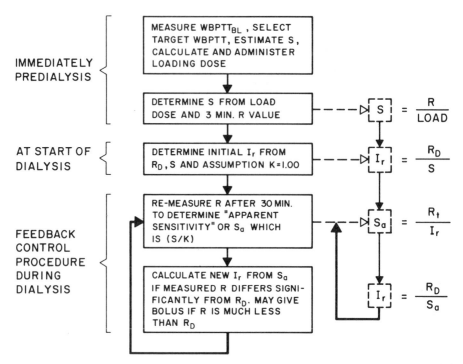

Fig. 3-19. Nursing procedure flow diagram for controlled minimal level heparinization.

Step 1. Initial Estimate of Heparin Requirement. The initial step is to measure the baseline $WBPTT_{BL}$ and then select a target WBPTT. Using Actin FS reagent, we have found $\sim$35 second prolongation over $WBPTT_{BL}$ to be adequate and to pose no increased risk for hemorrhage. The average $WBPTT_{BL}$ is 70 seconds, so the target WBPTT is usually 105 $\pm$ 5 seconds. In the occasional instance where $WBPTT_{BL}$ is markedly prolonged (i.e., 110 sec), associated with acute uremia for example, a minimal prolongation of 10–15 seconds may still be targeted because the $WBPTT_{BL}$ may drop rapidly during the first $\frac{1}{2}$ to 1 hour of hemodialysis. On the other hand, if $WBPTT_{BL}$ is less than 70 seconds, particularly in a high-risk situation, our practice is to prescribe no more than 35 seconds prolongation in WBPTT to a level of 90–95 seconds.

In order to select a reasonable loading dose it is necessary to have some estimate of S, since $D_L = R_d/S$. If there are previous S measurements available for the patient, these can be used to calculate the D_L. If not, a facility-derived mean S can be used to calculate the D_L. Whichever approach is used, it is advisable to not exceed 1000 U for the initial load. If the initial D_L falls significantly short of the target (i.e., more than 10 sec) another dose can be given to achieve the desired level of anticoagulation using the S determined from the initial dose and the additional increment in R desired. The additional loading dose is calculated from the additional increment in R desired divided by S.

Step 2. Calculate S from the Loading Dose. The technique described under regular-dose heparin should be followed.

Step 3. Calculate Initial Infusion Rate. A K_e of 1.0 is initially assumed so that the initial infusion rate is calculated from R_d/S [see Figure 3-10 and Equation (3-26)]. An important technical consideration is to assure that the volumetric infusion rate is at least 1.5 to 2.0 ml/hr. A heparin solution of 250 U/ml is usually flexible enough to meet the volumetric requirement, although concentrations ranging up to 1000 U/ml may be required depending on the hourly rate of heparin infusion required. After the Ir is calculated, dialysis and the heparin infusion are started and the time recorded.

Step 4. Determine Apparent Sensitivity (S_a). The WBPTT is measured every 30 minutes during dialysis and S_a calculated from Equation (3-33) as shown in Figure 3-19. If WBPTT is off-target, the S_a is used to adjust the Ir (see Step 5) and 30 minutes later S_a is remeasured. In this way, Steps 4 and 5 constitute a 30-minute feedback loop used to tightly control the level of anticoagulation.

Step 5. Adjust the Ir. In most instances the WBPTT will not deviate from target by more than 10 seconds, and serial S_a values are used to adjust the Ir as depicted in Figure 3-19. Occasionally WBPTT will deviate from target by more than $\pm$15 seconds. This is most likely to occur in the first hour and suggests a significant change in sensitivity or a K_e substantially different from 1.00. If the value is confirmed by repeat measurement to be 15 seconds or more below target, a bolus dose calculated to increase R to target level using the initial S (which should assure against overshooting the target) should be given and a new S calculated and used to calculate a new Ir. If the value is confirmed to be 15 seconds or more above target, the heparin pump should be turned off and S_a calculated from the value just measured. The WBPTT should be followed at 15-minute intervals until it reaches the targeted range and a new Ir calculated from the S_a measured just before the pump was turned off. In this case it is most likely that K_e is substantially less than 1.00, while WBPTT values which tend to drift below target (resulting in decreasing S_a) result from K_e substantially greater than 1.00.

Technical errors should also be considered when WBPTT deviates more than ± 15 seconds from target. The commonest technical errors are erroneous heparin pump calibration, which can be spotted by recording syringe readings every half hour, and errors in heparin dilution. In the case of a very low target R of 10–15 seconds, the WBPTT measurement error may result in unrealistic predicted changes in Ir. In this situation clinical judgment is used to prescribe smaller, empirical adjustments of the Ir.

The average D_L and Ir required for the low-level anticoagulation described here are ~750 U and 600 U/hr, respectively. This indicates K_e is ~0.8 and that the average dose of heparin circulating in plasma is held constant at ~750 U during the dialysis. However, patients at the extremes of the S and K_e range may require loading doses and infusion rates ranging from 200 to 2000 U to maintain equivalent WBPTT target values. This underscores the importance of individualizing low-level anticoagulation if maximum safety and effectiveness are to be achieved.

Reversal of Anticoagulation with Protamine

Occasionally there is a need to rapidly return the WBPTT to normal in a fully heparinized patient. It usually requires ~0.01 mg of protamine per unit of heparin circulating in the plasma to return the WBPTT to $WBPTT_{BL}$. Therefore, the most rational way to determine the dose of protamine required is to estimate the dose of heparin in the plasma. This can be done by solving Equation (3-26) for dose (D, units):

$$D = \frac{R}{S} = \frac{WBPTT - WBPTT_{BL}}{S} \tag{3-35}$$

In order to estimate the circulating dose of heparin, $WBPTT_{BL}$ and S values are required. Either the average normal values can be used or, if available, previously measured values for the patient. The dose of protamine is then calculated as 0.01 (D).

An example can be given to illustrate calculation of protamine dose to reverse a WBPTT of 160 seconds. Assuming $WBPTT_{BL} = 70$ seconds and $S = 0.045$, the dose of heparin in plasma is $(160 - 70)/0.045 = 2000$ U. The dose of protamine would be 0.01(2000) = 20 mg. The adequacy of the protamine dose should be evaluated by measuring WBPTT ~5 minutes after the dose has been administered.

COMPLICATIONS OF DIALYSIS

Hypotension

The most serious frequent complication of dialysis is hypotension, which has been stated to occur in 30% of dialyses overall, but varies markedly between patients. Some patients rarely exhibit hypotension, while others may experience it in 60% of dialyses.

The pathophysiology of hypotension in dialysis is multifactorial and not fully understood. A major factor is acute decrease in circulating blood volume due to depletion of plasma volume by ultrafiltration at a rate which exceeds the rate of plasma refilling from the extracellular water. Sequential intradialytic measurements of change in plasma volume correlated to the incidence of hypotension indicate that hypotension is likely to occur during simultaneous dialysis and ultrafiltration when the plasma volume decreases by ≥15%, while during isolated ultrafiltration (without dialysis) a fall in plasma volume of 20% may be tolerated without hypotension.

The occurrence of acute hypotension with a 15% decrease in plasma volume over 2–4 hours during dialysis contrasts sharply with the ability of the normal person to compensate for a comparable acute decrease in blood volume to maintain a normal blood pressure. In the nonuremic healthy person, acute depletion of plasma volume results in powerful sympathetic vasoconstriction that supports blood pressure through three effects: arterial constriction greatly increases total peripheral resistance; the veins and venous reservoirs constrict and thereby help maintain venous return and cardiac output despite diminished blood volume; and the heart rate increases markedly. These sympathetic responses are considerably blunted during simultaneous dialysis and ultrafiltration: total peripheral resistance may fail to increase or actually decrease; cardiac output may fall substantially; and heart rate does not increase appropriately. The fall in cardiac output probably reflects primarily the failure of total peripheral resistance and venous constriction to occur with consequent sharp decrease in venous return to the heart. These effects can be attributed at least in part to the vasodilation effect of acetate ion and in part to the autonomic neuropathy of uremia.

The blood pressure is much better maintained in isolated ultrafiltration than during acetate dialysis combined with ultrafiltration. The sympathetic responses are more appropriate in that there is substantial increase in total peripheral resistance. However, cardiac output does fall substantially and heart rate does not increase significantly even when isolated ultrafiltration results in shock.

The blood pressure is also better maintained during ultrafiltration with bicarbonate dialysis compared to acetate dialysis and is not associated with a fall in total peripheral resistance. However, ultrafiltration during dialysis with dialysate Na^+ of 140–145 mEq/L results in a smaller decrease in blood pressure with either acetate or bicarbonate dialysis and appears to have a greater protective effect than bicarbonate compared to acetate. The amelioration of hypotension by higher dialysate Na^+ most likely results from a smaller decrease in plasma volume, since the ultrafiltrate will be isotonic or hypotonic to plasma. When dialysate Na^+ is less than plasma Na^+, the ultrafiltrate will be hypertonic to plasma and result in greater depletion of plasma and extracellular fluid volume.

Finally, there are a number of studies showing that if the decrease in plasma osmolality due to fall in urea is prevented by infusing mannitol, the fall in blood pressure during dialysis is ameliorated. Mannitol (or Na^+) is anatomically confined to the extracellular and plasma compartments and exerts an effective osmotic gradient promoting water transfer out of cells in contrast to urea, which is distributed throughout body water. If the rate of dialysis (K/V) is greatly reduced the incidence of hypotension is also reduced but not attributable to the change in urea and osmolality.

Volume-unresponsive hypotension may also result from acute arrhythmias or from pericardial tamponade, which should easily be identified by physical examination and auscultation of the heart rhythm. A rare cause of hypotension is acute hypersensitivity reaction to Cuprophane membrane, which may result in an anaphylactic-like reaction with acute dyspnea, wheezing, and hypotension. Therapy in this case is discussed below.

Evaluation and Therapy of Hypotension.   The degree of hypotension may range from a mild, asymptomatic decrease in blood pressure to profound shock with loss of consciousness. The clinical symptoms associated with mild to moderate hypotension (systolic blood pressure 90 to 110) include yawning, feeling hot, dizziness or lightheadedness, and nausea or vomiting. These symptoms tend to be reproducible in individual patients and an experienced dialysis nurse can often diagnose the onset of hypotension by observing a patient yawning or fanning himself. Severe hypotension with no obtainable pulse or blood pressure may seem to appear abruptly and simulate cardiac arrest. Hypotension usually occurs in the latter part of dialysis, particularly with high ultrafiltration rate, but may also occasionally occur shortly after initiation of dialysis. Hypotension early in dialysis may be primarily due to the vasodilation induced by acetate. Although high ultrafiltration rates increase the risk of hypotension, the occurrence of hypotensive episodes is quite variable. On one occasion hypotension may occur with a low ultrafiltration rate of 300 ml/hr, while on another occasion the same patient will tolerate an ultrafiltration rate of 1200 ml/hr without difficulty.

Careful attention to determination of the optimal dry body weight is very important to minimize hypotensive episodes. A number of factors must be evaluated to properly assess dry body weight. Increasing frequency or sudden appearance of hypotensive episodes often signal an increase in dry body weight due to unrecognized gain in body fat or lean tissue. Increasing predialysis blood pressure may signal a decrease in dry body weight due to unrecognized weight loss. Predialysis assessment of jugular venous pressure is extremely helpful to evaluate volume overload. An increase in resting jugular venous pressure (manifested by distension of the jugular veins above the clavicle in sitting position) is unequivocal evidence of right heart failure and usually reflects marked volume overload, particularly in patients with organic heart disease. Evaluation of less severe signs of volume overload and milder right heart failure can be achieved by examining for an hepatojugular reflux. This sign is best elicited by applying firm pressure in the right upper quadrant of the abdomen over the liver for 15–20 seconds with the patient sitting upright at 90 degrees. A positive test is manifested by sustained distension of the jugular above the clavicles due to a sudden increase in venous return from a congested liver. It is essential to instruct the patient to breathe normally and avoid straining during this test, since this will falsely elevate jugular venous pressure due to an abrupt increase in intrathoracic pressure. Ideally this test should be negative predialysis in patients with optimal dry body weight and average interdialytic weight gain of ~2.5 kg. The test should certainly be negative postdialysis at dry body weight unless there is severe chronic heart failure.

Excessive volume depletion can also be assessed by orthostatic blood pressure measurements and to some extent from examination of the jugular veins. In supine position the jugulars should be filled. If there is marked reduction in circulating blood volume the jugular will be flat in supine position. It is very instructive to observe the jugular during the course of dialysis in supine position. They are well filled at the start of dialysis but become progressively flatter during dialysis with ultrafiltration, providing a visible bedside manifestation of blood volume depletion. Hypotension with supine distention of the jugulars suggests that the hypotension is not due to simple depletion of blood volume. If the veins remain collapsed postdialysis after blood return, the dry weight may be too low, particularly if associated with intradialytic hypotension or postdialysis postural hypotension.

Peripheral edema is infrequently seen unless there is extreme overhydration or other local factors such as varicose veins or stasis. In adults edema is not usually seen with an isotonic volume overload of <4.5 L. In patients who have very high 5–6 kg weight gains, the fluid loading is often hypotonic resulting in low predialysis sodium (125–130 mEq/L) and resultant sequestration of the fluid load in both intracellular and extracellular compartments. This further reduces the likelihood of observing edema, since this sign results only from expansion of extracellular water.

A very simple but important precaution against hypotension is to dialyze the patient in fasting state if at all possible. Intake of food just before or during dialysis results in increased gastrointestinal blood flow and secretion of isotonic intestinal juices at a brisk rate which can be considered additive to the extracorporeal ultrafiltration rate. Several years ago meal trays were routinely served to patients in our facility and when this was discountinued the incidence of hypotension dropped abruptly from 30% to 10%. Oral intake during dialysis should be limited to ~250 ml of ice, which most patients crave because of hypovolemia-mediated thirst.

Moderately severe anemia is characteristic of the chronic dialysis patient population, and the average hematocrit is 25–27 vol%. The decreased red cell mass is typically replaced by plasma and total blood volume is relatively normal in chronic uremia. However, in some dialysis patients when the hematocrit falls to 20 vol% or below, there is a sharp increase in hypotension during dialysis, which is corrected by transfusion of packed red cells. Thus, worsening of anemia must also be considered as a treatable mechanism of increased incidence of poor ultrafiltration tolerance and hypotension.

There are also a number of technical errors, which may result in hypotension. A common error is incorrectly weighing the patient due to variation in clothing weight and contents of pockets or simply reading the scales incorrectly. Weight errors are especially common when the patient returns as a fully clothed outpatient after a period of pajama-clad inpatient dialyses. Calibration errors in pressure monitors and high K_{UF} dialyzers (see Chapter 1) may cause substantial errors in Q_F with excessive (or inadequate) fluid removal.

After careful assessment of dry body weight, exclusion of technical errors or sudden worsening of anemia, there is still a significant residual incidence of hypotension which in our experience occurs in about 10% of dialyses overall but varies considerably in individual patients. In the patient with a high incidence of hypotension the treatment should be analyzed with respect to dialysate sodium, K/V, and Q_F. As discussed earlier, as a general rule hypertonic ultrafiltration should be avoided and the dialysate sodium should be equal or somewhat higher than the predialysis plasma sodium.

If the patient has frequent hypotension associated with very high ultrafiltration rate, intensive counseling for improved compliance with dietary sodium and water intake may be helpful, or some increase in treatment time to lower K/V and Q_F may be required.

If dialysate sodium has been optimized and frequent hypotension persists, some patients may be benefited by conversion to bicarbonate dialysis. This may be particularly helpful if a relatively high K/V is prescribed and if morbidity is associated with plasma acetate accumulation.

Some authors recommend infusion of mannitol to prevent or treat hypotension. This can be done during the initial dialyses but is not suitable for chronic therapy because mannitol accumulation would occur.

When severe hypotension does occur, it requires immediate treatment. The first step is to immediately put the patient flat and elevate the legs to increase venous return and improve cardiac output. The TMP should also be reduced temporarily. This may be all that is required for management of a mild hypotensive episode.

For more severe episodes of hypotension with systolic blood pressure < 80 mmHg or signs of impaired cerebral circulation, additional emergency therapy is required. These episodes are usually treated with 100–200 ml bolus doses of saline administered over a minute or two into the negative pressure segment of the dialyzer blood circuit. With profound hypotension multiple saline injections totaling 500–1000 ml may be used. A disadvantage of saline therapy is that it leads to greater difficulty in reaching dry body weight when repeated boluses of saline are administered.

An alternative therapy more attractive to us is administration of metaraminol (Aramine) in bolus doses of 0.1–0.5 mg up to a total of 2 mg per dialysis into the venous blood line. The rationale for vasopressor therapy is that, although there is almost always some plasma volume depletion due to ultrafiltration, major factors in the hypotensive reaction to moderate volume depletion are impaired sympathetic responses. Metaraminol nearly instantaneously effects arteriolar constriction, increasing peripheral resistance and venous constriction, which increases venous return and improves cardiac output.

The patient with profound hypotension may clinically simulate cardiac arrest. In the pulseless, apneic patient, cardiopulmonary resuscitation along with volume replacement should be instituted immediately by disconnection of the arterial line and rapid return of the blood volume in the extracorporeal circuit with saline.

Blood Gas Abnormalities

It has long been known that acetate dialysis induces moderate hypoxemia with fall in Pao_2 of 5–20 mmHg, which is variably associated with a modest fall in $Paco_2$ ranging from 0 to 10 mmHg. When bicarbonate dialysate is used, the $Paco_2$ is unchanged or increased, and many studies have shown less marked or no decrease in Pao_2. The arterial pH rises in both acetate and bicarbonate dialysis, but the increase is greater in bicarbonate dialysis.

The mechanism of hypoxemia during acetate dialysis remains controversial and may be multifactorial. One major mechanism, hypoventilation related to decreased pulmonary CO_2 excretion, appears to be well established. Total CO_2 production remains constant during acetate dialysis, but pulmonary excretion falls by 2–3 mmol/min (1/4 to 1/3 of the total) because of CO_2 loss as HCO_3^- across the dialyzer. The first step of acetate metabolism results in uptake of an H^+ in formation of acetyl-CoA. The major source of the H^+ is hydration of CO_2 to H_2CO_3, which then leaves HCO_3^-. The HCO_3^- to a great extent is dialyzed out. Thus, 2–3 mmol of CO_2 per minute no longer flow to the pulmonary circulation for excretion, causing hypoventilation with hypoxemia. Hypoxemia has also been reported by some observers with bicarbonate dialysis in association with unchanged or mildly increased $Paco_2$ by unknown mechanisms.

Alternative mechanisms proposed to result in hypoxemia are embolization of tiny fibrin clots from the dialyzer and pulmonary embolization of leukocyte aggregates resulting from complement activation by Cuprophane membrane. It has been possible to clearly dissociate the neutropenia from hypoxemia, suggesting this is not a common mechanism, although it may well be operative in the rare patient with a severe hypersensitivity reaction to Cuprophane. Studies of the alveolar-arterial oxygen gradient with increasing fraction of inspired oxygen have shown a linear increase in the gradient as oxygen tension increases. These results were considered to be highly indicative of shunting in the lungs and suggest that abnormalities of the pulmonary circulation induced by dialysis may also play some role in hypoxemia.

The clinical significance of dialysis-induced hypoxemia is uncertain. It can readily be prevented by administration of nasal O_2 at 2–5 L/min. In patients with coexisting lung disease and borderline Pao_2 oxygen therapy is indicated. Routine administration of supplemental oxygen would seem also desirable for patients who experience chest pain, shortness of breath, and extrasystoles or who develop electrocardiographic abnormalities during dialysis.

Neuromuscular Abnormalities

Acute central nervous system disturbances may develop during dialysis, constituting what is described as the *disequilibrium syndrome*. Milder symptoms of this entity include headache, nausea, vomiting, restlessness, and asterixis. Severe manifestations consist of confusion, stupor, coma, seizures, and fatality. Severe manifestations of disequilibrium occur almost exclusively in acute renal failure or the acutely ill chronic patient. Predisposing factors include hyperazotemia (BUN > 150 mg/dl), hypernatremia, severe metabolic acidosis and preexisting brain disease. In this setting there is often acute toxic encephalopathy from uremia or associated illness, which may result in many of the symptoms described above; thus, identification of superimposed disequilibrium manifestations may be difficult if not impossible at times.

The severe manifestations of disequilibrium described above may persist for 2 or 3 days beyond the dialysis session and thus blend into other causes of altered states of consciousness and seizures, particularly in older patients. The differential diagnosis of confusion, stupor, coma, and seizures developing during or accentuated by dialysis includes subdural hematoma, cerebrovascular accidents, and, particularly, drug-induced encephalopathy. Renal excretion is the primary route of elimination for many drugs and their metabolites, and unless dosages are carefully adjusted to the reduced elimination rates (see Chapter 6), there is a high risk of drug accumulation and toxicity.

The management of the disequilibrium syndrome should be based primarily on prevention by avoiding high rates of dialysis therapy in patients at high risk for these problems. This will be considered quantitatively below in the discussion of acute renal failure.

Severe painful and recurrent *muscle cramping* may occur and compromise dialysis therapy. The frequency of painful muscle cramping is similar to that for hypotension, but in our experience they do not usually occur simultaneously. Muscle cramping is generally believed to be mediated by some combination of hypovolemia and hyponatremia. It is of interest that most papers on this complication report patients treated with dialysate Na^+ of 130 mEq/L, which would result in both greater plasma volume depletion and hyponatremia. The incidence is sharply reduced with a dialysate Na^+ of 140 mEq/L but still occurs in ~10% of dialyses.

Prompt treatment of muscle cramps is required because they are extremely painful and can compromise treatment. The patient may be driven to stand up for relief with risk of separating the blood lines, infiltrating the fistula needles and fainting. The most effective treatment is injection of a bolus of hypertonic saline into the venous return blood line. Ampuls of 23.4% sodium chloride are commercially available for this purpose. Hemolysis with mildly elevated plasma hemoglobin is observed occasionally at the end of dialysis when 23.4% NaCl is injected for cramps. A 1:1 dilution is safe, and the effective dose usually ranges from 12 to 24 ml of the diluted NaCl solution, constituting a dose of 24–48 mEq NaCl. A bolus injection of 50% dextrose in a dose of 1 ml/kg has also been reported to provide effective relief of cramps. The effectiveness of 50% dextrose would suggest cellular overhydration and/or plasma volume depletion to be the major causative factors for cramping, since this therapy would transiently depress sodium concentration. Hypertonic NaCl is effective in substantially smaller injection volumes and is less viscous and considerably easier to administer.

Hemolysis

Severe hemolysis during dialysis can occur from a variety of causes attributable to improperly maintained or designed equipment. Fortunately, these events are rare now because of fail-safe monitoring systems, purification of water used to prepare dialysate, and use of nontoxic materials in the construction of delivery systems.

Oxidant hemolysis can occur from exposure to dialysate containing copper, chloramine, or nitrate. Copper-induced acute hemolysis was described 15 years ago, resulting from release of copper from copper piping in the dialysate inflow stream, which was exposed to low pH consequent to exhaustion of the deionizer anion resin bed. Copper has since been completely eliminated from delivery system circuits. Chloramine is an oxidant increasingly used as a bactericidal agent in city water supplies. It results in methemoglobinemia and acute hemolysis when present in dialysate. Charcoal filtration is the method of choice to remove chloramine from water supplies. Nitrates present in the water supply used for dialysate preparation (described only in well water) can cause methemoglobinemia.

Formaldehyde is a potent reducing agent that can inhibit red cell glycolysis and cause severe hemolysis. This has been reported with water filters releasing formaldehyde at a concentration of 400 ppm into the dialysate preparation stream.

Thermal red cell injury can occur from overheated dialysate but marked dialysate temperature elevation to >47°C is required to produce hemolysis. This should virtually never happen with bypass alarms set at 42°C.

Mechanical hemolysis can occur if high negative pressures are created in any segment of the extracorporeal circuit. Red cells can withstand massive positive pressure but can be ruptured with negative pressure due to dissolved gases coming out of solution. Hemolysis may be induced in the negative pressure prepump segment of the blood circuit between the blood access and the blood pump when the negative pressure becomes high enough to result in partial tubing collapse. Pressure in this segment of the blood circuit should always be monitored with limits set to alarm and shut down the blood pump when negative pressure exceeds − 250 mmHg. This is frequently not done in clinical practice and may contribute significantly to the degree of anemia in some patients dialyzed with high negative prepump pressure.

Failure of the dialysate proportioning pump and conductivity monitors could result in delivery of pure water or extremely hypotonic dialysate to the dialyzer with consequent acute hemolysis and water intoxication. This rare event has virtually always resulted from human error and has essentially been eliminated by the incorporation of conductivity monitors with fixed limits in individual and central dialysate delivery systems.

The symptoms presented by the patient experiencing severe hemolysis may include initial localized burning and pain in venous fistula or cannula insertion site, dyspnea and chest pain which may proceed to loss of consciousness and cardiac arrest. The most striking visual effect in the extracorporeal circuit is an unusual deep burgundy color in the venous blood line, which is translucent when viewed with a light source from behind. The color will be significantly different from the arterial blood line when the comparison is made.

Immediate treatment of this complication is to promptly stop the blood pump and apply clamps on the blood lines. The kidney and blood lines are removed without returning the blood to the patient. Supportive measures include oxygen, and Trendelenberg position may be useful if the patient is hypotensive. Significant hemolysis may cause cardiac arrest requiring appropriate cardiopulmonary resuscitation. The degree of hemolysis may necessitate transfusion of packed cells, depending on the patient's hematocrit measured after the hemolytic episode.

Fever-Pyrogen Reactions

The most common cause for febrile episodes occurring during dialysis are host infection and "pyrogen reactions." The differential diagnosis may be assisted by the time at which the episode occurs. When fever occurs just after the initiation or termination of dialysis, one may suspect infection resulting from contaminated equipment used in the procedure. Access infections may also produce chills and fever during dialysis.

Pyrogen reactions are assumed to be a result of endotoxemia. The source may be an improperly sterilized reused dialyzer or contaminated water supply used for dialysate preparation. Theoretically, the dialyzer membrane contains pores too small to allow passage of endotoxins from dialysate to blood. However, there are data to suggest that this does, in fact, occur at times.

Pyrogen reactions almost always occur about 45–75 minutes after the start of dialysis. The initial patient complaint is of feeling cold or chilled. It is important to determine that low dialysate temperature is not, in fact, the cause of this symptom. Chills will usually appear and will range from mild to severe shaking. The chills are likely to last 20–30 minutes. If the patient's temperature is taken during the chilling period, it is unlikely to be elevated. To accurately assess the maximum fever, the temperature should be obtained 5–10 minutes after chilling has ceased. The chills may be accompanied by nausea and/or hypotension. Once the chill has ended, and the temperature has reached the maximum level, the patient will feel somewhat better, although not well. Maximum temperature rarely exceeds 39°C, although, with heavily contaminated dialyzers, temperature may rise to 40°C accompanied by severe hypotension and shock. A severe episode such as this may require termination of dialysis. However, in most instances, dialysis can continue and symptoms be treated appropriately, since the pyrogenic material has already been cleared from the dialyzer when the reaction occurs. When a pyrogen reaction occurs, there will be a significant clotting in the dialyzer. As described in Chapter 1, this may compromise ultrafiltration and, if severe, may reduce transport unacceptably. These results may warrant replacement of the dialyzer.

It is important to obtain outlet blood and inlet and outlet dialysate samples for bacterial culture during the early course of the reaction. The samples should be collected using the appropriate culture technique. The blood cultures are usually negative because the pyrogen reaction is due to dead bacterial degradation products rather than viable bacterial contamination. A positive blood culture indicates either gross contamination of an improperly sterilized dialyzer or septicemia already present. Dialysate cultures are usually negative or show low colony counts, <1000 col/ml. The source of the pyrogenic material may be in the water used to prepare the sterilant, or it may be formed after storing due to slow sterilization caused by low sterilant concentration. Very high colony counts in the dialysate indicate gross breakdown in sterilization technique. Untreated water used for dialysate preparation may also yield high colony counts; if this is the cause, a high colony count will be present in the dialysate inflow sample.

The organism most frequently found in the positive cultures is *Pseudomonas,* infrequently *Escherichia coli,* and rarely staphylococci. One group of organisms that is occasionally found in tap water, the nontubercular acid-fast mycobacteria, are very resistant to formaldehyde and may remain viable for several days in 1.5% formaldehyde concentration. This is a serious potential cause of septicemia.

Treatment consists of administration of antipyretics, usually acetominephen, and intravenous Solu-Cortef in the event of a severe reaction. If possible, one should avoid adding extra blankets for warmth during the chill. This will only result in further elevation of the patient's temperature. Increasing the dialysate temperature to >37°C should also be avoided for the same reason.

Membrane Hypersensitivity Reactions

Chest pain and back pain of variable severity occur at the *start* of dialysis in ≤15% of patients when a new dialyzer is used. The incidence of these symptoms decreases to about 5% with properly processed reused dialyzers and indicates greater biocompatibility of the membrane after the first use of the device. It has also been shown that the leukopenia and complement activation which occur early in dialysis are low with the reused dialyzer. Although the mechanism of improved biocompatibility in the reused dialyzer is not well understood, it would seem most likely due to either the leaching of some toxic membrane chemical component or protein coating of the membrane surface during the first dialysis.

These startup symptoms are conventionally treated by transient slowing of the blood pump although it is difficult to assess the value of this maneuver since these symptoms are always transient and rarely last more than 5 or 10 minutes. Slowing of the blood pump for an extended period (30–45 min) will reduce the amount of treatment provided (*Kt/V*) and should be avoided.

A much rarer event occurring at the start of dialysis is a reaction similar to *anaphylaxis*, which occurs almost exclusively with Cuprophane membrane. These acute hypersensitivity reaction symptoms begin with 15 minutes of the start of dialysis and begin with a feeling of uneasiness, agitation, tightness in the chest, and nausea. These initial symptoms are very quickly followed by shortness of breath, coughing, wheezing, urticaria, facial edema, flushing, and either hypertension or hypotension. Therapy consists of immediate termination of dialysis without return of blood and injection of epinephrine intramuscularly, diphenhydramine intravenously, and if necessary, Solu-Cortef intravenously. This type of reaction typically occurs the first time a patient is dialyzed with a Cuprophane membrane and consequently is an absolute contraindication to subsequent use of Cuprophane dialyzers for the patient. It is estimated to occur in 3–5% of patients.

Air Embolism

With the almost universal application of blood pumps in the extracorporeal circuit, the possibility of air embolism remains a risk for hemodialysis patients. As described in the monitoring section in Chapter 1, air may be drawn into the circuit at any point before the blood pump, that part of the blood circuit where the pressure is subatmospheric.

The amount of air required to cause mortality or significant morbidity is variable and may be dependent on rate and type or size of air bubbles introduced. It is thought that a slow infusion of microbubbles may not cause significant morbidity in patients.

As described by Blagg, the signs and symptoms of air embolism are dependent in large part on the position of the patient. Air enters the systemic circulation through the venous return line and if the patient is sitting, air entering an arm vein will travel through the axillary and subclavian vein and then retrograde up the jugular vein to the cerebral venous system. The air then obstructs venules and blood flow to cerebral tissue stops in a patchy pattern with resultant convulsions, coma, and possibly death. The patient may cry out in alarm from the sound of air rushing through the venous system to the brain.

If the patient is lying flat, air travels directly to the right ventricle where it forms foam and interferes with the ability of the heart to pump blood. If the patient is lying on the right side air may pass through to the pulmonary capillary bed and cause obstruction with acute pulmonary hypertension. Some air may pass through the pulmonary circulation and be pumped into the systemic circulation where arterial embolization may occur. In these circumstances the patient develops acute dyspnea, cough, and tightness in the chest, becomes agitated and cyanotic, and may lapse into coma. The syndrome may present as cardiopulmonary arrest, and ausculatation may reveal a churning sound caused by foaming of the blood of the heart.

When air embolism is detected, the blood pump should be immediately stopped and the venous line clamped. The patient should immediately be positioned with head and chest down and turned on the left side, which will trap air at the apex of the right ventricle and away from the outflow tract. In this way the right ventricle can act as a bubble trap and allow blood flow through the dependent portion of the ventricle to the pulmonary arteries and lungs. If the patient is conscious, 100% oxygen by mask should be administered, and, if unconscious, an endotracheal tube should be placed and assisted respiration started with 100% oxygen.

In the event of massive air embolism simulating cardiopulmonary arrest and auscultation signs of foam in the right heart, percutaneous aspiration of foam may be necessary using a long needle and large syringe. In this extreme situation foam should be aspirated prior to cardiac massage, which will drive foam into the pulmonary bed and left heart.

Other measures include intravenous dexamethasone to reduce cerebral edema and heparin and low molecular weight dextran to improve the microcirculation.

ACUTE HEMODIALYSIS

The patient with acute renal failure and the chronic renal failure patient with superimposed acute illness often presents additional volume, electrolyte, acid-base, circulatory, and nutritional problems that may substantially complicate dialysis therapy. Mortality remains high in patients with acute renal failure (50–70%) and is probably largely determined by the prognosis of the underlying surgical or medical problems causing the renal failure.

Indications for Dialysis

Although mortality continues to be high with acute renal failure, particularly after surgery or trauma, there is evidence that adequate dialysis can significantly reduce mortality. The artificial kidney was used in the management of acute renal failure for nearly 20 years before it became an established therapy for chronic renal failure. The development of the "Scribner shunt" in 1960 made it possible to initiate dialysis therapy in acute renal failure before the patient was in far advanced uremia and to dialyze as often as necessary to achieve adequate control of uremia.

The indications to initiate dialysis in acute renal failure encompass a broader range of acute uremic abnormalities than is usually the case in chronic renal failure. Azotemia is a primary indication, and dialysis is usually indicated at BUN levels of 80–100 mg/dl. In the patient with acute multisystem abnormalities and azotemia in this range, acute toxic or metabolic encephalopathy is manifested by variable confusion or obtundation; asterixis is often present or likely to develop. Although these altered states of consciousness can and do frequently appear in multisystem disease without azotemia, the contribution of untreated uremia to these abnormalities should be avoided by institution of adequate dialysis. Since uremia may not be the sole mechanism of acute encephalopathy, gross central nervous system abnormalities may continue despite dialysis therapy.

Acute volume, electrolyte and acid-base abnormalities may constitute primary indications for acute dialysis and/or ultrafiltration therapy. Massive, iatrogenic fluid overload commonly occurs in the course of management of trauma and shock and may result in pulmonary edema or contributes to the acute respiratory distress syndrome. Acute hyponatremia and hypernatremia may contribute to encephalopathy and require correction by dialysis. Uncorrectable serum potassium levels greater than 7 mEq/L and bicarbonate values less than 10 mEq/L are urgent indications for dialysis. In the past, frequent dialysis to control severe metabolic alkalosis was occasionally required, but the advent of cimetidine to sharply reduce gastric acid secretion has greatly reduced the incidence of this acid-base problem.

The following sections deal with the special considerations of the dialysis prescription in a patient with acute renal failure.

The Rate (K/V) and Magnitude (Kt/V) of Dialysis

Both of these parameters of treatment should be reduced during the initial dialyses to minimize the disequilibrium syndrome in both acute and chronic renal failure, particularly with BUN levels >125 mg/dl. A number of authors have provided empirical recommendations with regard to these parameters, but often these recommendations have addressed either rate or magnitude but not both. One author recommends that the prescribed dialyzer urea clearance not exceed 1–2 ml/min · kg body weight for the first one to four dialyses. Assuming the V is 58% of body weight, the K/V resulting from this prescription would be very low: 0.001/0.58 to 0.002/0.58 or 0.0017 to 0.0034. Another author recommends standard dialyzer clearances for the initial dialyses in chronic renal failure but a short treatment time of 2 hours. Thus, assuming that the K/V is 0.0055, this recommendation results in a Kt/V of 0.0055(120) or 0.66, which would result in a 40–50% decrease in BUN in 2 hours.

It would seem more rational to consider both rate and magnitude of dialysis when targeting the initial and maintenance dialysis requirements. Our empirical initial therapy is to prescribe $K/V = 0.0040$ and $Kt/V = 0.80$ for the first two dialyses on successive days followed by the maintenance prescription, unless the predialysis BUN is still substantially greater than 100 mg/dl. This initial prescription will result in a 50% decrease in BUN over 3 hours for each dialysis and has not been associated with excessive morbidity in our experience, particularly if careful attention is also paid to ultrafiltration, Na^+ and K^+. In patients with very high initial BUN and high pcr, it may require 3 or 4 daily dialyses with K/V of 0.0040 and Kt/V of 0.80 to result in predialysis BUN levels of approximately 100 mg/dl, after which K/V values can be increased to the range of 0.0060.

The steps in calculating the dialysis prescription have been described above for chronic renal failure therapy. The process is the same for initial therapy except for the restrictions on K/V and Kt/V. Measurement of serial pre- and postdialysis BUN is essential to determine V and pcr and to guide the dialysis prescription.

Although this empirical initial prescription with $K/V = 0.0040$ and $Kt/V = 0.80$ is generally safe, for unstable patients with very high BUN levels greater than 200 mg/dl it may be desirable to scale the rate and magnitude of initial dialyses even lower. This can be done quantitatively by the use of Figure 3-20 where Kt/V is shown as a function of the ratio of post-dialysis BUN (BUN_t) to predialysis (BUN_o). This curve provides a simple method to determine the Kt/V required for any specified target value of BUN_t/BUN_o that the physician may

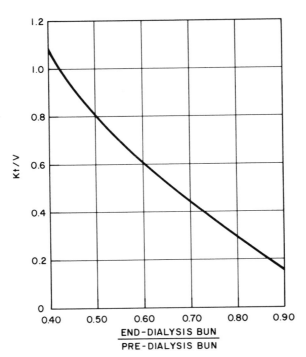

Fig. 3-20. Relationship between fractional dialyzer urea clearance (Kt/V) and the ratio of end-dialysis BUN to predialysis BUN.

choose. For example, if the BUN is 250 mg/dl and the physician elects to prescribe a 30% decrease in BUN of 75 mg/dl or BUN_t/BUN_o of 0.70, the Kt/V to be prescribed is 0.42. If the time elected to do this was 180 minutes, the K/V required can be calculated by rearrangement of Equation (3-22), which results in $K/V = (Kt/V)/t$ so $K/V = 0.42/180 = 0.0023$. The dialyzer clearance required is $(K/V)(V)$. If V were estimated to be 40 L, the K would be 0.0023(40) or 0.092 L/min. The use of Figure 3-20 and these simple relationships permit precise individualization of the initial dialyses with respect to clinically desired rates and magnitudes of BUN decrement.

The maintenance dialysis requirement for acute renal failure can be determined as for chronic renal failure using the modeling lines in Figures 3-5 and 3-6 if pcr is not excessive. If there is hypercatabolism with pcr substantially greater than 1.4 g/kg/day, more frequent daily or every other day dialysis will often be required to maintain predialysis BUN levels at 80–100 mg/dl. Relationships between the magnitude of dialysis (Kt/V) and interdialytic interval and the ΔBUN or pcr are shown in Figure 3-21 for two levels of predialysis BUN, 80 and 100 mg/dl.

The curves in Figure 3-21 are helpful to determine both the magnitude and frequency of dialysis required to control predialysis BUN between 80 and 100 mg/dl in the hypercatabolic patient. It is apparent from Figure 3-21A that when pcr exceeds 1.3 g/kg/day, it is impossible to maintain predialysis BUN of 80 mg/dl even with every other day dialysis, while in Figure 3-21B, it can be seen that predialysis BUN can be maintained at 100 mg/dl at pcr of 1.7 g/kg/day with

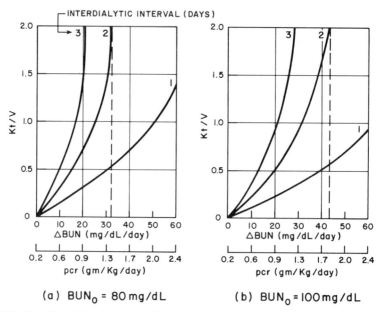

(a) BUN_0 = 80 mg/dL   (b) BUN_0 = 100 mg/dL

Fig. 3-21. Relationships between the magnitude of dialysis (Kt/V), daily change in BUN or protein catabolic rate (pcr), and interdialytic interval for two levels of predialysis BUN: (A) 80 mg/dl; and (B) 100 mg/dl.

Kt/V of 1.6 with dialysis every 2 days. Assuming $K/V = 0.0060$ is prescribed, this would require every other day dialysis with t = 1.6/0.0060 = 4.4 hours.

As pcr rises above 1.7 g/kg/day, it is apparent from Figure 3-21A,B that daily dialysis is required to maintain predialysis BUN between 80 and 100 mg/dl. At pcr = 2.4 g/kg/day, Kt/V values of 1.4 and 0.9 would be required for pre-dialysis BUN levels of 80 and 100 mg/dl (assuming $K/V = 0.0060$), and daily treatment times required would be 3.9 and 2.5 hours, respectively.

Dialysate Sodium

When hypernatremia is present at the initiation of dialysis therapy, particularly if the BUN is greater than 125 mg/dl, care should be taken to avoid rapid reduction of the serum Na^+ simultaneously with reduction of BUN. Simultaneous reduction of Na^+ and BUN greatly increase the likelihood of severe manifestations of disequilibrium syndrome due to cerebral edema. The following guidelines can be recommended for initial dialysis therapy of the hypernatremic patient with acute renal failure. If the serum Na^+ is greater than 160 mEq/L (a rare occurrence) and not associated with volume overload, a reasonable approach would be to infuse 5% dextrose solution in an amount calculated to *slowly* reduce serum Na^+ to ~160 mEq/L prior to dialysis, followed by dialysis with a high dialysate Na^+ to prevent further decrease in serum Na^+ as BUN is reduced. If marked hypernatremia is associated with volume overload, a rational approach would be to remove several liters by isolated ultrafiltration followed in sequence by infusion of 5% dextrose in water and dialysis. If the initial serum Na^+ is between 145 and 160 mEq/L, dialysis with dialysate Na^+ adequate to prevent a decrease in serum Na^+ (see Figure 3-12) would be recommended until the predialysis BUN has been reduced to ~100 mg/dl and hypernatremia corrected in subsequent dialyses.

Hyponatremia can be corrected simultaneously with reduction of BUN, since the rising serum Na^+ concentration will protect the patient from the disequilibrium syndrome. The relationships in Figure 3-12 can be used to select a dialysate Na^+ that will effect increase in serum Na^+ of 10–15 mEq/L per dialysis.

Dialysate Potassium

Hyperkalemia is commonly present at the initiation of dialysis therapy for acute renal failure. A dialysate K^+ should be chosen that will effect reduction of serum K^+ to 4.0 mEq/L, using Figure 3-13. If the patient is extremely acidotic at the start of dialysis, correction of the acidosis during dialysis may result in rapid decrease in serum K^+, which substantially exceeds the reduction predicted in Figure 3-13. Consequently, if the initial dialysis is associated with severe acidosis, serial intradialytic measurement of K^+ at hourly intervals is recommended to guard against hypokalemia and possible arrhythmias. If the patient is digitalized, and particularly if the digoxin blood levels are high (not uncommon in acute renal failure), the postdialysis serum K^+ should be targeted somewhat higher, in the range of 4.5 to 5.0 mEq/L.

Occasionally hypokalemia will be present initially due to excessive K^+ losses during the pathogenesis of the renal failure. In this circumstance, net K^+ flux into the patient during dialysis is indicated to correct hypokalemia. The dialysate K^+ required can be determined from Figure 3-13. Hypokalemia is very common later in acute renal failure due to restriction of intake below losses. Probably one of the commonest errors in the dialysis prescription is continued routine use of low dialysate K^+ in the presence of K^+ depletion during the course of acute renal failure. Careful attention to serum K^+ values and appropriate adjustment of dialysate K^+ using Figure 3-13 will prevent this unnecessary metabolic complication.

Acetate vs. Bicarbonate Dialysate

As discussed earlier, hypotensive episodes during dialysis are more frequent with acetate than bicarbonate dialysate probably due to the vasodilation effect of acetate ion. In patients with marked hemodynamic instability due to sepsis or other causes, particularly patients requiring a vasopressor such as dopamine for circulatory support, bicarbonate dialysate would be preferable over acetate. In patients with lactic acidosis and impaired oxidative metabolism, metabolism of acetate is likely to also be impaired, and bicarbonate dialysate should be used. However, in the majority of patients with acute renal failure, acetate dialysate is not associated with any increase in morbidity, as compared with bicarbonate, and is technically simpler to use and less expensive.

Ultrafiltration

Marked volume overload is commonly encountered in acute renal failure, often due to excessive parenteral fluid administration. When there is associated hemodynamic instability, simultaneous dialysis and ultrafiltration may be difficult due to frequent episodes of hypotension. The use of dialysate Na^+ high enough to prevent diffusive Na^+ loss in addition to convective removal (see above) and the use of bicarbonate dialysate in many instances will permit adequate ultrafiltration without inducing hypotension. In patients with extremely low cardiac output, particularly after open heart surgery, a high left ventricular filling pressure may be required to maintain adequate cardiac output. In such circumstances continuous monitoring of the left atrial or pulmonary capillary pressure may be required to guide the rate of ultrafiltration and avoid shock due to severe reduction in cardiac output.

In some patients because of severe hemodynamic instability and large ultrafiltration requirements it may be necessary to remove fluid by isolated ultrafiltration completely separated from dialysis. In such circumstances, isolated ultrafiltration may have to be performed on separate days so that the frequency of treatment doubles and essentially becomes daily.

A conventional dialyzer can be used for isolated ultrafiltration operated with Q_B of 100–200 ml/min without dialysate flow. The transmembrane pressure required for the desired ultrafiltration rate is calculated from the ultrafiltration coefficient of the dialyzer and achieved by some combination of suction on the dialysate compartment and/or a clamp on the venous outflow line (see Chapter 1). Some dialysate delivery systems can be operated in isolated ultrafiltration mode and used to control TMP. The simplest system is to connect the dialysate compartment to a Gomco-type suction apparatus for negative pressure. Although stable patients often tolerate 3–4 liters of fluid removal with isolated ultrafiltration at a rate as high as 2.0 L/hr, the patient with acute renal failure and hemodynamic instability in some instances requires much lower rates of fluid removal to avoid hypotension.

An alternative approach to management of the ultrafiltration requirement in acute renal failure is the use of a very small ultrafiltration device containing only ~0.2 m² of membrane and an ultrafiltration coefficient 10 to 20 times that of conventional dialysis membranes. These small ultrafiltration devices are often called arteriovenous hemofilters because they can provide slow continuous ultrafiltration with blood flow driven only by an arteriovenous pressure gradient without a blood pump. Operation in this mode requires either a Scribner shunt with arterial and venous cannulas or inlying arterial and venous catheters. An advantage of such a device is that ultrafiltration can be undertaken at a slow rate (100–400 ml/hr) over many hours independent of dialysis without the complexity of a blood pump. The passive blood flow and absence of dialysate greatly simplifies the extracorporeal circulation so that this therapy can be monitored in the intensive care unit or by specially trained ward nursing staff. A disadvantage is that anticoagulation is required for very extended intervals of time, which may pose a problem for patients at high risk for bleeding.

Recently arteriovenous hemofilters have been used to replace dialysis by providing ultrafiltration rates high enough to convectively remove urea and other solutes at an adequate rate. When used in this mode, the ultrafiltration rate is maintained at ~7–15 ml/min which will yield 10–20 L of ultrafiltrate per day. A balanced acetate or bicarbonate solution similar to dialysate is continuously infused at a rate equal to the ultrafiltration rate minus the desired volume of fluid loss. This therapy provides continuous solute and fluid removal and should in theory reduce both dialysis and ultrafiltration related morbidity. Disadvantages are continuous heparinization and the need to accurately control quite large input and output volumes. This approach has been used primarily in extremely high-risk patients with very high mortality so that it is not yet possible to evaluate its utility. It could not be recommended for routine management of acute renal failure at present.

Effects of Hyperalimentation on the Dialysis Prescription

In some patients associated hypercatabolism complicates dialysis therapy and rapidly results in energy deficits and protein malnutrition. This complication is more likely to occur with surgical complications, trauma, sepsis, and prednisone therapy. Although the role of hyperalimentation in acute renal failure remains somewhat controversial, there is evidence that mortality is higher for patients whose energy intakes are inadequate. There is also evidence that the pcr can be reduced, and nitrogen balance can become less negative or positive by adequate intake of both calories and amino acids.

The basic goals of hyperalimentation are to provide adequate energy in the form of carbohydrate and fat to approximate energy expenditures and adequate amino acid nitrogen to achieve nitrogen balance or at least to reduce the magnitude of negative nitrogen balance. Depending on the catabolic response, the energy expenditures may range from 25 to 70 kcal/kg/day and amino acid nitrogen intake requirements from 0.13 to 0.32 g/kg/day (equivalent to pcr of 0.8 2.0 g/kg/day). The pcr can readily be determined from the rate of rise in BUN between dialyses using Equation (3-16), and the effectiveness in an individual patient of increased caloric intake to reduce pcr can be quantitatively determined by serially increasing calories over 3 to 4 days with daily measurement of pcr. The level of pcr also provides an index to the amount of amino acid nitrogen required to achieve nitrogen balance (not always feasible) or at least to reduce the magnitude of negative nitrogen balance.

If an optimal caloric intake is successful in substantially reducing a markedly elevated pcr, it may be possible to decrease from daily to thrice weekly dialysis. However, substantial rates of glucose, amino acid and fat infusions require the administration of substantial quantities of fluid ranging from 1 to 3 L/day. This, of course, greatly increases the ultrafiltration requirement.

Another complication of high caloric parenteral nutrition is respiratory acidosis due to CO_2 retention in patients maintained on mechanical ventilation. If the caloric loading substantially exceeds energy expenditure and glucose is utilized for fat synthesis, there is a markedly increase in CO_2 production. The usual molar ratio of CO_2 production to O_2 consumption is ~ 1. With high levels of fat synthesis this ratio can increase markedly to levels as high as 8 and result in increased P_{CO_2} when alveolar ventilation is relatively fixed with mechanical ventilation. Serial monitoring of blood gases should guard against this complication.

The sodium, potassium, acetate, phosphorus, calcium, and magnesium content of the hyperalimentation fluid must all be carefully monitored in the patient with renal failure. When body protein stores are catabolized, K^+ is liberated at a rate of 3 mEq potassium per gram of nitrogen catabolized and contributes to recurring hyperkalemia. Net K^+ liberation may go to zero when K^+-free amino acid infusion equals pcr, and may even become negative if anabolism is achieved with net formation of body protein. Thus, as noted earlier, the likelihood of hypokalemia is as great as hyperkalemia and requires attention to the K^+ content of infusions as well as of dialysate. Similar considerations apply to phosphorus and magnesium which may be required in substantial quantities in the infusions despite renal failure. The catabolism of some of the amino acids results in the formation of hydrogen ions so that acetate buffer is required to minimize the magnitude of interdialytic acidosis.

The Na^+ content of hyperalimentation fluid is usually hypotonic relative to body fluids. The resulting fluid overload is distributed between both cell and extracellular water and is associated with a mild decrease in serum Na^+ between dialyses. If the dialysate Na^+ is selected to regularly restore serum Na^+ to 140 mEq/L (see Figure 3-12), the tonicity of the ultrafiltrate will be equal to the infusate resulting in net zero Na^+ and water balance for each dialysis cycle. If the infusate is isotonic or hypertonic with respect to Na^+, substantially larger swings in extracellular fluid volume will occur between and during dialyses and could result in a higher incidence of hypotensive episodes.

Heparin Dosage

In many patients with acute renal failure there is a substantially increased risk of hemorrhage due to fresh operative wounds, sites of recent trauma and gastrointestinal bleeding from stress ulcer. When increased bleeding risk is identified, the level of heparin anticoagulation should be low and tightly controlled using the kinetic feedback control algorithm discussed previously under heparin administration.

PEDIATRIC DIALYSIS
(Donald E. Potter)

The principles and techniques of dialysis are similar in children and adults. However, there are some differences, related to the adaptation of dialyzer characteristics to children of varying sizes, vascular access, and problems concerning the physical and emotional growth of children undergoing chronic dialysis.

The characteristics of a dialyzer which must be matched with the size of the child are efficiency, as measured by urea clearance, extracorporeal volume, and ultrafiltration coefficient. Children have a higher metabolic rate and food intake in relation to body weight than adults and therefore have a greater generation relative to body size of urea nitrogen and other metabolites when renal function is decreased. To accommodate this burden, high-efficiency dialyzers are used; for a child of any given size a dialyzer is selected that will provide a urea clearance three times the child's weight in kilograms at a blood flow of 100 ml/min in a child of <15 kg and 150–200 ml/min in a larger child. If the V of a child is ~65% body weight, then the equivalent Kt/V for a typical 4-hour dialysis is: $3(wt)(240)/0.65(wt) = 1.1$. The K/V is $0.003/0.65 = 0.0046$. With this efficiency the BUN level will decrease by ~65% during a 4-hour dialysis, and when dialysis is performed three times a week, the predialysis BUN level will usually be maintained below 100 mg/dl.

The extracorporeal volume of the dialyzer and blood lines should not exceed 8–10% of the child's blood volume. The ultrafiltration capacity of the dialyzer should be sufficient to remove 6–8% of the child's weight during a 4-hour dialysis using 400 mmHg of transmembrane pressure. Examples of dialyzer characteristics appropriate for a small child and a larger child are given in Table 3-2. The Grambro Mini Minor and Gambro Minor are commonly used dialyzers

Table 3-2. Dialyzer Characteristics for a Small Child and a Larger Child

Body Weight (kg)	K_{urea} (ml/min)	EBV* (ml)	K_{UF} (ml/hr/mmHg)
15	45	100	0.75
30	90	200	1.50

* Extracorporeal blood volume, which includes pediatric blood lines with a volume of 60–75 ml.

that meet these specifications. Adult dialyzers are used in children larger than 35 to 40 kg.

Because children require more efficient dialysis for removal of solutes and fluid than adults, they are more subject to the effects of osmotic disequilibrium and rapid contraction of extracellular fluid volume during a dialysis procedure. A high incidence of convulsions has been reported from one center. Mannitol infusions, 1 g/kg over the course of dialysis, have been used routinely in the dialysis of infants but are seldom necessary in older children. Hypotension usually responds to 5% saline, 1–2 ml/kg, repeated as often as necessary.

REFERENCES

Azancot I, Degoulet P, Juillet Y, et al: Hemodynamic evaluation of hypotension during chronic hemodialysis. Clin Nephrol 8:312–316, 1977

Bergstrom J: Ultrafiltration without dialysis for removal of fluid and solutes in uremia. Clin Nephrol 9:156–164, 1978

Blagg CR: Acute complications associated with hemodialysis. pp. 611–630. In Drukker W, Parsons FM, Maher JF (eds): Replacement of Renal Function by Dialysis. Martinus Nijhoff, Boston, 1983

Borah MF, Schoenfeld PY, Gotch FA, et al: Nitrogen balance during intermittent dialysis therapy of uremia. Kidney Int 14:491, 1978

Delano BG: Regular dialysis treatment. pp. 391–410. In Drukker W, Parsons FM, Maher JF (eds): Replacement of Renal Function by Dialysis. Martinus Nijhoff, Boston, 1983

Gotch FA, Keen ML: Precise control of minimal heparinization for high bleeding risk hemodialysis (HRHD). Trans Am Soc Artif Intern Organs 23:168–175, 1977

Gotch FA, Kreuger KK (eds): Adequacy of dialysis. Kidney Int 7(Suppl 2):51–5263, 1975

Gotch FA, Lam MA, Prowitt M, Keen ML: Preliminary clinical results with sodium—Volume modeling of hemodialysis therapy. Proc Clin Dial Transplant Forum 10:12, 1980

Gotch FA, Sargent JA: Modeling of middle molecules in clinical studies. Proceedings of the Symposium on Present Status and Future Orientation of Middle Molecules in Uremia and Other Diseases. Artif Organs 4(Suppl):133–137, 1980

Gotch, FA, Sargent, JA: A mechanistic analysis of the National Cooperative Dialysis Study (NCDS). Kidney Int., In press, 1984.

Kjellstrand CM, Pru CE, Jahuke WR, Dovin TD: Acute renal failure. pp. 536–569. In Drukker W, Parsons FM, Maher JF (eds): Replacement of Renal Function by Dialysis. Martinus Nijhoff, Boston, 1983

Lazarus JM: Complications in hemodialysis: An overview. Kidney Int 18:783–796, 1980

Lazarus JM, Kjellstrand CM: Dialysis: Medical aspects. pp. 2490–2544. In Brenner BM, Rector FC (eds): The Kidney. 2nd Ed. Saunders, Philadelphia, 1981

Lindsay RM: Practical use of anticoagulants. pp. 201–223. In Drukker W, Parsons FM, Maher JF (eds): Replacement of renal function by dialysis. Martinus Nijhoff, Boston, 1983

Lowrie EG, Laird NM (eds): Cooperative dialysis study. Kidney Int 23(Suppl 13):51–522, 1983

Novello AC, Kjellstrand CM: Commentary: Is bicarbonate dialysis better than acetate dialysis? Am Soc Artif Intern Organs 6:103–108, 1983

Sargent JA, Gotch FA: Bicarbonate and carbon dioxide transport during hemodialysis. Am Soc Artif Intern Organs 2:61–72, 1979

Sargent JA, Gotch FA: Mathematical modeling of dialysis therapy. Kidney Int 18:510, 1980

Sargent JA, Gotch FA: Nutrition and treatment of the acutely ill patient using urea kinetics. Dial Transplant 10:314, 1981

Shaldon S, Deschodt G, Beau MG, et al: The importance of serum osmotic changes in symptomatic hypotension during short hemodialysis. Proc Clin Dial Transplant Forum 8:184–188, 1978

Walzer M: Conservative management of the uremic patient. pp. 2383–2425. In Brenner BM, Rector FC (eds): The Kidney. 2nd Ed. Saunders, Philadelphia, 1981

Wehle B, Asaba H, Castenfors J, et al: The influence of dialysis fluid composition on the blood pressure response during dialysis. Clin Nephrol 10:62–66, 1978

4

CARE OF THE PATIENT ON
PERITONEAL DIALYSIS

Patricia Schoenfeld

Peritoneal dialysis (PD) has been used for the treatment of acute renal failure since 1923, antedating hemodialysis by 20 years. In 1962 Boen was first to apply the technique of intermittent peritoneal dialysis (IPD) for the therapy of chronic renal insufficiency, and in 1968 Tenckhoff convinced his peers of the practicability of the permanent indwelling peritoneal dialysis catheter. The efforts of these two pioneers advanced this modality as a long-term alternative to hemodialysis. In 1976 Popovich described the possibility of continuous, long-dwell time peritoneal dialysis, and by 1978, as a result of his collaboration with Moncrief, the clinical implementation of continuous ambulatory peritoneal dialysis (CAPD) was a *fait accompli*. During the past 20 years, only a small percentage of patients with end-stage renal disease (ESRD) have been treated with chronic peritoneal dialysis as their primary renal replacement therapy. However, the promising clinical results of CAPD has resulted in rapid development of this modality, and it is estimated that approximately 10% of chronically dialyzed patients in the United States and 27% of patients in Canada are currently being treated with chronic peritoneal dialysis.

The relative advantages of peritoneal dialysis in contrast with hemodialysis have been debated for many years, and these advantages have been dynamically modified in accordance with refinements in the technology and clinical quality of chronic peritoneal dialysis. Until recently, a majority of nephrologists have considered peritoneal dialysis to be primarily an acute therapy or a holding modality for maturation of access for chronic hemodialysis. However, with the development of automated intermittent peritoneal dialysis equipment and continuous ambulatory peritoneal dialysis techniques, many physicians now offer their patients chronic peritoneal dialysis as a choice that is equivalent or superior to hemodialysis.

The choice between peritoneal dialysis and hemodialysis is often based on individual exigencies in both the acute and the chronic settings, but some of the basic reasons that make peritoneal dialysis more attractive than hemodialysis are listed in Table 4-1 and are summarized as follows. (1) Peritoneal dialysis is technically less complicated than hemodialysis, and thus can be learned easily by nonspecialized medical personnel as well as by most patients. (2) If sterile technique is practiced strictly, peritoneal dialysis is a very safe mode, with fewer potential life-threatening complications than hemodialysis. This feature allows it to be readily adapted for home and self-care use. (3) While portable devices for hemodialysis have been designed, they are more complex and difficult to carry than the peritoneal dialyzer, expecially the CAPD apparatus, which requires primarily disposable supplies. The capability for travel and a more flexible lifestyle are two of the most powerful attractions of peritoneal dialysis that determine the preference of many patients for this mode of therapy. (4) Since peritoneal dialysis can be performed without the use of specialized equipment, it can be used in almost any hospital setting. (5) Most patients on peritoneal dialysis have fewer dialysis-related symptoms that those on hemodialysis. Continuous ambulatory peritoneal dialysis, which is the only form of dialysis that achieves steady-state biochemical status, is associated with the fewest symptoms related to solute and water removal. (6) For dialysis patients in whom bleeding as a complication of anticoagulation would pose serious or life-threatening risk, peritoneal dialysis offers a safe alternative without this hazard. Common clinical situations in which avoidance of anticoagulation is desirable include ocular and intracranial bleeding.

Admittedly, there are some disadvantages of peritoneal dialysis, as compared with hemodialysis. These are listed in Table 4-1 and are summarized here. (1) Peritoneal dialysis is relatively slow and inefficient, providing only 20% of the solute clearance achieved with hemodialysis, although it is more effective at clearing high molecular weight substances. More dialysis time is usually required to compensate for this lack of efficiency, which may cause inconvenience and may be less cost-effective than hemodialysis. In those circumstances where rapid correction of abnormalities or clearance of solute is critical, peritoneal dialysis is inappropriate and hemodialysis should be used. (2) Effective peri-

---

Table 4-1. Peritoneal Dialysis vs Hemodialysis

Advantages of peritoneal dialysis
1. Ease of performance
2. High safety margin
3. Portability
4. Availability
5. Fewer dialysis-related symptoms
6. No anticoagulation

Disadvantages of peritoneal dialysis
1. Low efficiency
2. Immobilization
3. Pulmonary compromise
4. Protein loss
5. Metabolic complications

Table 4-2. Average Protein Losses During Peritoneal Dialysis

Protein (g)	Intermittent PD (10 h)	CAPD (24 h)	Acute PD (36 h)
Total protein	12.9	8.8	22.3
Albumin	8.5	5.7	13.3
IgG	1.3	1.2	2.5
IgA	0.4	0.2	0.6
Transferrin	0.3	0.3	—

toneal dialysis in the acute setting often requires 24–48 hours of continuous cycling, which confines the patient to bed or chair during that time. This limitation may be less severe with chronic peritoneal dialysis, in that the intermittent peritoneal dialysis sessions usually last only 10 hours or overnight; continuous ambulatory peritoneal dialysis, as the name implies, is not restrictive of movement, except for short periods of bag exchange during the day. (3) In the acutely ill patient with pulmonary disease, distention of the abdomen by peritoneal dialysis fluid may compromise pulmonary function by causing basal atelectasis, or, in rare circumstances, by causing pleural effusion where a leak occurs between the peritoneal space and the pleural space. (4) Peritoneal dialysis, especially in the acute setting, is associated with significant loss of protein across the peritoneal membrane. The older literature documents protein losses of up to 1 g/L dialysate, or 20–200 g total protein loss per 24–28 hours of dialysis. More recent data, as shown in Table 4-2, indicate that the average amount of protein lost in a single acute peritoneal dialysis is 22 g, of which 60% is albumin. Consequently, in patients who are acutely ill and already compromised by nutritional insults, peritoneal dialysis may add significantly to the nutritional deprivation of these patients. When peritonitis is present, the loss of protein is striking—as high as 50 g per dialysis. (5) Both hemodialysis and peritoneal dialysis can result in metabolic derangements, especially if dialysate composition is not carefully evaluated for the specific needs of the patient. However, peritoneal dialysis more frequently results in metabolic disturbances, including hyperglycemia, which may necessitate insulin therapy in some patients. Hypernatremia and hyperosmolar states can result from aggressive ultrafiltration when serum sodium and glucose concentrations are not adequately monitored.

PERITONEAL MEMBRANE FUNCTION AND TRANSPORT CHARACTERISTICS

Peritoneal dialysis involves the transfer of solute and water from the peritoneal capillary blood to the dialysate in the peritoneal space, as well as the absorption of glucose and other solutes from peritoneal fluid into the blood. In order to authenticate the efficacy of this system and to determine the optimal manner of administration, it is necessary to understand peritoneal membrane blood supply and flow characteristics, the structure and function of the membrane that serves as the main barrier to the transport of substances, and the effects of large dialysate and blood fluid film layers on the dialysis process. The physiology of peritoneal dialysis is thus more complex than that of hemodialysis and less well understood, especially with regard to those factors that can be modified to optimize the efficiency of solute and water transport.

Peritoneal Capillary Blood Flow

The source of most solute and water removed by peritoneal dialysis is probably the capillary blood supply. A variety of indirect clinical evidence supports this theory, although it does not exclude the possible transport of solute from intracellular sites as well. Certain disease states and factors that adversely affect peritoneal blood supply are known to decrease peritoneal transport; also the concentrations of solute removed do not exceed the concentration in the blood, indicating that intracellular loss of solute does not significantly contribute to the solute removal.

Peritoneal capillary blood flow rates through vessels participating in peritoneal dialysis are not known, but these flow rates are estimated to be considerably less than total splanchnic blood flow. In vivo studies in the rat indicate that, under normal conditions, the mesentery is not very vascular, and only a fraction of capillaries may be actually perfused at a given time. Despite these potential limitations of capillary blood flow, clearance measurements in animal models and humans indicate that peritoneal blood flow is not a limiting factor in the transfer of solute across the peritoneal membrane. Evidence for this comes from the observation that even under conditions of severe hypotension and shock, resulting in marked decreases in peritoneal capillary blood flow, clearance of urea is only modestly reduced, disproportionate to the reduction in blood flow; conversely, when agents that cause vasodilatation and increased flow through the peritoneal capillary are used, only small (20%) increases are noted in urea clearance. Gas exchange across the peritoneal membrane is nearly three times greater than urea. These data therefore would indicate that the peritoneal capillary membrane acts as the major barrier to transport; thus, efforts to improve peritoneal clearances should be directed toward altering the permeability of this membrane.

Peritoneal Membrane Structure and Permeability

The structure of the peritoneal membrane is illustrated in Figure 4-1, which schematically depicts the various layers and relative sizes of these barriers to solute transport, expressed as resistances R_1 to R_6. In addition to these anatomical considerations, the functional state of the peritoneal membrane barrier may be affected by variation in number and size of the pores, by the hydration state of the matrix, and by the effects of disease states and other factors that may influence the metabolism and physical structure of this system. The relative importance of each of these barriers to peritoneal mass transport is not known with certainty, but available evidence indicates that the peritoneal membrane

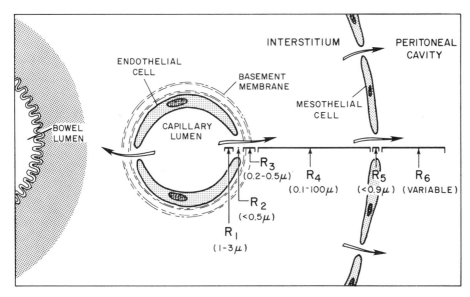

Fig. 4-1. Schematic representation of the resistances to solute and fluid movement from capillary to peritoneal cavity. R_1 through R_6 represent the mass transfer resistances of the capillary blood fluid film layer, (R_1), the capillary endothelium (R_2), the capillary basement membrane (R_3), the interstitium (R_4), the mesothelial cell layer (R_5), and the peritoneal cavity fluid film layer (R_6). (Nolph KD: Peritoneal anatomy and transport physiology. p. 441. In Drukker W, Parsons FM, Maher JF (eds): Replacement of Renal Function by Dialysis. 2nd Ed. Martinus Nijhoff, The Hague, 1983)

capillary acts as a major resistance to solute passage, especially for the high molecular weight substances, such as proteins.

Nolph and coworkers have hypothesized that permeability of the peritoneal capillary varies according to the anatomic site of the vessel, as illustrated in Figure 4-2. The proximal portion is an area of high ultrafiltration favored by high hydrostatic pressure and high glucose osmotic pressure, but has low permeability to solute because of relatively small pore sizes. In the more distal, or venular, segment, the capillary is more permeable as a result of larger pore size, while hydrostatic and osmotic pressures would tend to decrease water transport.

Pharmacologic agents and other factors that cause vasodilatation and increase vascular permeability seem to affect preferentially the venular segment of the capillary, thereby escalating protein transport, but only modestly influencing urea clearance. This is clinically exemplified by the effects of peritoneal inflammation, which conduces to vasodilatation and enhanced protein loss, but no increase in the clearance of low molecular weight compounds.

Vasodilatation of the peritoneal capillary network, and presumably an attendant elevation of blood flow rate, results in the perfusion of an increased number of capillaries, and thus increases the surface area available for solute transport. Such vasodilatation may also alter vascular permeability by enlarging membrane pore size or by dilating more permeable capillaries. The action of

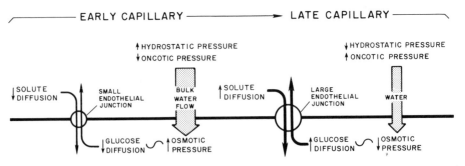

Fig. 4-2. Schematic representation of solute and fluid fluxes into the peritoneal cavity along the length of the capillary. Solute diffusion is less, while bulk water flow is greater, in the early (proximal) segment of the capillary, compared to the late (distal) segment. Axial flux heterogeneity exists because of differences in junctional permeability and relative driving forces for fluid movement.

vasoactive drugs that affect peritoneal clearances is probably mediated by these mechanisms, either through systemic effects, or by direct action on the peritoneum when administered by the intraperitoneal route.

Peritoneal Clearance and Factors Affecting Dialysis Efficiency

Measurements of peritoneal clearance are most commonly obtained by dividing the amount of solute removed per unit time, the mass transfer rate, by the concentration of solute in the serum. Unlike hemodialysis, in which solute removal is continuous, peritoneal dialysis involves cyclical inflow and outflow of dialysate into the peritoneal cavity. This sequence results in varying rates of peritoneal clearance; the greatest clearance occurs at the beginning of the dialysis cycle, when the dialysate diffusion gradients are maximal, and the rate diminishes gradually, as the concentration of the solute increases in the dialysate. One complete cycle of peritoneal dialysis is called an exchange. Clearance (K_{PD}) is usually measured over a period of one cycle and is expressed in milliliters per minute, as follows:

$$K_{PD} = \frac{C_{dialysate} \cdot V_{exchange}}{C_{plasma} \cdot t_{exchange}}$$

where $C_{dialysate}$ is the concentration of solute in the dialysate, $V_{exchange}$ is the exchange volume in time $t_{exchange}$, and C_{plasma} is the concentration of solute in the plasma. For example, if the blood urea nitrogen (BUN) is 68 mg/dl and the dialysate urea nitrogen is 26 mg/dl in an exchange volume of 2660 ml that required 42 minutes, then

$$K_{PD} = \frac{(26 \text{ mg/dl})(2660 \text{ ml})}{(68 \text{ mg/dl})(42 \text{ min})} = 24 \text{ ml/min}$$

Table 4-3. Factors Affecting Peritoneal Dialysis Clearance

Factors that can be modified with clinical technique
    Dialysate volume
    Dialysate temperature
    Dialysate composition
    Capillary permeability

Factors not easily changed
    Peritoneal membrane area participating in dialysis
    Peritoneal capillary blood flow
    Thickness of fluid film in peritoneal cavity (stirring, mixing, etc.)

While independent of serum concentration, the peritoneal clearance rate is affected by many factors (Table 4-3), including the total membrane area participating in the exchange, the blood flow rate to that area, the composition and temperature of the dialysate, the thickness of fluid films adjacent to the peritoneal membrane and endothelium, and permeability characteristics of the membrane itself. Some of these factors can be influenced favorably by adjusting peritoneal dialysis techniques; these factors are discussed in the following sections with special attention to their effect on dialysis efficiency.

Dialysate Volume. It has been clearly shown by many investigators that increasing the volume of peritoneal dialysate per exchange, or increasing the flow rate, will yield enhanced dialysis efficiency or clearance. Figure 4-3 illustrates the work of Boen, in which he demonstrated the relationship between dialysate volume in liters per hour and peritoneal urea, creatinine, and potassium clearance, using a single catheter and alternating gravity inflow and outflow. This

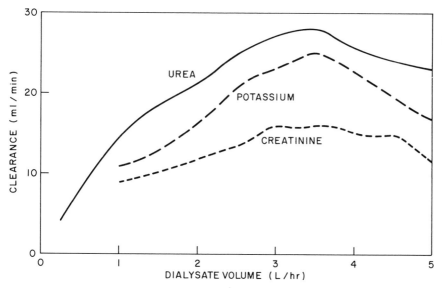

Fig. 4-3. Peritoneal dialysis clearance of urea, potassium, and creatinine as a function of dialysate volume.

work shows that when the dialysate flow rate reaches the level of 3.5 L/h, the urea clearance rate will rise to a maximum of 26 ml/min. With dialysate volumes greater than 3.5 L/hr, the proportion of inflow-outflow exchange time increases, thereby comprising the dwell time for solute transport, which precludes any further improvement in clearance rate. Subsequent to Boen's research, other investigators, using dual peritoneal catheters and continuous flow, producing large volumes of dialysate—up to 12 L/h—observed that urea clearance can be further augmented to ~40 ml/min. In the routine clinical setting, however, such a rapid flow rate is often extremely uncomfortable for the patient, and commercial dialysate is very expensive, so that the therapeutic benefits of this alternative procedure must be clearly established to justify its use rather than the more manageable flow of 3.5 L/h.

The classical technique for acute manual peritoneal dialysis is to achieve 2-L exchanges every hour. This is a compromise between maximum dialysis efficiency and the cost of dialysate and staff time required for more rapid cycles. Urea clearance with this technique will average 18–20 ml/min. With automated peritoneal dialysis systems, such as cyclers, shorter cycles (30–40 minutes), removing 4 L dialysate per hour, is standard procedure, thus obtaining more efficient dialysis, with an average urea clearance of 26 ml/min.

Temperature. Dialysate should always be warmed to body temperature, using dry heat, because better clearances are obtained than at room temperature (probably due to the vasodilatory effect of the warm solution), and it is usually more comfortable for the patient.

Ultrafiltration. The ultrafiltration of fluid during peritoneal dialysis is accomplished by the use of hypertonic dialysate containing dextrose monohydrate in concentrations ranging from 1.5 to 4.25%. The removal of fluid is very efficient in peritoneal dialysis, thus making it an effective procedure for treatment of severe volume overload and for control of extracellular volume. Table 4-4 and Figure 4-4 summarize the net removal of fluid, using various concentrations of glucose. Table 4-4 shows typical cycle lengths for acute dialysis and longer dwell times used in continuous ambulatory peritoneal dialysis. As shown in Figure 4-4, ultrafiltration is maximal when the dialysate is introduced into the peritoneal cavity, and after 2–3 hours of dwell time, it begins to decrease as the dialysate

Table 4-4. Ultrafiltration Volume (ml) Using 2-L Exchanges in Peritoneal Dialysis

Glucose Concentration	Dwell Time		
	1 Hour	4 Hours	
		Range	Mean
1.5%* (76 mmol/L)	50–100	−40 to 600	130
2.5% (126 mmol/L)	100–200	200–300	250
4.25% (215 mmol/L)	300–400	150–1100	750

* Glucose monohydrate or 1.36% glucose.

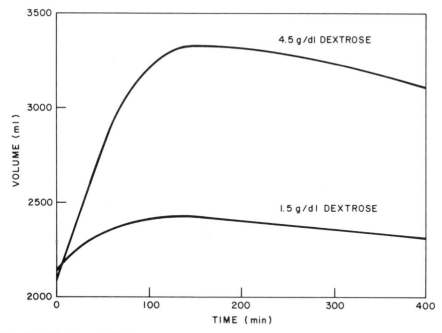

Fig. 4-4. Peritoneal dialysate volume as a function of time for two different concentrations of dialysate glucose.

is slowly absorbed concomitant with glucose absorption and loss of the osmotic gradient.

Ultrafiltration increases peritoneal clearance through convective transport of solute. However, most solutes do not accompany the bulk flow of water in the same concentration in which they are present in the extracellular fluid compartment. This sieving effect of the peritoneal membrane has been ascribed to several mechanisms, including (1) ultrafiltration through very small pores in the arteriolar end of the capillary wall, (2) surface charges on the endothelial and mesothelial cells, as well as in the interstitial gel layer, which can retard the movement of charged solute, analogous to the charge barrier in the glomerulus, and (3) the movement of glucose from dialysate to blood, which may cause molecular interactions in the peritoneal membrane that modify the sieving properties of the membrane.

Figure 4-2 schematically describes those factors that favor ultrafiltration of water in the proximal segment of the peritoneal capillary and greater transport of solute in the distal, venular segment. The high osmotic gradient and narrow pores of the proximal end of the capillary provide a sieving mechanism for water removal. The lower vascular osmotic pressure and wider pores of the distal end of the capillary accommodate transport of the large molecules of the solute.

Fluid Films and Stagnant Layers. Two sites of resistance to solute transport, as described in Figure 4-1, are fluid films in both the capillary lumen (blood) and the peritoneum (dialysate). The dialysate, which is probably stagnant in most parts of the peritoneal cavity during equilibration phase of dialysis, forms a very large fluid film resistance, which solute must traverse before it is removed. This system, when compared with the more efficient hollow fiber artificial kidney geometry, which has a relatively thin dialysate film adjacent to hollow fibers through which blood flows at rapid rates, demonstrates the adverse effects of this design on solute and water transport. In an attempt to decrease peritoneal dialysate stagnation, clinicians have used a rapid continuous delivery of fresh fluid procedure (semicontinuous peritoneal dialysis technique), in which small quantities of dialysate (100 ml) are exchanged every minute with a continuous reservoir of 1.5–2 L. With this technique, ~50 L of dialysate is used every 8 hours, and urea clearance can be increased to nearly 40 ml/min. Although effective, this mode of peritoneal dialysis remains investigational, and the cost-benefit ratio, as well as long-term clinical results, require further study.

Augmentation of Peritoneal Transport. A variety of approaches to modify the factors discussed above in order to augment peritoneal transport have been described in the past few years. Large increases in creatinine (244%) and urea (166%) clearance were demonstrated when dioctyl sodium succinate was added to the dialysate. It is possible that this compound, which has surfactant properties, induces some alterations in membrane surface lipids and other resistances in the peritoneal membrane structure, thereby enhancing transport.

Nitroprusside, prostaglandins, and many other vasoactive pharmacologic agents have been shown to increase peritoneal transport. Unfortunately, most of these drugs have undesirable side effects, such as increased protein loss, or only transient benefits, so that continued or chronic use may not be justified. It is important, however, for the clinician to understand the activity of these frequently prescribed drugs, expecially their effects on peritoneal blood flow and permeability, in order to establish a rationale for the optimal administration of these agents, both in patients receiving acute peritoneal dialysis and in the chronic outpatient setting.

TECHNICAL ASPECTS OF PERITONEAL DIALYSIS

Manual Peritoneal Dialysis

With the introduction of commercially prepared dialysate and the stylet percutaneous peritoneal catheter in the late 1950s, manual peritoneal dialysis rapidly became widely used as an easily performed, safe, and effective treatment for acute renal failure. The basic procedure for performing acute peritoneal dialysis using these materials is as follows:

1. Insert acute peritoneal dialysis catheter (See Chapter 2).
2. Instill 2 L warmed (37°C) dialysate (bag or bottle) into the peritoneal cavity as rapidly as gravity permits (5–10 minutes).
3. Allow the fluid to dwell for 20–30 minutes.
4. Drain the dialysate by gravity until flow stops or becomes very slow (20–30 minutes). Changing the patient's position may augment dialysate outflow.

5. Disconnect the used dialysate container and attach a new bag or bottle and repeat steps 1 to 4.

6. Measure drainage volume by weight or in a volumetric cylinder, and record the total outflow and the difference between inflow and outflow volumes as net outflow volume. Cumulate net outflow volumes to calculate net fluid balance to the patient.

Note: Dialysate containers are usually slightly overfilled (~80 ml per 2-L bag); thus, inflow volumes should be adjusted to obtain more accurate fluid balances during peritoneal dialysis.

When performing manual peritoneal dialysis, the dialysate must be heated to 37°C to optimize clearance and improve patient comfort during instillation of the solution. Dry heat should be used to warm the plastic bags or, alternatively, the bags may be placed in a microwave oven for 2–3 minutes. Water baths should not be used because of possible contamination of the bag port by unsterile water when the protective cap is removed. Caution: Do not overheat the dialysate, which can result in thermal injury to the peritoneum.

Automated Peritoneal Dialysis

Automated peritoneal dialysis machines are used in several clinical settings: (1) for in-hospital patients with acute renal failure (acute perioneal dialysis), (2) for patients with end-state renal disease who are beginning dialytic therapy following chronic peritoneal catheter placement, and (3) for chronic intermittent peritoneal dialysis, which is usually performed in the home setting.

The technique of chronic intermittent peritoneal dialysis usually involves 3 to 4 dialyses per week, each dialysis of 10 to 12 hours duration. Because of the length of treatment time, overnight dialysis is usually most convenient.

In the acute setting, intermittent peritoneal dialysis can be performed daily or continuously for 24 hours or more for inpatients who have had new catheters placed or are beginning chronic peritoneal dialysis.

Reverse Osmosis Machines. In 1962 Boen and coworkers introduced an automatic cycler for peritoneal dialysis that used a large reservoir of premixed sterile solution and offered the significant advantages of a closed system for a single peritoneal dialysis. Because of the cumbersome dialysate containers, however, this system was subsequently modified and incorporated with reverse osmosis (RO) water treatment equipment to become the automated reverse osmosis peritoneal dialysis system. This system can produce high-quality pyrogen-free water, automatically combine it proportionally with peritoneal dialysis concentrate, and heat it to body temperature. Some models of these machines can variably adjust the dextrose concentration of the prepared dialysate by incorporating additional hypertonic dextrose. The prepared fluid is continuously produced and delivered to the patient by pump; drainage from the patient to the waste drain is drawn by gravity. Separate timers for inflow rate and volume, dwell or dialysis time, and outflow are included and can be adjusted for individualization of patient treatment.

There are several diadvantages of reverse osmosis peritoneal dialysis machines. The complexity of the design necessitates regular maintenance and repair. Of all the peritoneal dialysis equipment currently available, these machines require the highest initial capital investment. Much greater space is needed to accommodate the large, bulky size, and often plumbing modifications are necessary for installation. The time claimed by setup and shut down, including sterilization, is substantial, which adds to the overall extensive time demands of intermittent peritoneal dialysis therapy. For the home dialysis patient, these machines require the most time for training, maintenance, and troubleshooting, and the most space for installation and plumbing hookup.

The advantages of reverse osmosis machines are significant. They are almost completely automated, and once the patient has started dialysis, the machine can operate for many hours without any necessity for changing dialysate or any contingencies requiring interruption of the system. They are economical to operate, since staff time is minimal during operation, and the concentrate is less expensive than premixed dialysate solutions. Several models are equipped with automated sterilization and rinsing cycles, which saves considerable time while ensuring safety and good performance. Finally, the reverse osmosis machine provides many hours of trouble-free dialysis, is safe, and with correct use, has a very low potential for causing peritonitis.

Cyclers. Peritoneal dialysis cyclers are semiautomated systems that use premixed dialysate, which is automatically heated and delivered to the patient. Two currently available cycler systems and their operations are schematically illustrated in Figures 4-5 and 4-6. A series of timers can be adjusted for inflow, dwell, and drainage time. Dialysate inflow and outflow is conducted by gravity, thus eliminating the need for pumps. Newer cycler systems also feature electronic monitoring of the number of cycles, of outflow volume, and of cumulative ultrafiltration volume. They also feature pressure alarms to protect against overfilling of the peritoneal cavity and to detect mechanical problems with dialysate inflow and outflow. These machines demand a sizeable quantity of disposable equipment and supplies; the entire sterile dialysate pathway, from bag to outflow dialysate collection, is used once and then is discarded. From 5 to 12 bags of dialysate (2–3 L) can be attached to the machine at one time, thus permitting 5–18 hours of dialysis without a break in the system, assuming a schedule of 2-L hourly exchanges. The dextrose concentration of the dialysate is somewhat less flexible than that used with reverse osmosis machines, and must be adjusted by selecting an appropriate mixture of dextrose concentrations at the time the bags are attached to the machine.

The major advantage of cyclers is their inherent simplicity; they have a minimum of mechanical functions, which makes it easy for staff and patients to setup and operate. Low initial capital expense, minimal maintainence requirements, and relatively trouble-free performance make these machines attractive for many programs, especially for patients who wish to do home peritoneal dialysis without the complexity of the reverse osmosis systems.

The major disadvantage of cycler systems has been their high cost of op-

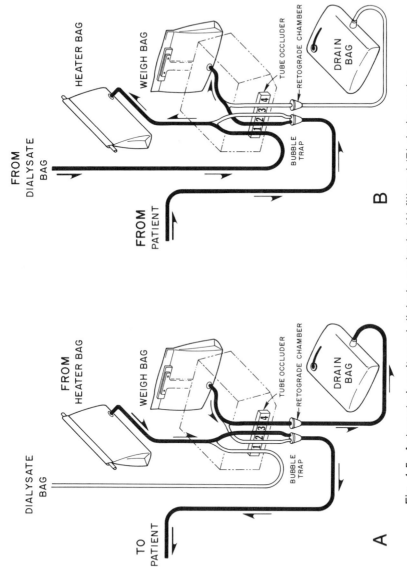

Fig. 4-5. Automated peritoneal dialysis cycler in (A) fill and (B) drain modes.

157

PATIENT FILL

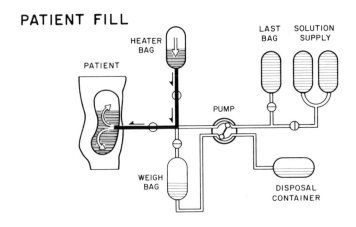

DWELL

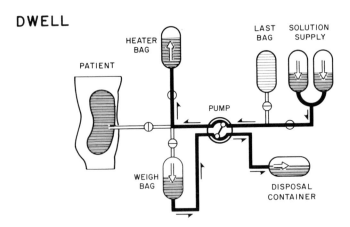

PATIENT DRAIN

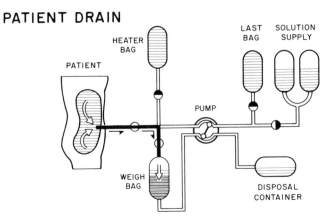

Fig. 4-6. Automated peritoneal dialysis cycler in fill, dwell, and drain modes.

eration, this owing to the prerequisite large quantities of disposable supplies and the higher cost of premixed dialysate. For acute dialysis, this cost differential has not been critical, but in the chronic setting, these costs have made the cycler the most expensive form of chronic peritoneal dialysis. Currently, however, in order to make cyclers attractive within the framework of composite reimbursement rates, several major manufacturers of peritoneal dialysis supplies are committed to the development of new equipment and supplies designed to reduce the overall cost of cycler peritoneal dialysis.

Continuous Ambulatory Peritoneal Dialysis

Continuous ambulatory peritoneal dialysis (CAPD) is the newest and most successful peritoneal dialysis technique yet devised and is attracting a significant number of patients to this modality. In the late 1970s Popovich and coworkers developed the theoretical basis for continuous ambulatory peritoneal dialysis, which argued that the low clearance rates of peritoneal dialysis can be compensated by continuous peritoneal transport, accomplished by a few long-dwell time exchanges performed daily. Popovich, in conjunction with Moncrief, first demonstrated the clinical efficacy of this theory, which quickly led to its use by several other investigators, who have advanced our knowledge of this technique and contributed to many technical and clinical improvements over the past several years.

The basic technique of continuous ambulatory peritoneal dialysis is extremely simple, and, as a form of manual peritoneal dialysis, is an example of recidivism in the complex world of dialysis technology. This unique simplicity partly answers for the allure of this modality and makes it the most versatile and manageable of dialysis techniques. The fundamental continuous ambulatory peritoneal dialysis system is schematically depicted in Figure 4-7.

The bag exchange procedure as depicted in Figure 4-7 illustrates the simple inflow and outflow of dialysate by gravity, which require ~10 and 15–20 minutes, respectively. Usually 2 L of dialysate are used per exchange; most patients require 4 exchanges per day, with a total outflow volume of ~10 L/day (including ultrafiltrate), providing a continuous urea clearance of about 7 ml/min. Some patients require as few as 3, and others as many as 5, exchanges per day for adequate biochemical control. It has recently been established that up to one third of patients can tolerate 3 L of dialysate per exchange, which can be used either to increase the efficiency of dialysis or to decrease the number of exchanges required. Dialysate volume and schedules for CAPD in children are different; see the last section in this chapter.

Sterile Techniques in Continuous Ambulatory Peritoneal Dialysis. Success or failure with CAPD is strongly dependent on the rigid adherence to aseptic technique when performing bag exchanges in order to prevent peritonitis. Specific procedures and techniques for performing CAPD vary considerably among dialysis facilities; however, the following guidelines are generally con-

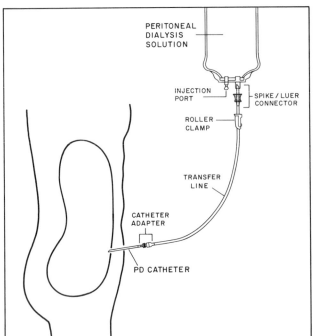
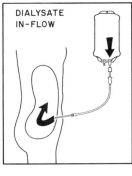
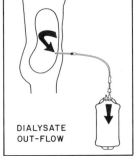

Fig. 4-7. Schematic representation of continuous ambulatory peritoneal dialysis components (left) and techniques of inflow (top right) and outflow (bottom right). A catheter adapter made of lightweight titanium securely connects the Silastic peritoneal dialysis catheter to the transfer line, which is inserted by means of a spike or leur-type adapter into a bag of dialysate. The connection site between the transfer line and the bag is protected by a plastic connection shield with a sponge lining that can be soaked with a povidone-iodine solution.

sidered effective in preventing contamination:

1. Follow specified techniques carefully without deviation.
   a. Perform bag exchanges in a clean area and wear a mask.
   b. Exclude pets, birds, and other animals from this area.
   c. Restrict traffic and other activities in the area during a bag exchange.
   d. Close off the area if possible.
2. Good personal hygiene is obligatory.
   a. Wash the hands scrupulously for 5 minutes with soap or other bacteriostatic cleansing agents after setting out supplies and draining the peritoneal cavity.
   b. Shower daily.
3. Observe and inspect supplies and dialysate outflow regularly.
   a. Examine new bag, ports, line, etc. for possible defects or leaks.
   b. Examine outflow bag for cloudy appearance, fibrin, or blood.
   c. Examine catheter exit site and palpate the tunnel tract for signs of tenderness.

4. Known contamination of the spike during a bag exchange must be reported to the dialysis center staff immediately, and established procedure must be followed strictly (emergency line changes, soaking of the spike in povidone-iodine solution, etc.).

Despite apparent careful attention to techniques, many motivated and conscientious patients will develop peritonitis, which probably occurs as a result of accidental contamination during the bag exchange. In order to prevent this inapparent contamination, several new sophisticated systems have been devised to reduce the incidence of peritonitis.

In-line filter. A 0.22-μm filter (Peridex) has been made commercially available by Millipore Corporation. This filter is interposed between the transfer line and the bag, which provides a dual pathway for inflow of dialysate through the filter and outflow of dialysate bypassing the filter. Several European and United States studies have reported the success of this device in reducing the incidence of peritonitis. The effectiveness of the filter has been demonstrated by the presence of bacteria on its surface after removal from use, while the patient remained infection-free.

Peridex has some serious disadvantages. First, these filters are very expensive and, under optimal conditions, must be changed every 2 weeks; sometimes, however, because of the slow flow rate, the filter becomes clogged and must be changed oftener than 2-week intervals. Second, the filter apparatus adds bulk to the CAPD system. Finally, dialysate inflow and outflow rates are slower, requiring even more time to perform this time-demanding procedure. Still, the effectiveness of Peridex is inarguable, and may be critical in allowing some patients to receive the benefits of CAPD without being subjected to the complications of infection.

Ultraviolet light sterilization. Baxter Travenol has designed a portable box containing an ultraviolet light sterilization system, which is utilized during the routine bag exchange procedure to treat possible contamination as soon as it occurs. Operation is simple, but adds approximately 5–10 minutes to the bag exchange procedure. The device can operate with a rechargeable battery or directly through an electric outlet.

Further clinical trials, with large numbers of patients, are needed to confirm the effectiveness of ultraviolet light sterilization in reducing infection. Disadvantages of the system include a relatively high cost, which can be amortized over a period of several years, the addition of equipment and "machines," which CAPD is designed to avoid, and the extra time required to do a bag exchange. If this device can successfully eliminate or reduce infection, then these disadvantages are only relative, the cost being outweighed by the expense of treating peritonitis in the hospital setting or by the loss of a catheter due to peritonitis.

Sterile connection device. E. I. Du Pont de Nemors and Company have developed an instrument that accomplishes bag exchanges by thermally welding an extension tubing from the dialysate bag to the patient transfer line (Fig. 4-

8). This device thus eliminates the connection procedure in an open system and allows the patient to maintain a continuously closed system. The single connection device is slightly larger than a cigar box (12 cm × 23 cm × 23 cm) and operates with a rechargeable battery. The major advantages of this system are the elimination of the open system and the impossibility of "shortcutting." It is fast, requiring only 15 seconds to make the new connection; the weld is strong, retaining 90% of the original tubing strength. The major disadvantages are, again, the high cost and the introduction of additional equipment into an otherwise simple procedure.

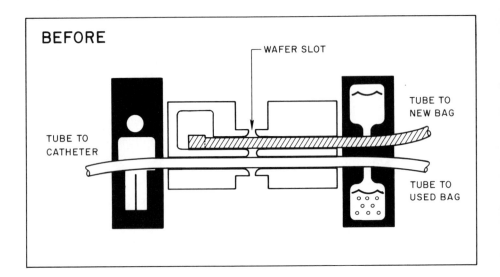

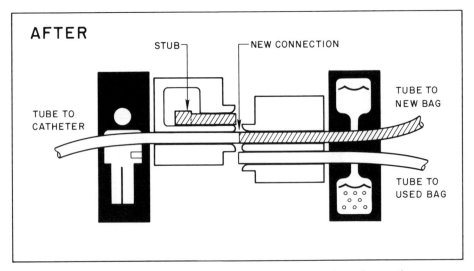

Fig. 4-8. Sterile connection device for changing tubing to bags in continuous ambulatory peritoneal dialysis shown before and after connection.

Mechanical devices for bag exchange. Mechanical devices to guide the removal of the spike from the used bag and insert it into a new bag have been developed to assist patients with physical disability (e.g., hand weakness, visual impairment) and to reduce the risk of accidental spike contamination. While helpful for some patients, it is still possible for spike contamination to occur with this type of apparatus, especially if used improperly. The major drawback is that patients do not have to use them, and therefore are able to "shortcut" by eliminating the device. Such tracking devices have been most helpful for blind or severely visually impaired patients to enable partial self-care with CAPD. These patients, of course, still require assistance to inspect the dialysate outflow for abnormalities and to assist with catheter and exit site inspection and care.

New connection systems. Several vendors have developed modifications of the connection between the transfer set and the bag, which are designed to decrease bacteriologic contamination of the site by continuous bathing with povidone-iodine-soaked material and protective sheaths to prevent exposure to air or touch by contaminated surfaces. Such systems are currently being tested for efficacy in reducing the incidence of peritonitis.

Continuous Ambulatory Peritoneal Dialysis Schedules. Most patients adapt their CAPD schedule to fit daily activities, and perform the last exchange at bedtime for the long overnight dwell period (8–10 hours). Since each exchange requires about 30–40 minutes, or a total of 3–4 hours daily, planning is required to accommodate exchanges to work schedules and to enable patients to perform exchanges opportunely and in the safest environment. Daily logs should be kept in which each exchange is documented and weight, blood pressure, and symptoms are recorded. Diabetic patients should record insulin dosage for each bag and document results obtained from self-monitoring of blood glucose.

Modification of CAPD: Continuous Cycling Peritoneal Dialysis (CCPD). Because of the constraining time commitment required throughout the day for CAPD, a hybrid of long-dwell peritoneal dialysis and cycler-assisted dialysis was developed to allow patients to reverse the diurnal rhythm of CAPD from three daytime exchanges and one long overnight dwell to three or four short overnight exchanges and one long exchange during the day. The night exchanges are performed by a cycler to automate the process and allow the patient to sleep. A further attraction of this system is that the risk of peritonitis should be reduced, since the peritoneal catheter is opened only twice a day instead of four times with CAPD. This type of dialysis is indicated for patients who require assistance to perform peritoneal dialysis, such as the elderly, the visually impaired, and children, where CAPD would require greater demands of time and scheduling than the use of the cycler each night. The major disadvantages of this modality are the increased costs of disposable supplies for the cycler each night and the relative inconvenience of introducing a machine to the otherwise simple CAPD system. However, as mentioned above, manufacturers are now committed to the production of cost-effective cycler systems, which should make continuous cycling peritoneal dialysis cost-competitive with CAPD in the near future.

With this modality, it is also theoretically possible for patients to alternate between continuous cycling peritoneal dialysis and continuous ambulatory peritoneal dialysis as their daily activities dictate. Thus, some patients may perform CCPD routinely, but switch to CAPD for traveling.

Dialysate

Composition. Peritoneal dialysate is supplied commercially in two major forms: (1) premixed, ready to use; and (2) concentrate, requiring dilution with an automated peritoneal dialysis delivery system.

Premixed dialysate is available from several vendors with varying electrolyte and mineral composition; the most widely used formulations are listed in Table 4-5. While some manufacturers supply dialysate with a sodium concentration of 141 mEq/L, most clinicians, respectful of the sieving effect on solute removal with peritoneal dialysis, prefer to use the lower sodium concentration of 132 mEq/L, hoping to reduce the incidence of systemic hypernatremia.

The dialysate concentration of ionized calcium is relatively high (3.5 mEq/L) so as to maintain a positive calcium balance in the patient and to prevent calcium losses during continuous cycling. When this high calcium concentration is used in combination with 1.5% dextrose solution, the net calcium balance or mass transfer is positive, but with higher percentages of dextrose the calcium balance is less positive or even negative. The lower positive calcium balance attained with hypertonic dextrose has been attributed to a greater convective removal of calcium during ultrafiltration, which counterbalances the diffusion of calcium from dialysate to patient.

Magnesium concentration in the dialysate has been generally maintained at the low normal serum level; however, some studies, using this formulation with 1.5% dextrose solution, found the magnesium mass transfer in peritoneal dialysis patients to be slightly positive, despite the finding that in these patients the mean serum magnesium level was 2.5 mEq/L, which was higher than the dialysate level. Other studies have shown magnesium flux to be negative, especially with 4.25% dextrose. Because of these observations dialysate is now available with a low magnesium formulation containing 0.5 mEq/L, and studies of a zero magnesium dialysate are currently being conducted.

Table 4-5. Composition of Peritoneal Dialysis Solutions

Dialysate	Standard	Low Magnesium	Concentrate (diluted 1 : 19 H₂O)
Dextrose monohydrate	1.5–4.25%	1.5–4.25%	1.5–2.5%
Sodium	132 mEq/L	132 mEq/L	132 mEq/L
Calcium	3.5 mEq/L	3.5 mEq/L	3.5 mEq/L
Magnesium	1.5 mEq/L	0.5 mEq/L	1.5 mEq/L
Chloride	102 mEq/L	96 mEq/L	101 mEq/L
Lactate	35 mEq/L	40 mEq/L	37 mEq/L (acetate)

The lower magnesium-containing dialysate also contains a higher lactate concentration of 40 mEq/L, rather than the 35 mEq/L present in the standard formulation. The higher lactate level is clearly advantageous for those patients who achieve suboptimal correction of systemic acidosis with the standard formula, and studies have demonstrated that mean plasma bicarbonate levels are significantly higher with lactate concentration of 40 mEq/L. The lower magnesium and higher lactate levels may be favorable to preventing or retarding the progression of osteodystrophy in chronic peritoneal dialysis patients, since both hypermagnesemia and chronic acidosis may be deleterious to skeletal composition and metabolism.

Concentrated dialysate is commercially prepared for use with automated peritoneal dialysis machines which contain reverse osmosis equipment for sterile water preparation. The concentrate is automatically proportioned in a ratio of 1 part concentrate to 19 parts sterile, nonpyrogenic water. The composition of the dialysate prepared in this fashion is listed in Table 4-5. It is available in two glucose concentrations, 30% and 50%, which, when diluted, contain 1.5 and 2.5 mg/dl, respectively.

Premixed dialysate, originally packaged in 1- and 2-L glass bottles, is now most commonly used in flexible plastic bags, ranging in size from 250 to 750 ml for pediatric use to 1.0, 1.5, 2.0, and 3.0 L for adult dialysis. Most adults can tolerate 2 L of dialysate at a time without overdistention; occasionally small adults with tight muscular abdominal walls may be able to use only 1.5 L with comfort. Recent studies suggest that up to one third of adults can use 3 L of dialysate at one time, which allows fewer exchanges for continuous ambulatory peritoneal dialysis, and possibly a reduction in the incidence of peritonitis, which is the major complication of chronic peritoneal dialysis.

Ultrafiltration volumes with a standard 2 L exchange range from 100 to 800 ml or more with hypertonic dextrose. The compliance of the bags is such that 3 L of total volume can be contained in the bag, thus allowing adequate volume for removal of ultrafiltrate. However, for patients who have larger outflow volumes or feel that they are incompletely drained of dialysate, underfilled bags are available (2 L in a 3 L bag) to allow for greater outflow capacity.

Glucose Concentrations. Premixed dialysate is available in three standard dextrose concentrations: 1.5, 2.5, and 4.25%. These concentrations represent dextrose monohydrate; actual concentration of anhydrous dextrose is somewhat lower, for example, 1.5% dextrose monohydrate equals 1.36 g/dl of anhydrous dextrose (180 daltons) or 75.6 mmol/L.

All dialysate solutions are hypertonic to normal plasma osmolality, ranging from 347 mosm/L for 1.5% dextrose to 486 mosm/L for 4.25% dextrose.

Appearance. Normally, dialysate is clear or very slightly amber colored. Concentrate is usually light to medium amber in appearance. Dialysate that is cloudy or contains precipitated material should not be used. Bags should be squeezed slightly to check for leaks.

Additives. Heparin. Heparin is frequently added to dialysate in a dose of 1000 U/bag in the following situations:

1. Following placement of a new catheter, when small quantities of blood may be present in the peritoneal cavity
2. Whenever blood is present in the peritoneal fluid
3. During peritonitis
4. When fibrin formation is noted in the dialysate outflow

Insulin. Insulin may be added to the dialysate during acute intermittent peritoneal dialysis to correct hyperglycemia resulting from absorption of glucose. This is commonly required in nondiabetic, as well as in diabetic, patients, especially when continuous cycling with hypertonic dextrose results in absorption of large quantities of dextrose. The quantity of insulin required in the acute setting must be determined specifically for each patient by titrating the dose of insulin with the blood glucose concentration. As a guide, in addition to the patient's regular dose of insulin, the following amounts of insulin may be added and adjusted according to response:

Glucose Concentration	Additional Insulin Dose
1.5%	4–5 U/L
2.5%	5–7 U/L
4.25%	7–10 U/L

During acute or intermittent peritoneal dialysis, postdialysis hypoglycemia is a potential complication of adding insulin to the dialysate; it may be avoided by omitting insulin from the last several exchanges or by leaving 500 ml of dialysate in the peritoneal cavity before terminating the dialysis.

Insulin may also be added to concentrated dialysate when used with automated reverse osmosis machines. Much larger quantities are required, ranging from 200 U/2 L of 30% concentrate to 400 U/2 L of 50% concentrate. If supplemental glucose is added to increase the final concentration of dextrose, then additional insulin may be added to these containers as well (50U/500 ml of 50% dextrose).

Management of insulin therapy in diabetic patients on continuous ambulatory peritoneal dialysis has been evaluated by many investigators, and it is now established that significant reduction of daily blood sugar variations can be achieved using continuous intraperitoneal insulin via the dialysate with no subcutaneous insulin administration. Recent studies in continuous ambulatory peritoneal dialysis patients found that 65% of the insulin injected into the bag was retained, indicating some adsorption to the surface of the bags and tubing. Of the remaining insulin, an average of 37% was absorbed across the peritoneal membrane (or only 13% of the amount originally injected into the bag), with the percentage absorbed proportional to the length of dwell time. Mean absorption of insulin was 21, 28, and 46% at 2, 4, and 8 hours, respectively. Despite the fact that in these patients the administered dose of insulin was 2.5 times greater than the prior dose of insulin, the amount absorbed corresponds to only 46% of the previous subcutaneous dose before continuous ambulatory peritoneal dialysis. This suggests that better utilization of insulin and glucose is obtained with the intraperitoneal route and clearly demonstrates that patients can be well managed without the use of additional exogenous insulin.

To develop a schedule of intraperitoneal insulin for continuous ambulatory peritoneal dialysis patients, it is suggested that the prior insulin dose be divided into four exchanges, allowing more for the morning exchange and less at night to avoid noctural hypoglycemia. A typical 24-hour pattern might be 1/3, 1/4, 1/4, and 1/6. For example, a patient who required 35 U NPH insulin and 10 U regular insulin prior to continuous ambulatory peritoneal dialysis, or 45 U total, could be started on the following regimen:

8 AM exchange: 15 U
12 PM exchange: 11 U
5 PM exchange: 11 U
11 PM exchange: 8 U

The amount of insulin would then be adjusted upward according to the blood glucose levels obtained during the midpoint of each exchange. It is desirable to have chronic peritoneal dialysis patients monitor their own blood glucose levels using chemical strip reagents and an Autolet finger stick device. This permits a permanent record of glucose control and allows more intelligent adjustment of insulin dosage.

Potassium. Commercial dialysate does not contain potassium, since it is not customarily used in chronic peritoneal dialysis to allow for greater removal of ingested potassium in these patients.

However, during acute peritoneal dialysis, especially with long periods of continuous cycling (24–48 hours), potassium is usually added to the dialysate at a concentration of 3–4 mEq/L or at the serum level one wishes to achieve at the end of the dialysis. When hyperkalemia is present at the start of acute peritoneal dialysis, it is customary to use potassium-free dialysate for the initial exchanges, and then to add potassium to the dialysate as the serum potassium reaches the normal range.

Bicarbonate. Sodium bicarbonate may be added to dialysate to raise pH in those patients in whom the standard pH of 5.5 causes abdominal discomfort on inflow. Empirically, the addition of 10 ml of 7.5% NaHCO$_3$ has been found to be effective in most patients. This quantity of NaHCO$_3$ added to a 2-L bag of dialysate will raise the pH sufficiently to remove discomfort, but will not result in precipitation of calcium in the container.

Antibiotics. Antibiotics are frequently added to dialysate for treatment of peritonitis. This route of administration is extremely useful, since it achieves therapeutic concentrations of drug quickly at the site of the infection, is easier than parenteral administration in many patients, and allows treatment of infection on an outpatient basis. The most frequently used antibiotics are listed in Table 4-6, along with the currently recommended loading and maintenance doses. This list is a composite of recommended dosage from several major centers;

Table 4-6. Concentrations of Additives to Peritoneal Dialysate

Additive	Loading	Maintenance (mg/L)
Antibiotics		
Ampicillin	500 mg/L	50
Amikacin	5 mg/kg/bag	50
Cloxacillin	1000 mg/L	100
Cephalothin	500 mg/L	50–250
Gentamicin	1.7 mg/kg/bag	5–8
Methicillin	1000 mg/L	100
Sulfamethoxazole/trimethoprim	400/80 mg/L	25/5
Ticarcillin	1000 mg/L	100
Tobramycin	1.7 mg/kg/bag	5–8
Vancomycin	1000 mg IV	25
5-Fluorocytosine	—	100
Amphotericin	—	5
Heparin	1000 U/bag	

generally there is good agreement, except cephalothin, for which there is some variation in maintenance dosage.

Often only a single drug is used to treat peritonitis. However, some facilities prefer to start therapy with two antibiotics, pending culture results. It is important to be certain that there are no incompatibilities before drugs are combined. A known incompatibility between penicillin and aminoglycosides—the aminoglycoside is inactivated—makes this combination ineffective. An incompatibility between heparin and aminoglycosides has been suggested because of a visible formation of precipitate in the container. Studies of in vivo antibiotic effectiveness with the combination, however, indicate that the antibiotic does not lose its efficacy; heparin activity is also retained, although it has been recommended that these additives be injected separately in a dilute solution. Loss of antibiotic efficacy secondary to decomposition on standing in an electrolyte dextrose solution is not a problem with continuous ambulatory peritoneal dialysis or manual peritoneal dialysis where additives are placed in solution just prior to administration. But during automated dialysis using concentrate or with reverse osmosis cyclers where dialysate is hung for 8 hours of dialysis, some loss of activity may occur with the use of penicillin, cephalothin, gentamicin, and nafcillin.

Most antibiotics are well tolerated intraperitoneally; an exception may be amphotericin, which has been reported to cause abdominal pain at recommended dosage.

CHRONIC PERITONEAL DIALYSIS

Indications for Choice of the Chronic Peritoneal Dialysis Modality.

The choice of chronic peritoneal dialysis (CPD) is now very attractive for patients as well as dialysis professionals because, by virtue of its varied techniques, it offers a flexible approach to treatment of end-stage renal disease. The availability of automated intermittent peritoneal dialysis, continuous ambulatory peritoneal dialysis, and continuous cycling peritoneal dialysis make this form of dialysis adaptable to the medical needs and lifestyles of a wide range of patients. Of the numerous parameters that must be considered in selecting a dialysis modality, perhaps the most important are medical factors, age, and psychosocial criteria, including patient and physician preferences. Because of current economic pressures, the alternative of chronic peritoneal dialysis, which is basically a home or self-care modality, must be considered seriously as a means of controlling costs and as a potentially more attractive fiscal program for dialysis providers.

Medical criteria for chronic peritoneal dialysis initially singled out patients who were judged poor candidates for hemodialysis, such as patients with diabetes mellitus, unstable or severe cardiovascular disease, and/or limited vascular access sites. Today these indications are still valid, but, in addition, many physicians offer patients a choice of chronic peritoneal dialysis as part of a broad policy to utilize all modalities for therapy of renal failure. The patient should be actively included in the selection and planning process. There are currently few firmly established medical indications for chronic peritoneal dialysis, but, in addition to those mentioned above, several medical situations would favor a choice of peritoneal dialysis; these are summarized in Table 4-7.

Lack of vascular access sites or severe difficulty in maintaining patent vascular access is probably the most compelling indication for chronic peritoneal dialysis. This complication is not uncommon in patients with diabetes mellitus and older individuals with severe vascular disease; it also occurs in younger patients and in those with prior intravenous drug abuse.

Patients with diabetes mellitus have been frequently selected for chronic peritoneal dialysis because of their generally poor prognosis on hemodialysis and the risk of systemic anticoagulation. It has been argued that chronic peritoneal dialysis is better for diabetic patients with retinopathy, since it does not require systemic heparinization and is associated with a lower incidence of dialysis related hypotension, which perhaps protects the patient from retinal hemorrhage and other ocular complications. However, experience has not clearly established that diabetics on chronic peritoneal dialysis are less prone to pro-

Table 4-7. Situations in Which Peritoneal Dialysis May Be Preferable to Hemodialysis

Medical
   Lack of vascular access
   Diabetes mellitus
   Coronary artery disease
   Age
      Small children
      Older adults
   Patients unwilling to accept blood transfusions
   Severe anemia
   Severe hemodialysis-related symptoms or disequilibrium
Social
   Residence remote from dialysis center
   Self-dialysis for patients who live alone or have no home helper
   Patients who wish to travel frequently

gressive retinopathy. In contrast to the earlier experience with therapy in diabetic patients, recent studies indicate that progressive retinopathy, resulting in blindness, is now less common, perhaps due to better management of hypertension, the metabolic control of diabetes, and the widespread use of photocoagulation therapy. Perhaps the best indication for chronic peritoneal dialysis in diabetics, however, is the evidence that significantly better control of blood glucose concentration can be achieved with the intraperitoneal administration of insulin, and with continuous ambulatory peritoneal dialysis, eliminating the need for subcutaneous insulin. Despite the frequent requirement for larger doses of insulin because of dialysate dextrose, it is possible to maintain blood glucose in the normal range without the sharp fluctuations seen in patients on one or two daily subcutaneous doses of insulin.

Patients with clinically significant coronary artery disease and angina frequently have better progress on chronic peritoneal dialysis because it avoids the rapid fluctuations in fluid and electrolyte concentrations that occur with intermittent hemodialysis. In addition, as a result of continuous ultrafiltration associated with continuous ambulatory peritoneal dialysis, fluid accumulation does not occur, resulting in less hypertension and fewer demands on cardiac performance. Higher hemoglobin levels are seen in many CAPD patients without the need for transfusion, which is beneficial in patients with significant angina. Finally, although no data from controlled studies are available, clinical experience suggests that significant arrhythmias and the need for cardiac drug therapy may be reduced in patients on chronic peritoneal dialysis.

Chronic peritoneal dialysis has been shown to be better tolerated and technically easier in infants and small children. Similarly, many elderly patients, because of multiple associated medical problems, often are intolerant of hemodialysis, but progress well on either intermittent or continuous peritoneal dialysis. In a small percentage of patients of any age, hemodialysis symptoms associated with hypotension and disequilibrium are so severe that chronic peritoneal dialysis may result in a substantial reduction in symptoms and thus may promote better rehabilitation of the patient.

Anemia is often less severe in patients on chronic peritoneal dialysis, in part due to the avoidance of blood loss associated with hemodialysis, but perhaps also due to better removal of uremic toxins. For this reasons, peritoneal dialysis may be advantageous for those patients who refuse blood transfusions because of religious beliefs, and for those who sustain severe asymptomatic anemia on hemodialysis. Patients may also choose chronic peritoneal dialysis for a variety of social reasons. Patients who are self-reliant and prefer not to come to the hospital or dialysis facility three times a week often choose peritoneal dialysis as the least troublesome mode of home therapy. This is particularly appropriate for patients who live alone or have no suitable home helper but wish to do home dialysis. Transportation to a dialysis facility, especially if the patient lives in a rural area may be a significant motivating factor for home care and peritoneal dialysis. Those patients who desire the freedom or flexibility to vary daily schedules or to travel frequently because of business are probably best served by continuous ambulatory peritoneal dialysis therapy, which allows maximum flexibility of scheduling.

Considerations for the Selection of the Chronic Peritoneal Dialysis Modality

Patients who select chronic peritoneal dialysis as a therapeutic modality for end-stage renal disease have a choice of three scheduling options: continuous ambulatory peritoneal dialysis, (CAPD), continuous cycling peritoneal dialysis (CCPD), and intermittent peritoneal dialysis (IPD). The selection of technique for an individual patient is usually based on the following considerations.

Time and Scheduling Demands. Continuous ambulatory peritoneal dialysis requires the least amount of time when evaluated on a weekly basis, as shown in Table 4-8. However, it must be performed every day, throughout the day, and therefore may be more difficult for patients who work or may be inconvenient for those who require assisted CAPD (children, the blind, the disabled). The steady, daily demands of CAPD also cause some patients to complain of "dialysis fatigue," or the desire to have a period of time without constant dialysis.

Unlike CAPD, where dialysis and regular activity occur simultaneously, both continuous cycling peritoneal dialysis and intermittent peritoneal dialysis require dedicated time for actual dialysis because of the use of the cycler, though when done at night, it should not detract from daytime activities. In addition to dialysis time, the use of the cycler or reverse osmosis machine requires time for setting up and dismantling the equipment, which adds significantly to time expenditure for the total effort on a weekly basis.

Assistance. Patients who require assistance with their dialysis are usually most efficiently managed with intermittent peritoneal dialysis or continuous cycling peritoneal dialysis; these techniques allow greater freedom to the helpers in organizing their time and effort than is possible with CAPD. For example, the service of a helper is necessary only once or twice a day to perform exchanges with IPD or CCPD, as opposed to four times a day with CAPD. Also, helpers who are employed during the day, or have other constraints, can conveniently perform the dialysis at night.

Table 4-8. Chronic Peritoneal Dialysis Schedules

	Procedures: Setup, Bag Exchange (Hours/Day)	Time on Machine		Total Time (Hours/Week)
		Hours/Day	Hours/Week	
CAPD	2–3 (30–45 minutes per exchange)	0	0	21
CCPD	1–1.5	8–9	56	63
IPD	2 (3–4 times per week)	8–12 hours 3–4 times per week	30–40	36–46

CAPD, continuous ambulatory peritoneal dialysis; CCPD, continuous cycling peritoneal dialysis; IPD, intermittent peritoneal dialysis.

Peritonitis. Many patients who are especially disposed to peritonitis on continuous ambulatory peritoneal dialysis have been transferred to continuous cycling peritoneal dialysis or intermittent peritoneal dialysis with better results. The incidence of peritonitis is lower with IPD and CCPD, probably because the peritoneal dialysis catheter is opened less frequently. This consideration currently makes these modes of therapy more attractive for those patients who may be at increased risk of peritonitis at the outset (those who have visual impairment, physical weakness, suboptimal physical hygiene, and other disabilities).

Equipment. Many patients are attracted to continuous ambulatory peritoneal dialysis because it does not require the presence of a machine or specialized equipment, which is of particular advantage when living space is very limited. Cyclers and, to an even greater extent, reverse osmosis machines require space for storage and operation, and the latter requires a plumbing connection for tap water.

Complications of Chronic Peritoneal Dialysis Therapy

The most aggressive complication of chronic peritoneal dialysis is peritonitis, which becomes the limiting factor in the success of this technique for many patients, especially those on continuous ambulatory peritoneal dialysis. However, there are other potential problems of chronic peritoneal dialysis, which can be classified as catheter-related, mechanical, and medical. These complications are listed in Table 4-9 and are discussed in the following sections.

Peritonitis Peritonitis accounts for nearly half of the treatment failures with continuous ambulatory peritoneal dialysis and has been implicated as a factor in 25% of the deaths of patients managed by this modality. Consequently, research and development programs throughout the dialysis industry are unified in distinguishing peritonitis as the focal point in the ongoing pursuit of a technological design that will drastically reduce the incidence of this pathology.

Diagnosis. The diagnostic features of peritonitis in continuous ambulatory peritoneal dialysis are listed in Table 4-10. The diagnosis of peritonitis is usually made by observation of cloudy dialysate outflow, which contains an increased number of leukocytes (>100/ml in CAPD and >500/ml in IPD), with a predominance of polymorphonuclear forms (>50%). Abdominal pain and other symptoms, while often present, may be absent in the early stages of infection. Gram stains of peritoneal fluid will often reveal organisms in patients with fungal and more severe bacterial infections, but these are positive only about 50% of the time in the more typical case of gram-positive infection. Cultures are almost always positive if the techniques used enable identification of low numbers of organisms in dialysate solution. In most centers with experience in CAPD, so-called "culture-negative" peritonitis is extremely uncommon.

Table 4-9. Complications of Chronic Peritoneal Dialysis

Peritonitis
Catheter-related
  Infection
      Exit site
      Tunnel
  Cuff extrusion
  Malposition
  Pain
  Bleeding
  Catheter obstruction
  Visceral perforation
Mechanical
  Dialysate leaks
      Pericatheter
      Pleural
      Abdominal wall, genitalia
      Vaginal
  Hernias
      Incisional
      Ventral
      Periumbilical
      Catheter tract
      Inguinal
  Back pain
Medical
  Hypotension
      Peripheral vascular insufficiency
  Nutritional
      Hypoalbuminemia
      Obesity
      Hyperlipidemia
  Peritoneal dialysate eosinophilia
  Loss of peritoneal ultrafiltration or transport capacity

Incidence. The frequency of the various pathogens causing peritonitis is listed in Table 4-11. From 65 to 75% of all infection is caused by gram-positive bacteria, with *Staphylococcus epidermidis* or coagulase-negative *Staphylococci* being the most frequent offenders. Gram-negative infection occurs in about 25–30% of cases. Fungal and mycobacterial peritonitis accounts for ≤5% of cases and may be associated with treatment of previous bacterial infections or prolonged use of antibiotics for recurrent peritonitis.

The diagnosis of peritonitis caused by multiple organisms, especially with mixed aerobic and anaerobic forms, is almost always diagnostic of bowel perforation, with or without abscess formation. Fecal peritonitis is a very serious

Table 4-10. Diagnostic Features of Peritonitis in CAPD

Cloudy outflow
Peritoneal fluid white blood cells >100/ml with >50%
    polymorphonuclear leukocytes
Gram stain positive for organism ~50% of time
Culture positive in 95% of cases
Abdominal pain and bowel symptoms (mild to moderate severity) in
    about 75% of cases

Table 4-11. Organisms Causing Peritonitis and Frequency of Occurrence

Gram-positive pathogens: 65–75%
Staphylococcus epidermidis
Staphylococcus aureus
Streptococcus species
Gram-negative pathogens: 25–30%
Enterobacteriaceae
Proteus species
Escherichia coli
Klebsiella species
Enterobacter cloacae
Acinetobacter species
Pseudomonas species
Other pathogens: ≤5%
Candida albicans
Nocardia asteroides
Aspergillus species
Fusarium species
Mycobacterium tuberculosis
Actinomyces species
Pityrosporum ovale
Nontuberculous mycobacteria

complication, which carries a high rate of morbidity and mortality. Analysis of this problem by investigators in Toronto revealed that it was a major cause of continuous ambulatory peritoneal dialysis failure secondary to peritonitis and had a 22% mortality. Fecal peritonitis was associated with diverticulosis or diverticulitis in 78% of the cases, which has raised the issue of whether diverticulosis should be regarded as a relative contraindication to chronic peritoneal dialysis therapy. Despite the severity of this complication, one third of patients with fecal peritonitis were successfully treated without catheter removal and returned to CAPD therapy.

The frequency of peritonitis in patient populations on various forms of chronic peritoneal dialysis has been intensely scrutinized in an effort to develop strategies for better treatment and prevention. Incidence rates have significantly changed as peritoneal dialysis technology has evolved, and the general trend reflects a steady decrease in peritonitis with respect to changes in technique. In the United States, when CAPD was initially performed with solution in glass bottles, infection rates were very high, averaging one episode every 2–3 months of patient time on dialysis. With the introduction of dialysate in plastic bags and improved connection techniques, the results are much better, with many centers now reporting a peritonitis incidence of one episode every 12–18 patient months. With the newer devices designed to prevent accidental spike contamination, incidence rates should decline even further. Not all patients will sustain peritonitis; several reports indicate that 40–50% of patients can remain free of infection for long periods of time (1–2 years). The risk of peritonitis is probably greater in the first 6 months when the technique is still new to the patient. Canadian data show a diminished risk of peritonitis for new patients, ~25% in 1981, compared with ~50% in 1978 when the technique was less mature. Analysis of failure of patients on CAPD secondary to peritonitis indicates two patterns of infection: (1) frequent, recurrent episodes, and (2) sporadic episodes that are very severe or complex, such as fecal peritonitis or fungal infection. The incidence of technique failure rates from peritonitis has remained stable at 6–7% of patients in the Toronto program from 1978 to 1982, suggesting that this outcome may be dependent on nontechnical factors. Some programs have arbitrarily removed patients from CAPD when they experience more than three infections per year or a predetermined excessive rate of infection, while others allow patients to continue as long as peritoneal dialysis remains effective and clinical status is satisfactory. The potential adverse effects of recurrent peritonitis include fibrosis and loculation of the peritoneal cavity, which may result in mechanical interference with dialysis as well as in thickening and sclerosis of the peritoneal membrane, in turn resulting in loss of transport formation, as described below. Also, of course, each episode of peritonitis places the patient at potential risk of sepsis, abscess formation, and possible mortality. At the present time, there are few generally accepted criteria for stopping peritoneal dialysis therapy secondary to peritonitis, but many centers would include (1) fecal peritonitis secondary to diverticulosis, (2) mycobacterial peritonitis, and (3) severe fungal peritonitis, which often can result in peritoneal fibrosis.

Treatment. The management of peritonitis in chronic peritoneal dialysis includes the following therapeutic maneuvers: (1) lavage, (2) antibiotic treatment, and (3) catheter removal. Protocols for treatment of peritonitis vary widely; a sample treatment protocol used at this center is summarized in Table 4-12. While most centers teach all patients how to recognize and initiate therapy for peritonitis, it is critically important that patients notify the center as soon as symptoms are noticed and bring samples of dialysate to the laboratory for cell count and culture. Unless the patient lives remote from the center, it is usually recommended that patients be seen and evaluated prior to initiation of antibiotic treatment for peritonitis.

Lavage. Continuous peritoneal dialysis provides mechanical lavage of the peritoneal cavity with dialysate, which may aid in the treatment of peritonitis by increasing removal of bacteria and cellular exudate. It may also help to maintain

Table 4-12. Protocol for Treatment of Peritonitis in CAPD Patients

Organism	Clinical Status of Patient	Antibiotics	Route	Setting
1. No organisms or gram positive organisms	Mild symptoms	Cephalosporin or vancomycin	IP and PO IV (Loading) then IP	Home
2. Gram negative organisms	Mild symptoms; afebrile	Tobramycin	IV (Loading) then IP	Home
	Severe symptoms	Tobramycin	IV and IP	Hospital;? Lavage
3. Fungal organisms	Variable	Amphotericin	IP	Hospital; continuous lavage
4. Mixed organisms	Moderate to severe	Cefoxitin	IV and IP	Hospital; lavage and remove catheter

IP, intraperitoneal; PO, oral; IV, intravenous.

patency of the peritoneal catheter by removal of fibrin that rapidly forms in the presence of peritonitis. Lavage frequently mitigates abdominal pain in patients who present with acute peritonitis. The possible negative consequences of this therapy include the deleterious effects of low dialysate pH and hyperosmolality on leukocyte function, an increased loss of protein secondary to increased vascular permeability associated with inflammation, and the need for hospitalization to perform continuous peritoneal dialysis. For patients on intermittent peritoneal dialysis, lavage is usually performed for 24 hours or until the dialysate has cleared; then the patient may return to the usual dialysis schedule and continue oral as well as intraperitoneal antibiotic therapy. Continuous lavage was frequently employed in patients receiving continuous ambulatory peritoneal dialysis during the early years of the technique. However, because many patients can detect infection early and have minimal or no symptoms, they are able to continue a regular CAPD regimen and thus achieve successful treatment of peritonitis in the outpatient setting. As an alternative to continuous lavage, some centers instruct patients to perform several rapid CAPD exchanges (in and out) when peritonitis is diagnosed, to flush out the peritoneal cavity as noted above and to reduce abdominal pain if present. Most programs now treat peritonitis in CAPD patients by initial continuation of the outpatient regimen and reserve hospital admission and continuous lavage for those patients who present with any of the following:

1. Infection has not responded to appropriate therapy after 24–48 hours of outpatient treatment.

2. Unusually severe peritonitis and/or infection with unusual organisms, including fungal peritonitis.

3. Catheter removal is anticipated, prior to which continuous dialysis may be performed for 24–48 hours to treat the acute infection and ensure that the patient is well dialyzed before surgery.

Antibiotic therapy. Antibiotics may be administered for treatment of peritonitis by the intraperitoneal route, systemically, or by a combination of these methods. The choice of route of administration has resulted in wide variations from facility to facility; currently, no universally accepted treatment regimen has been developed. The use of intraperitoneal administration either initially or exclusively has become the major route of treatment, however, because the medical characteristics of continuous ambulatory peritoneal dialysis-related peritonitis, patient convenience, and economic factors all favor this approach. Peritonitis in patients on chronic peritoneal dialysis is often mild and is usually confined to the peritoneal space; therefore intraperitoneal antibiotic administration makes sense and is usually effective. It is easy to instruct patients to add antibiotics to the dialysate bags, and intraperitoneal administration is much simpler and more cost-effective than frequent trips to the outpatient center or hospitalization.

Many clinicians choose to use intraperitoneal antibiotics combined with systemic administration, especially during the initial 4–5 days of infection. Following clearing of the peritoneal fluid, intraperitoneal antibiotics may then be discontinued and the course of treatment completed with systemic drug therapy.

The choice of antibiotics for initial treatment of peritonitis is guided by the Gram stain if positive, by the clinical severity of infections, and by the observed incidence of bacterial organisms in this group of patients (Table 4-12). Because gram-positive organisms are the most frequent cause of peritonitis, initial treatment with a cephalosporin or vancomycin is most commonly employed in patients with typical symptoms and no evidence of gram-negative or unusual infection. Alternatively, some centers prefer to cover patients initially for gram-negative infection with a combination of cephalosporin and aminoglycoside, and then stop one drug when culture results and patient response are established. Currently, the broad-spectrum, third-generation cephalosporins are being evaluated as possible agents that would provide wider coverage with a single antibiotic. A loading dose, followed by a maintenance antibiotic for 10 days, is commonly employed, with the usual doses as summarized in Table 4-6.

Treatment of mycobacterial and fungal peritonitis poses additional challenges to antibiotic therapy. *Mycobacterium tuberculosis* as well as nontuberculous mycobacteria have been documented to cause peritonitis in patients on CAPD and intermittent peritoneal dialysis. The treatment of *M. tuberculosis* peritonitis includes catheter removal and standard systemic antituberculosis therapy. However, the treatment of nontuberculous mycobacterial infection has been difficult and, in several reported instances, unsuccessful, despite therapy with appropriate antibiotics at adequate levels.

Treatment of fungal peritonitis in chronic peritoneal dialysis patients remains controversial with respect to the issues of catheter removal and antifungal therapy. Both intraperitoneal and systemic antibiotics have been advocated, each with reported success. The presence of a foreign body (catheter), which can be colonized by fungal organisms, and the tendency for *Candida,* a common fungal agent, to form thick secretions, which may cause bowel adhesions and mechanical loculation of peritoneal space, make sterilization of the peritoneal cavity a significant challenge with this category of infection. While many *Candida* species are sensitive to both amphotericin and 5-fluorocytosine, many clinicians believe that amphotericin is the drug of choice for initial therapy, and that it should be given both systemically and intraperitoneally. The optimal dose of intraperitoneal amphotericin is not established; the dosage of 5 mg/L listed in Table 4-6 may cause abdominal irritation in some patients, thus necessitating a reduction to 3 mg/L. There are currently no guidelines for initiation of combined therapy with 5-fluorocytosine. However, the significant bone marrow toxicity that can occur with the accumulation of this drug would favor cautious use.

Catheter removal. In some cases of peritonitis, despite prompt recognition and appropriate antibiotic therapy, the infection fails to improve and necessitates the final therapeutic maneuver available, that of catheter removal. Since there are a limited number of sites for placement of catheters, and since many patients are dependent on peritoneal dialysis for treatment of renal failure, the removal of the catheter is not undertaken lightly. However, in some circumstances, catheter removal can be life-saving and frequently results in rapid improvement in peritonitis; this maneuver, must be performed when the appropriate circumstances are present and clinical judgment dictates it is necessary.

The primary indications for catheter removal are listed in Table 4-13. Infection occurring between the two catheter cuffs may form an abscess or, if the external cuff is not sealed, a chronically infected sinus tract. These infections may respond initially to antibiotic therapy but usually relapse when therapy is discontinued; they can be eradicated only by removal of the catheter. Tunnel abcesses can be difficult to detect and will occasionally form a sinus tract to the skin, which will not heal until the catheter is removed.

The most urgent situation requiring catheter removal is severe peritonitis that fails to respond to antibiotic therapy, especially when fecal peritonitis with bowel perforation is present. These patients are frequently very ill with sepsis and require emergent catheter removal which may be life-saving. A few patients have severe peritonitis secondary to the commonly encountered bacterial agents that responds very slowly and smolders for days despite adequate doses of appropriate antimicrobials, even when continuous peritoneal dialysis lavage is administered. *Staphylococcus aureus* and some gram-negative infections are the chief perpetrators in these situations, but the reason for poor resolution of infection is usually not apparent, although intraperitoneal abscess formation or catheter colonization are often suspected. The timing for catheter removal must be individualized, but if after 2–3 days of continuous ambulatory peritoneal dialysis and 48 hours of continuous lavage with antibiotics there is still active peritonitis with cloudy fluid and positive dialysate cultures, then catheter removal may be necessary to cure the infection. Removal should be performed sooner if the patient's clinical status deteriorates rapidly with signs of sepsis.

For the resolution of most cases of mycobacterial peritonitis, and fungal infection that does not respond to therapy, catheter removal is obligatory.

Catheter-Related Complications

Infection. In addition to peritonitis, two distinct types of infection can occur in patients on chronic peritoneal dialysis, both of which are catheter-related: exit site infection and tunnel abscess.

Exit site infection. Localized infection can occur with consequent inflammation characterized by induration and drainage around the catheter exit site. These infections may be associated with poor care of the exit site (failure to take daily showers or to remove crusting that occurs around the catheter), with trauma or traction on the catheter, and possibly with chemical irritation secondary to overuse of topical antimicrobials or other cleansing agents. Failure to change

Table 4-13. Indications for Catheter Removal

Tunnel infection
Peritonitis that fails to respond to appropriate antibiotic therapy
Mycobacterial peritonitis
Fungal peritonitis that fails to respond to appropriate antifungal therapy
Fecal peritonitis

dressing and tape regularly may also predispose to these infections. Exit site infections are usually caused by staphylococci and respond well to good skin care and oral antibiotics such as cloxacillin or dicloxacillin. The major sequelae include accidental contamination during bag exchange or dialysis, resulting in peritonitis or progression to tunnel infection. The frequency of exit site infections has not been shown to be influenced by the use of occlusive dressing instead of leaving the catheter open. However, securing the catheter to avoid excessive movement, especially in patients who are obese or physically active, is recommended. The catheter exit site should not be located under the belt line or tight clothing as this may cause significant irritation.

Tunnel abscess. Tunnel abscess is a closed space infection occurring between the two Dacron catheter cuffs, typically presenting with tenderness, erythema, and induration along the catheter tract. If unrecognized, a sinus tract to the skin over the catheter may develop, or it may drain through the exit site if the external cuff is not tightly sealed. Many of these infections may be clinically inapparent and present as recurrent episodes of peritonitis with the same organism. Recently, the use of indium-111 labeled leukocyte scanning has been described as an effective technique to detect localized collections of leukocytes along the catheter tract. Such scans have been found to be uniformly negative in patients without tunnel infection, including patients with active peritonitis. The management of tunnel infection includes antibiotic treatment, followed by catheter removal; a new catheter can be placed in a distant site after an interval of several days to 2 weeks depending on the degree of inflammation and cellulitis surrounding the old tunnel.

Catheter cuff extrusion. With the use of double-cuffed peritoneal dialysis catheters, it is not uncommon for the distal cuff to be gradually extruded through the catheter exit site. This extrusion is often in consequence of positioning the distal cuff too superficially or of a tunnel that is too short. Ideally, the distal cuff should be positioned at least 2 cm beneath the skin. Distal cuff erosion is more frequent in individuals who are thin and lack adequate subcutaneous fat tissue to anchor the cuff. When the cuff has been completely externalized, it may be removed or secured to prevent retraction and the catheter left in place, provided infection does not develop around the catheter or peritonitis does not recur. Development of such infection suggests patency of the catheter tract down to the peritoneum. Patients should be advised not to attempt reinsertion of the cuff, since this will usually result in tunnel infection.

Catheter malposition. A major management problem with some peritoneal catheters is migration of the catheter out of the pelvis to another position, usually pointing laterally or cephalad in the peritoneal cavity. The diagnosis of catheter migration can be made radiographically with a flat plate of the abdomen, since most catheters are now impregnated with a radiopaque stripe. While some catheters continue to function well under these circumstances, many do not and the patient presents with outflow drainage problems and occasionally pain if the catheter tip is irritating other abdominal structures. The cause of this shift in catheter position is usually not evident but may include normal bowel motility, with traction on the catheter or entanglement in omentum. A variety of maneuvers have been advocated for repositioning the catheter, which should be attempted only if mechanical function is a problem. Such maneuvers include the following:

1. Laxatives should be administered to stimulate bowel motility and, it is hoped, to induce the return of the catheter to a more dependent portion of the peritoneal cavity, thereby enhancing its function. This procedure is not often rewarding, but it is the most benign therapy and should be attempted before more invasive maneuvers are considered.

2. A trocar or a specialized instrument can be placed through the catheter, under radiographic guidance, in an attempt to reposition the catheter in the pelvis. Physicians experienced with this technique report some success.

3. In many cases, an improperly positioned catheter will require surgical replacement. A technique for limited surgical replacement of the distal segment of the catheter only, leaving the proximal tunnel segment in place, was described many years ago by Tenckhoff and would seem to offer some advantages over total catheter removal and replacement.

Well-functioning catheters should be left alone even when aberrantly positioned.

Pain. Pain during peritoneal dialysis can result from a variety of causes, which are summarized in Table 4-14. The chronic peritoneal catheter may cause pain under the following circumstances.

Peritoneal irritation. Frequently when catheters are newly placed, the patients will experience pain in the perineum, rectum, or genitalia, which is probably due to irritation by the catheter tip. Such pain is usually self limited and disappears after several days to a week. In an occasional patient, this pain persists in a continuous fashion, but more often it is intensified when the peritoneal cavity is drained of fluid. In such cases, the catheter may be too long for the patient, causing continuous irritation by pressing against pelvic structures. While this symptom is usually benign, there are reports of late development of transvisceral erosion, necessitating at least a temporary interruption of chronic peritoneal dialysis and catheter removal. In at least one patient in our experience, a catheter was replaced for the amelioration of chronic pain, with good results. Catheters are available in various lengths to meet the individual size requirements of patients, and a catheter with a curled tip would seem to be potentially less irritating than the straight-tipped type.

Inflow of dialysate. Pain associated with inflow of dialysate occurs in some patients in consequence of peritoneal irritation caused by the low pH of the fluid. This is often a limited phenomenon in new patients, but it may persist and require the addition of sodium bicarbonate to the dialysate.

Table 4-14. Diagnosis of Peritoneal Dialysis-Related and Peritoneal Dialysis Catheter-Related Pain

Symptom	Possible Cause	Treatment
Pain on inflow of dialysate	Low dialysate pH	Add HCO_3^- to dialysate
	Catheter tip irritation	Observation
Pain during dwell	Overdistention of abdomen	Longer drain time Decrease cycle volume in small patients
	Low dialysate pH	Add HCO_3^- to dialysate
Pain following dialysis	Peritonitis	Antibiotics, lavage
	Free abdominal air	None Recumbent position
Constant pain Diffuse	Peritonitis	Antibiotics, lavage
	Other abdominal pathology	Diagnosis and appropriate therapy
Pelvic area	Perineal, rectal, bladder irritation by catheter tip	Observation; consider catheter replacement if present longer than 6–8 weeks
Shoulder pain	Air under diaphragm	None Recumbent position

Bleeding. Spontaneous bleeding into the peritoneal fluid occurs in some patients, usually lasting for a few exchanges and resolving without intervention. This self-limited appearance of bloody dialysate is of unknown cause in most situations, but some patients report prior accidental catheter irritation or traction on the catheter, or unusual physical activity. Rarely, during menstruation, women will have small quantities of blood in the dialysate. However, blood in the dialysate has been equally frequent in both sexes in our patient population. Since the presentation is a cloudy outflow, even though it has a pigmented appearance and does not look like peritonitis, a peritoneal fluid cell count and differential should be obtained to exclude peritonitis with inflammation as the cause.

Catheter obstruction. Mechanical dysfunction of the peritoneal catheter not due to malposition is most frequently a one-way outflow obstruction due to partial occlusion of the catheter by fibrin, omental trapping in the catheter drainage holes, or encasement of the distal catheter with a fibrous sheath. Fibrin occurs commonly in chronic peritoneal dialysis, especially during peritonitis, but also without obvious reason in some patients. Patients who have recurrent peritonitis, particularly when infection is not promptly diagnosed and treated, may develop gradual fibrosis around the catheter, which limits mechanical exchange of dialysate. Similarly, the omentum will tend to wrap around the catheter during inflammation and become entrapped in the catheter openings. Fibrin obstruction of the catheter can often be cleared with vigorous flushing of the catheter and the institution of heparin therapy, 1000 U/bag. Obstruction of the lumen by omentum or fibrous encasement will usually require catheter replacement.

Visceral perforation. There are several reports of delayed perforation of the colon by erosion of the chronic catheter. These complications were preceded by peritonitis, suggesting that inflammation of the bowel wall may have been a predisposing factor. There exists a case report of the development of a perito-neovaginal fistula, 18 months after insertion of a Tenckhoff catheter.

Mechanical Complications. Dialysate leaks. Unfortunately, dialysate does not always remain in the peritoneal cavity where it belongs. The most frequent site of fluid leakage is around the dialysis catheter, usually within 1 to 2 weeks of catheter placement, before the tunnel has become tightly sealed. Occasionally, leakage will occur along the catheter tract months after the catheter is placed, suggesting either delayed adherence of the catheter cuffs or traumatic injury to the catheter, resulting in patency around the cuffs. Pericatheter dialysate leaks, frequently associated with overdistention of the peritoneal cavity with fluid, are the major reason for the use of small exchange volumes for several days to a week after catheter placement. Similarly, the use of hypertonic dialysate should be minimized with new catheters to reduce the volume of ultrafiltrate. The management of pericatheter leak, like other forms of dialysate leak described below, includes discontinuation of peritoneal dialysis for several days to several weeks, followed by cautious reinstitution of dialysis with smaller volumes. This maneuver, presumably by decreasing pressure on the leak site for a period of time, will often seal the tract and allow dialysis to be resumed successfully.

There are now many case reports of dialysate leaks into the pleural space, often resulting in massive hydrothorax, which is most often right-sided. Frequent presenting symptoms include shortness of breath associated with decreased dialysate outflow volume. Onset of symptoms is usually abrupt, appearing during the first few days of peritoneal dialysis, although there are reported cases of late occurrence after initiation of chronic peritoneal dialysis. The administration of greater amounts of hypertonic dialysate exacerbates abdominal distention secondary to ultrafiltration, which suggests that new pleural-peritoneal communications result from increased intraabdominal pressure. That dialysate is the source of the pleural fluid has been documented by utilizing methylene blue, radionuclide imaging as well as chemical analysis. When sudden, massive hydrothorax occurs in a patient on chronic peritoneal dialysis, there is usually little doubt that the origin is peritoneal fluid. The use of intraperitoneal methylene blue has been reported to cause peritoneal irritation in several patients and thus perhaps should be avoided as a diagnostic agent.

There are several approaches to the treatment of dialysate leaks:

1. Discontinue peritoneal dialysis and transfer the patient to hemodialysis on a permanent basis.

2. Temporarily discontinue peritoneal dialysis, for 2–4 weeks, then cautiously resume peritoneal dialysis. This has been successful with several patients in our experience, especially with late onset.

3. Use therapeutic interventions to seal the leak with either pleural talc insufflation (talcage) or adhesion pleurodesis. These procedures are not without risk or morbidity; they should probably be undertaken only in those patients who have compelling reasons for continuing peritoneal dialysis and for whom waiting 2–4 weeks does not result in spontaneous healing.

4. In those cases where the pleural fluid collection is relatively small, it may be clinically acceptable to follow the patient on continued peritoneal dialysis, avoiding hypertonic dialysate and abdominal distention, in the hope that the leak may gradually resolve.

Dialysate can also leak into the scrotum and genitalia of patients with inguinal hernias or patent processus vaginalis. This type of leak usually requires hernia repair to prevent recurrent leakage of dialysate.

In a few patients, dialysate has been found to leak into the abdominal wall, presenting as a bulge over the anterior or lateral abdominal wall. The cause of these fluid dissections is not clearly established but may represent fluid leakage around a patent internal catheter cuff, or through a pressure-induced rent in the peritoneal membrane, with subsequent dissection of fluid into the subcutaneous tissue. Such leaks can often be managed with discontinuation of peritoneal dialysis for 1–2 weeks and restarting with lower volumes. If the leak recurs after several such attempts to seal it, then catheter replacement may be necessary.

In all types of late dialysate leakage, overdistention of the peritoneal cavity is an important predisposing factor; this should be guarded against by minimizing the use of hypertonic dialysate (4.25%) and by instructing patients to be sure they are draining completely at each exchange.

Hernias. Hernias of various types have become common complications in patients on chronic peritoneal dialysis, especially continuous ambulatory peritoneal dialysis, because of the chronic presence of intraabdominal fluid, which leads to increased pressure on the abdominal wall and other structures. Any preexisting weakness of the abdominal wall, such as a surgical incision, a patent catheter tract, or an inguinal defect, will be the most likely site of herniation. Numerous case reports and two series of hernia cases have described multiple sites of herniation; the two most common sites, in order of frequency, are incisional (often from the catheter placement) and inguinal (see Table 4-15). Several recent reports have documented herniation through the catheter tract itself, both with the catheter in place and after it had been removed. Most of these patients presented with bowel obstruction due to the tight anatomic features of the space. The incidence of hernias in several large CAPD programs ranges from 11.5 to 24% of patients, with a higher frequency in women, especially those who are older or multiparous. In the Toronto series a high percentage of hernia patients (68%) had dialysate leakage at the exit site at the time of catheter

Table 4-15. Location of Hernias in 37 Patients on Chronic
Peritoneal Dialysis

Incisional	20
Inguinal	11
Epigastric	5
Catheter tract	4
Umbilical	3
Diaphragmatic	1
Total	44

placement, suggesting a weak abdominal wall and a predisposition to hernia. While many incisional hernias present with painless swelling, and genital edema usually accompanies inguinal hernias, it has been observed that patients with catheter tract, epigastric, and incisional hernias often present with complete bowel obstruction and incarceration, some requiring resection for ischemic bowel. However, following successful surgical repair in most instances, a high percentage of these patients return to CAPD without further difficulty. Clinicians should be attentive to the possibility that some patients will come to dialysis with preexisting hernias, especially inguinal, that were not clinically detected, and that repair should be undertaken prior to starting chronic peritoneal dialysis, if possible. Avoidance of overdistention of the abdomen should also be emphasized in those patients at high risk. The Toronto investigators have suggested that new catheters be placed with a paramedial incision through the rectus muscle, rather than in the midline. Although the midline is less vascular, it is a weaker area of the abdominal wall, and over time may yield to increased intraabdominal pressure.

Back pain. Another mechanical consequence of the constant presence of 2–3 L of fluid in the peritoneal cavity is low back pain in some patients. Often this is an aggravation of prior chronic lumbar pain, perhaps due to exaggeration of the lordotic position from the extra weight of the abdominal fluid. In some elderly patients this complication has been severe enough to require discontinuation of CAPD.

Medical Complications. Hypotension. Symptomatic hypotension or orthostatic hypotension has been observed in patients treated with chronic peritoneal dialysis, usually in patients on continuous ambulatory peritoneal dialysis. The clinical evaluation of such patients indicates that this hypotension is probably due to a combination of factors, including (1) chronic depletion of extracellular volume, resulting from continuous ultrafiltration via peritoneal dialysis, with inadequate replacement of dietary salt and volume; (2) hypoproteinemia, which may further aggravate low extracellular volume and peripheral pooling of interstitial fluid; and (3) autonomic insufficiency secondary to uremia and/or atherosclerotic vascular disease. The effects of oral salt loading without concomitant gain in body weight have been evaluated with measurement of blood volume, extracellular volume, and total exchangeable body sodium, as well as by the clinical response of blood pressure and sympathetic tone. Oral salt loads of 85–170 mmol/day for several weeks have resulted in an increase in mean arterial pressure and even plasma norepinephrine levels in some patients despite a lack of increase in body weight. These results suggest that salt replacement by a more liberal diet may be clinically helpful in CAPD patients who develop hypotension.

In older patients with peripheral vascular disease, the development of hypotension has been associated with either worsening or newly recognized ischemic symptoms in the extremities. In appropriate cases, such patients require diagnostic studies and surgical repair. However, in those patients who are not surgical candidates, raising the blood pressure by salt administration or by decreasing ultrafiltration may be effective in reducing pain and other symptoms of peripheral vascular insufficiency.

Nutritional abnormalities. *Protein loss.* Chronic peritoneal dialysis is associated with loss of protein through the dialysate, which averages 9–10 g/day with continuous ambulatory peritoneal dialysis and 12–15 g/treatment with intermittent peritoneal dialysis (see Table 4-1). The majority of this protein is lost as albumin, though smaller quantities of immunoglobulins and other proteins are removed as well. The clinical consequence of this phenomenon is reflected in the serum protein concentrations of patients on chronic peritoneal dialysis, which are moderately depressed, compared with those of patients on chronic hemodialysis. However, during peritonitis, protein losses are sharply increased; this protein loss may persist for several weeks after successful treatment. If these losses are not compensated by a generous dietary protein intake, or if patients without infection do not eat an adequate diet, significant hypoalbuminemia may result. Such patients may then be at increased risk for nutritionally induced immunologic compromise and infection. To compensate for dialysate losses, patients on chronic peritoneal dialysis are usually prescribed a diet containing 1.5 g protein/kg body weight and sufficient calories to provide a total of 35 kcal/kg/day (diet plus dialysate calories from absorbed glucose). Patients who follow these dietary recommendations generally do well and have only moderately reduced serum protein concentrations.

Obesity. A relatively frequent sequela of continuous ambulatory peritoneal dialysis is significant weight gain. This results from absorption of calories from dialysate glucose, which can be as high as 600 or more calories per day when hypertonic dextrose is used systematically. Also, 10–15% of patients become obese because they are unwilling to restrict the usage of hypertonic dextrose, preferring a more liberal fluid allowance, or because they cannot or will not reduce dietary calories. Such patients require intensive and long-term dietary counseling by a dietitian to provide the necessary education, motivation, and correct dietary instructions to reduce calories without compromising protein intake. It is possible that dialysate containing nonglucose osmotic agents will be developed in the near future, which would provide a salutary alternative for those patients who need significant weight reduction.

Hyperlipidemia. Serum lipid abnormalities secondary to uremia are well documented in chronic hemodialysis patients and are regarded as a potential risk factor in the development of atherogenesis. Hypertriglyceridemia is the predominant abnormality, but some patients have hypercholesterolemia as well. Because of the carbohydrate absorption and its attendant effects on insulin metabolism, chronic peritoneal dialysis has been found to aggravate these changes in a significant number of patients, especially those on continuous ambulatory peritoneal dialysis. Mean serum triglyceride levels in patients on CAPD remain elevated, while total serum cholesterol is normal and high density lipoprotein (HDL) cholesterol is variably low or normal. The majority of patients, although not all (and usually not diabetics), have moderate elevation of triglycerides in the 200–300 mg/dl range, while a few patients will have extremely high levels above 1000 mg/dl. Most data on lipid studies in CAPD patients must be interpreted with the knowledge that these values may be obtained in the dietary fasting state, but with the constant presence of glucose-containing fluid in the peritoneal cavity. These conditions are thus not strictly comparable to values obtained in normal subjects or to patients on chronic hemodialysis.

Defective removal of triglyceride due to a deficiency or inhibitor of lipoprotein lipase has been documented by many investigators. The role of overproduction of very low density lipoprotein (VLDL) by the liver remains more controversial. Increased carbohydrate load and insulin production from CAPD may contribute to the increased clinical severity of hypertriglyceridemia and perhaps to an eventual increase in cardiovascular disease and mortality.

To date, the treatment of this problem remains a difficult challenge. Removal of glucose from the dialysate is an obvious solution, but this procedure is not yet available. Modification of the diet is more difficult because of the need to maintain adequate dietary protein and calories to compensate for dialysate protein loss. Exercise has been shown to be an effective means of reducing plasma triglyceride and cholesterol levels of hemodialysis and CAPD patients. It is difficult, however, for all patients to exercise, and patient dropout from a regular program is high. In one study, the addition of insulin to the dialysate sufficient to lower the blood glucose levels in nondiabetics was not associated with significant change in plasma lipids. Thus, effective treatment for hyperlipidemia is currently inaccessible.

Peritoneal dialysate eosinophilia. Peritoneal dialysate eosinophilia is a benign, usually self-limited condition of unknown etiology, which most commonly occurs in patients shortly after beginning dialysis. It is not associated with peritonitis, and thus the term eosinophilic peritonitis is a misnomer, although the peritoneal fluid is cloudy and must be carefully distinguished from bacterial infection. The clinical presentation includes cloudy fluid, with elevated leukocyte counts containing 40–95% eosinophils, and no associated symptoms. It appears unrelated to the type of dialysis catheter used or to the dialysate dextrose concentration. Studies of immunoglobulin E (IgE) levels in several patients revealed very low concentrations in the peritoneal fluid, thus making it unlikely that this potent eosinophilotactic agent plays a role in this disorder. It has also been demonstrated that peritoneal protein loss does not increase with eosinophilia, which is further evidence against inflammation as the etiologic agent. No treatment is currently indicated, but patients must be carefully followed because the primary signal of bacterial peritonitis, that is, cloudy dialysate outflow, has been obscured by the eosinophilia.

Peritoneal dialysis failure. As experience with chronic peritoneal dialysis has broadened, it has become evident that the peritoneal membrane may lose its ability to serve as a transport membrane (Table 4-16). Clinically, the most common cause of membrane failure is the loss of ultrafiltration, although the ability to remove solute remains intact. This usually presents as the need for increasingly higher hypertonic solutions, clinical volume overload, and low outflow volumes.

Another cause of peritoneal dialysis failure is loculation of the peritoneal cavity secondary to fibrosis and adhesions resulting from inflammation. In this situation, the peritoneal membrane may function adequately, but the mechanical restrictions to fluid movement are so severe that adequate dialysate volume cannot be achieved, thus severely limiting peritoneal clearance and effective therapy.

In 1983 a French group of investigators described for the first time a third pattern of peritoneal dialysis failure, in which there is progressive peritoneal membrane thickening; they named this condition "sclerosing peritonitis." This aberration occurs usually in patients who lose ultrafiltration capability and transfer to hemodialysis. The predominant symptoms are nausea, vomiting, malabsorption, and bowel obstruction. Laparotomy discloses an exceedingly thickened peritoneal membrane encasing all bowel loops in a dense mass. Despite the surgical lysis of adhesions, mortality has been high. Thus far, no correlation between this syndrome and the previous type of dialysis regimen, frequency of peritonitis, or drug therapy has been found. Only a few cases of this severe complication have been reported in the United States and Canada; none of these patients have been on continuous ambulatory peritoneal dialysis.

The pathogenesis of these three types of peritoneal dialysis failure remains incompletely understood. A respected theory is that the loss of peritoneal ultrafiltration with intact solute transport is the result of an increase in membrane or vascular permeability; thus glucose is rapidly absorbed, abolishing the water gradient while preserving or even enhancing the removal of high molecular weight solutes. This phenomenon frequently occurs as a transient event during

Table 4-16. Clinical Characteristics of the Major Causes of Peritoneal Dialysis Failure

Loss of ultrafiltration	Increasing need for hypertonic solution
	Fluid retention
	Solute removal intact
Loculation of peritoneal cavity	Sensation of distention
	Inability to tolerate previously used dialysate volumes
	Poor dialysate outflow
	Poor catheter function
Peritoneal membrane sclerosis	Nausea, vomiting
	Malabsorption
	Bowel obstruction

the course of acute peritonitis, with resultant clinical volume overload and decreased drainage volumes.

The reported incidence of peritoneal dialysis failure due to peritoneal membrane dysfunction has been as high as 25% of CAPD patients in France but is only 2.8% in Canada. A suggested cause for this considerable difference in frequency may be attributable to the predominant use of acetate as the dialysate buffer in France, while the majority of dialysate in North America contains lactate. However, many other factors including frequency of peritonitis, antibiotic treatment, and other dialysate additives must be considered in the pathogenesis of these cases of peritoneal dialysis failure.

ACUTE PERITONEAL DIALYSIS

Indications for Acute Peritoneal Dialysis

Peritoneal dialysis is the oldest form of dialytic treatment for acute renal failure and remains the treatment of choice in many situations today, despite the widespread availability of hemodialysis. The more commonly encountered indications for acute peritoneal dialysis are listed in Table 4-17. In many of these events, peritoneal dialysis may be clearly preferable to hemodialysis. However, the choice of modality in the individual patient must always rest on careful analysis of multiple factors, including (1) principal goals of dialytic therapy in

Table 4-17. Acute Peritoneal Dialysis

Relative indications
  Hemodialysis not available
  Difficulty with vascular access
    Children
    Adults with severe vascular disease or limitations of vessels for hemodialysis
  High risk of anticoagulation
  Unstable cardiovascular status
  Slower correction of severe azotemia
  Removal of edema
  Hemorrhagic pancreatitis
  Hypothermia
Relative contraindications
  Medical complications associated with limited effectiveness of peritoneal dialysis
    Hypercatabolism
    Severe hyperkalemia
    Diseased peritoneal vasculature (systemic lupus erythematosus, scleroderma, etc.)
  Abdominal complications that increase risks or technical difficulty with peritoneal dialysis
    Recent surgery/trauma
    Undiagnosed abdominal disease
    Aortic vascular graft
    Extensive adhesions
    Diaphragmatic defects and fluid extravasation
    Fistula/colostomy
    Large polycystic kidneys
  Need for rapid removal of solute
    Toxins
    Drugs
    Hypercalcemia

that patient, for example, fluid, solute, and toxin removal; (2) medical factors that may impact on the safety and efficacy of the dialysis modality; (3) availability of equipment and specialized dialysis staff; (4) experience and treatment philosophy of the medical facility. Frequently, either peritoneal dialysis or hemodialysis will be equally effective medically, and choice becomes a matter of other factors, such as economic considerations, convenience, and personal preference.

The use of peritoneal dialysis in special circumstances, such as hemorrhagic pancreatitis, hypotension, or hypothermia, is not frequently encountered, but the coexistence of one of these problems with acute renal failure could influence the choice of peritoneal dialysis as therapy of choice for an individual patient. Difficult blood access is a relatively frequent problem in some patient populations especially in children, adults with vascular disease, or adults with a history of intravenous drug abuse and obliteration of accessible vessels for dialysis access. The greater use of venous cannulation for hemodialysis, especially via the subclavian route, has somewhat tempered this indication for peritoneal dialysis and made hemodialysis feasible in many acute situations (see Chapter 2). It should be borne in mind, however, that central venous cannulation carries risks of trauma to large vessels and the lung, which may be a significant hazard to the acutely ill patient with multiple medical problems. Peritoneal dialysis may be a relatively safer approach to dialysis in such situations.

The availability of the acute Tenckhoff catheter and Deane's prosthesis makes repetitive peritoneal dialysis feasible without the need for recurrent puncture of the abdominal wall. The combination of acute Tenckhoff catheter and automated cycler dialysis offers a semiautomated, safe, and effective approach to therapy of acute renal failure. This system is easily learned and accepted by intensive care and ward nursing staff, reduces the risk of peritonitis through use of a closed system, and has relatively few mechanical complications associated with its use.

Contraindications to Acute Peritoneal Dialysis

There are few absolute contraindications to peritoneal dialysis. However, some medical contingencies create relatively strong factors that militate against the success of peritoneal dialysis or significantly increase the risk of its use. These contingencies fall into three major categories, which are listed in Table 4-17. Perhaps the most frequently encountered abnormality is hypercatabolism, particularly in the setting of trauma, sepsis, or acute rhabdomyolysis. Since severely catabolized patients generate urea and other metabolites at very high rates, exceeding the clearance capabilities of routine peritoneal dialysis, they are usually better managed with acute hemodialysis. The second potential problem with acute peritoneal dialysis is associated abdominal disease (see Table 4-17). Peritoneal dialysis can be performed in a patient shortly after abdominal surgery; however, there is a formidable risk of infection in such settings, as well as a greater likelihood of mechanical difficulty due to dialysate leakage, wound care, and healing, to cite a few.

Abdominal adhesions and a history of peritonitis are prominent among abdominal complications that are hazardous for blind peritoneal catheter placement; frequently these disorders are associated with reduced efficiency of peritoneal dialysis secondary to limitations of surface area and loculations. Diphragmatic defects and other sites of dialysate extravasation such as genital and abdominal wall edema, may not interefer with dialysis per se but can compromise respiratory function and cause extreme discomfort, which may preclude the continuation of peritoneal dialysis. Open abdominal wounds, bowel fistulas, and ostomies greatly increase the risk of bacterial contamination of the peritoneal dialysis catheter site, so that catheter placement becomes seriously problematic. In such cases, hemodialysis is generally preferable. Finally, peritoneal dialysis is usually contraindicated when there is a need for rapid removal of solutes, especially toxins and drugs. While it is possible to remove many substances with peritoneal dialysis, rapid clearance is generally superior with hemodialysis or hemoperfusion, the therapy of choice in this case; see Chapter 6 for discussion.

Emergent treatment of hyperkalemia and hypercalcemia is also best managed with hemodialysis.

Acute Peritoneal Dialysis Prescription

Peritoneal dialysis for acute renal failure is usually accomplished by performing continuous exchanges for ~48 hours (range 36–60 hours), or until the appropriate degree of biochemical and extracellular volume correction has been achieved, as discussed in Chapter 3. Dialysis is then terminated and restarted several days later or when clinical parameters dictate. Alternatively, if a Silastic catheter has been placed (Tenckhoff), and automated or cycler devices are available, the patient can be dialyzed for 10–12 hours, 3 times weekly, or every other day, on a regular schedule analogous to that for hemodialysis. One-hour cycles, with 2 L volumes, are most commonly employed, although the the efficiency of peritoneal dialysis can be influenced by increasing dialysate flow rates up to 3.5–4.0 L/h.

Dialysate composition and glucose concentration are determined by the clinical needs of the patient. In patients with significant acidosis, the high bicarbonate concentrate is preferred for better correction. Obviously, lactate-containing dialysate should not be used in patients with lactic acidosis. If hyperkalemia is present at the initiation of dialysis, potassium may be withheld from the dialysate during the first 6–8 cycles or until the serum potassium falls below 5.0 mEq/L, but then it should be added to all subsequent exchanges to achieve the desired serum concentration at the end of dialysis. Hypertonic dialysate is used for the correction of extracellular volume excess. Using the average ultrafiltration rates that can be expected from each glucose concentration (see Table 4-4), one can predict the hourly rate of fluid removal and thus estimate the total ultrafiltration volume over the projected course of dialysis. For example, if 1.5%

dextrose is used for 48 exchanges, and 150 ml is removed per exchange, then total volume loss should be ~7200 ml. This will, of course, be offset by oral and/or intravenous fluid intake during the period of dialysis, therefore the *net* negative fluid balance should be calculated to compensate for these factors. Continuous use of hypertonic dextrose (4.25%) requires careful observation of the patient, since large quantities of fluid (800–1000 L) can be removed with each exchange; such removal can rapidly result in extracellular volume depletion and other metabolic abnormalities (see below under Complications).

Monitoring Acute Peritoneal Dialysis

Clinical Status. The patient should be examined frequently during the course of peritoneal dialysis to look for possible catheter problems, such as leakage of dialysate, overdistention of the abdominal cavity, and signs of infection. Monitoring blood pressure and peripheral edema will facilitate the appropriate adjustment of the ultrafiltration rate. Evaluation of mental status and thirst are helpful in detecting clinical signs of hyperglycemia and hypernatremia that may result from rapid ultrafiltration and hypertonic dextrose. The onset of respiratory distress should suggest the possibility of dialysate leakage into the pleural space.

Abdominal Pain. Abdominal pain is common during acute peritoneal dialysis and can result from a variety of causes. The correct diagnosis of pain during peritoneal dialysis is usually dependent on careful assessment of the time of discomfort during the exchange cycle and the duration of the symptoms. Table 4-14 lists the various causes of abdominal pain during peritoneal dialysis and categorizes them according to cycle time.

Evaluation of Acute Peritoneal Dialysis. The following steps are essential in the evaluation of acute peritoneal dialysis:

1. Observe the dialysate outflow for cloudy appearance, which may be the earliest sign of peritonitis.
2. Check the outflow for blood and/or fibrin. If present, heparin should be added to the dialysate to prevent obstruction of the catheter. Continued bright red bleeding that does not clear after a few exchanges suggests either a possible bleeder in the abdominal wall catheter track, or coagulopathy.
3. Monitor the net patient fluid balance to guide ultrafiltration adjustment.
4. Weigh the patient with abdomen empty every 12 hours to confirm ultrafiltration results and to evaluate volume status.
5. If peritonitis is suspected:
   a. Do not rely on routine dialysate cultures for an accurate diagnosis in the absence of clinical symptoms or cloudy dialysate.
   b. Evaluate the peritoneal fluid overflow with a cell count and differential. If polymorphonuclear leukocytes predominate with >100 cells/mm^3, then make a presumptive diagnosis of peritonitis.
   c. Inaugurate appropriate measures for diagnosis and treatment.

Laboratory Studies. The following laboratory studies are recommended to evaluate the efficacy and safety of acute peritoneal dialysis:

1. Daily electrolytes, BUN, and creatinine. It may be necessary to monitor sodium and potassium more frequently, depending on the degree of catabolism, hypertonicity of the dialysate, and usage of insulin.

2. Blood sugar every 6–8 hours initially in all patients. Diabetics may require more frequent measurement initially, and perhaps throughout the dialysis, in order to monitor insulin therapy.

Complications with Acute Peritoneal Dialysis

The major complications of acute peritoneal dialysis are listed in Table 4-18. These fall into two categories of mechanical and catheter-related problems and medical disturbances. Of the catheter-related complications, the most common symptom is pain, which occurs in 50–60% of patients; it is usually mild

Table 4-18. Complications of Acute Peritoneal Dialysis

Mechanical/catheter-related
  Pain
  Bleeding
  Poor function, inflow or outflow drainage problems
  Dialysate leakage
    Around catheter
    Abdominal wall, scrotal edema
  Intraperitoneal catheter loss
  Bowel/bladder perforation
  Overdistention of peritoneum
  Peritoneal burn secondary to overheated dialysate
Medical
  Inflammatory
    Exit site infection
    Peritonitis
    Chemical irritation
    Eosinophilic peritonitis
  Cardiovascular
    Fluid overload
    Hypotension
    Arrhythmias
  Pulmonary
    Basal atelectasis
    Pleural effusions
  Metabolic
    Hypernatremia
    Hyperglycemia
    Hyperosmolar coma
    Postdialysis hyperglycemia
    Hypokalemia
    Protein loss
  Neurologic
    Seizures
    Postdialysis disequilibrium

Table 4-19. Diagnosis of Mechanical Catheter Dysfunction

Problem	Possible Cause	Treatment
Poor dialysate inflow	Fibrin/blood clot obstruction of catheter	Flush catheter, add heparin to dialysate, ? streptokinase
	Poor catheter position	Reposition catheter if still sterile or replace catheter
	Kinked external tubing	Correct
Poor dialysis outflow	Kinked external tubing	Examine line and correct
	Malposition of catheter	Reposition catheter if still sterile, or replace catheter
	Air in line	Flush line
	Fibrin obstruction	Flush catheter with heparinized saline; add heparin to dialysate
	Lack of vent in outflow container	Correct
	Catheter encasement by bowel, omentum, fibrous tissue	Replace catheter

to moderate in severity and can be managed with analgesics or minor catheter adjustment. Problems with dialysate outflow, occurring in 40% of all dialyses, are most frequently caused by poor catheter placement and loss of siphon effect. Typical causes and approaches to treatment are shown in Table 4-19. Bleeding, which is usually mild and does not require blood replacement, is experienced in 30% of dialyses.

Metabolic disturbances are the most frequently encountered medical complications, of which hyperglycemia (blood glucose >300 mg/dl) afflicts many patients, followed by hypokalemia (serum K <3.5 mEq/L) in about 20%. Hyperkalemia and metabolic alkalosis are each seen in 10% of dialyses. Appropriate monitoring and adjustment of the dialysate composition should prevent these metabolic complications.

Cardiovascular complications are usually not very common. A rather high incidence of arrhythmias (37%), of which most were tachyarrhythmias and required intervention, has been reported, although this may reflect more frequent cardiac monitoring. Arrhythmias, not unexpectedly, are correlated with the clinical status of the patient and with preexisting cardiac disease.

Peritonitis as a complication of acute peritoneal dialysis is relatively less prevalent; the incidence is quite variable in the literature, but 5–6% is typical of recent experience. When automated equipment and Tenckhoff-type catheters are used, this percentage should be even lower. The incidence of positive cultures not associated with clinical infection is always higher (30%), a further argument against the relevance of routine dialysate cultures. While peritonitis is not frequent, it is a potentially serious problem and can result in dialysis-related mortality. It is more often encountered in patients with mechanical or catheter problems requiring repeated manipulations. Leakage of dialysate around the catheter also predisposes to infection at the exit site. Peritonitis should be treated promptly by adding antibiotics to the dialysate in appropriate amounts (see Table 4-6) and by continuing peritoneal lavage until the dialysate has cleared.

Results of Acute Peritoneal Dialysis Treatment

It has been well documented that survival from acute renal failure is most dependent on the underlying cause of the renal insult and that mortality remains high, particularly in patients with trauma and multiple complications. Rarely does mortality in acute renal failure result from dialytic therapy per se. At this time there are no controlled studies that compare the clinical efficacy and safety of peritoneal dialysis with hemodialysis for acute renal failure. However, based on available data of a large series of patients receiving acute peritoneal dialysis, the overall mortality rate is about the same as that obtained with hemodialysis. These data lend support to the conviction that peritoneal dialysis is as effective as hemodialysis and can be readily employed in nearly any hospital setting for rapid and safe treatment of many patients with acute renal failure.

PERITONEAL DIALYSIS IN CHILDREN
(Donald E. Potter)

Continuous ambulatory peritoneal dialysis is exceptionally popular in the treatment of children; a number of pediatric dialysis units have more than 50% of their patients on this modality. The volume of dialysate used is determined by the peritoneal surface area and volume of the peritoneal cavity, which are roughly proportional to body surface area. The prescribed volume is 1200 ml/m^2 body surface area, but this is modified according to the available dialysate bag sizes as shown in Table 4-20. As with adults, most children perform four exchanges a day, and adequate ultrafiltration is commonly achieved with three cycles of 1.5% glucose and one cycle of 4.25% glucose. Infants, however, have a higher clearance in relation to body weight than older children and adults and absorb glucose more rapidly from the dialysate. This interferes with ultrafiltration, and some infants require five or more exchanges a day, all with 4.25% or 2.5% glucose. Infants and small children also lose more protein in the dialysate, 0.30 g/kg/day, than older children, 0.14 g/kg/day, and are more likely to have low serum levels of albumin.

The biochemical control of uremia is comparable with CAPD and hemodialysis, although children on CAPD have higher serum bicarbonate levels, lower blood pressure levels, higher hematocrit levels, and require fewer transfusions than children on hemodialysis. Children on CAPD absorb 2.0 g/kg/day of glucose

Table 4-20. Prescription for Dialysate Volume Based on Body Weight in Children

Body Weight (kg)	Dialysate Bag Volume (ml)
5–9	250
10–14	500
14–19	750
20–34	1000
35–49	1500
>50	2000

from the dialysate. There is evidence that children have better nutrition and growth with CAPD than with hemodialysis, but most children on CAPD do not grow normally.

The complications of CAPD in children are the same as those in adults. The peritonitis rate in children has varied from one episode every 3.1 patient-months to one episode every 13 patient-months in different centers. Skin erosion from the subcutaneous catheter cuff has been common in children, and the use of catheters with a single, preperitoneal cuff has been advocated. The primary advantage of CAPD is probably that it is easily performed in the home, without a machine, and allows children more freedom to perform normal activities. In addition, most children older than 12 or 13 years can perform their own bag changes, and this contributes to a sense of responsibility and independence. CAPD has been particularly advantageous in infants and young children, a group that tolerates chronic hemodialysis poorly. Normal, or almost normal, growth and development have been reported in infants maintained on CAPD and given gavage feedings for more than a year. Some nephrologists feel that CAPD is preferable to transplantation for children during the first 2 or 3 years of life.

Although the experience with CAPD in children has been extremely positive, it should be emphasized that this is a new form of treatment, and that the initial enthusiasm of patients, families, and medical staff may be tempered with time. A failure rate of 20% at one year from complications has been reported, and the ability of parents to withstand the stresses of performing CAPD in their children for prolonged periods has yet to be determined.

REFERENCES

Ahmad S, Shen FH, Blagg CR: Intermittent peritoneal dialysis as renal replacement therapy. p. 144. In Nolph KD (ed): Peritoneal Dialysis. Developments in Nephrology. Vol. 2. Martinus Nijhoff, The Hague, 1981

Blumenkrantz MJ, Gahl GM, Kopple JD, et al: Protein losses during peritoneal dialysis. Kidney Int 19:593, 1981

Boen ST: Peritoneal Dialysis in Clinical Medicine. Charles C Thomas, Springfield, IL, 1964

Boen ST: Review of the clinical use of peritoneal dialysis. p. 1. In Nolph KD (ed): Peritoneal Dialysis. Developments in Nephrology. Vol. 2. Martinus Nijhoff, The Hague, 1981

Baum M, Powell D, Calvin S, et al: Continuous ambulatory peritoneal dialysis in children: Comparison with hemodialysis. N Engl J Med 307:1542–1547, 1982

Diaz-Buxo JA, Walker PJ, Chandler JT, et al: Advances in peritoneal dialysis. Continuous cyclic peritoneal dialysis. Contemp Dial Nov 1981

Digenis GE, Khanna R, Mathews R, et al: Abdominal hernias in patients undergoing continuous ambulatory peritoneal dialysis. Peritoneal Dial Bull 2:115, 1982

Drukker W: Peritoneal dialysis: A historical review. p. 40. In Drukker W, Parsons FM, Maher JF (eds): Replacement of Renal Function by Dialysis. Martinus Nijhoff, The Hague, 1983

Firmat J, Zucchini A: Peritoneal Dialysis in acute renal failure. Contrib Nephrol 17:33, 1979

Gloor HJ, Nichols WK, Sorkin MI, et al: Peritoneal access and related complications in continuous ambulatory peritoneal dialysis. Am J Med 74:593, 1983

Miller RB, Tassistro CR: Peritoneal dialysis. N Engl J Med 281:945, 1969

Mion CM: Practical use of peritoneal dialysis. p. 457. In Drukker W, Parsons FM, Maher J (eds): Replacement of Renal Function by Dialysis. 2nd Ed. Martinus Nijhoff, The Hague, 1983

Nolph KD: Peritoneal anatomy and transport physiology. p. 440. In Drukker W, Parsons FM, Maher JF (eds): Replacement of Renal Function by Dialysis. 2nd Ed. Martinus Nijhoff, The Hague, 1983

Nolph KD, Sorkin, MI: The peritonal dialysis system. p. 21. In Nolph KD (ed): Peritoneal Dialysis. Developments in Nephrology. Vol. 2. Martinus Nijhoff, The Hague, 1981

Nolph KD, Sorkin M: Peritoneal dialysis in acute renal failure. p. 689. In Brenner BM, Lazarus JM (eds): Acute Renal Failure. Saunders, Philadelphia, 1983

Nolph KD, Sorkin MI, Rubin J, et al: Continuous ambulatory peritoneal dialysis: Three year experience at one center. Ann Intern Med 92:609, 1980

Oreopoulos DG, Khanna R: Complications of peritoneal dialysis other than peritonitis. p. 309. In Nolph KD (ed): Peritoneal Dialysis, Developments in Nephrology. Vol 2. Martinus Nijhoff, The Hague, 1981

Oreopoulos DG, Wu G, Khanna R, et al (eds): CAPD failures. Proceedings of a workshop. Peritoneal Dial Bull Suppl 3(3):S9, 1983

Popovich, RP, Pyle, WK, Moncrief, JW: Kinetics of peritoneal transport. p. 79. In Nolph KD (ed): Peritoneal Dialysis. Developments in Nephrology. Vol. 2. Martinus Nijhoff, The Hague, 1981

Rubin J, Ray R, Barnes T, et al: Peritonitis in continuous ambulatory peritoneal dialysis patients. Am J Kidney Dis 2:602, 1983

Tenckhoff H: Chronic Peritoneal Dialysis Manual. University of Washington School of Medicine, Seattle, WA, 1974

Valk TW, Swartz RD, Hsu CH: Peritoneal dialysis in acute renal failure. Analysis of outcome and complications. Dial Transplant. 9:48, 1980

Wideröe TE, Smeby LC, Berg KJ et al: Intraperitoneal (^{125}I) insulin absorption during intermittent and continuous peritoneal dialysis. Kidney Int 23:22, 1983

5

CARE OF THE PATIENT BETWEEN DIALYSES

Patricia Schoenfeld

HEMATOLOGIC ABNORMALITIES

Anemia

Despite optimal treatment with dialysis, the majority of patients with end-stage renal disease remain significantly anemic, and many are symptomatic. While a small percentage of patients are able to normalize their hematocrit with dialysis and adjunctive pharmacologic therapy, most patients have hematocrits in the 20–30% range. Anephric patients usually have even lower hematocrits and may be transfusion-dependent.

Pathophysiology of Anemia. The anemia in end-stage renal disease patients is normochromic and normocytic, unless iron deficiency, which is relatively common in chronic hemodialysis patients, occurs as well. The pathophysiology of anemia in dialysis patients is more complex than in chronic renal failure because of the additional risks and variables attendant to dialytic therapy. Table 5-1 lists the multiple pathophysiologic variables that cause and influence the severity of anemia in these patients, including disorders that result from the loss of functioning renal tissue, as well as dialysis-related complications. The major causes of anemia are (1) decreased erythropoietin production by the damaged kidney, (2) decreased erythrocyte survival, (3) retention of uremic toxins, which suppress bone marrow production of erythrocytes, and (4) blood loss from dialysis, regular sampling, and abnormal bleeding.

Decreased erythrocyte production, primarily due to insufficient erythropoietin, is the major defect in dialyzed patients. It has recently been shown by more sensitive assays that nonfiltering renal tissue retains the ability to produce small quantities of erythropoietin; the liver can contribute an additional small

197

Table 5-1. Pathophysiology of Hematologic Abnormalities: Anemia

Decreased erythrocyte production
    Decreased erythropoietin production
        Loss of renal mass by disease or nephrectomy
        Decreased hemoglobin oxygen affinity
    Nutritional deficiencies
        Folic acid
        Pyridoxine
        Histidine
    Inhibitors of erythropoiesis
        Uremic toxins
    Transfusion-induced marrow suppression
    Iron deficiency
        Dietary deficiency
        Blood loss
        Malabsorption of iron supplements secondary to phosphate binders
    Infection
    Hyperparathyroidism
Increased erythrocyte destruction
    Hemolysis
        Dialysis-related injury
            Copper
            Chloramine
            Nitrates
            Formaldehyde
            Overheated dialysate
            Hypoosmolar dialysate
        Drugs
        Hypophosphatemia
        Hypersplenism
        Mechanical injury due to high negative pressure in arterial line
        Associated disease producing hemolytic anemia (e.g., systemic lupus
            erythematosus, sickle cell disease, microangiopathy)
        Formalin-induced anti-N antibody
Blood loss
    Sequestration of blood in dialyzer
    Sampling for laboratory studies
    Accidental loss during dialysis
    Abnormal bleeding (gastrointestinal tract, vaginal, epistaxis, etc.)

amount, but this remains subnormal for the degree of anemia in most dialyzed patients. The second major cause of decreased erythrocyte production is iron deficiency, which occurs frequently in the hemodialysis population due to unavoidable blood loss associated with dialysis, including regular blood sampling for laboratory tests and occasional accidental blood loss. Gastrointestinal, vaginal, and other abnormal bleeding may also contribute to blood loss and iron deficiency in these patients. It has been conservatively estimated that the average dialysis patient loses about 800 ml of blood per year by way of the dialyzer; when other losses are superimposed, it is not surprising that most patients will become iron-deficient if iron stores are not routinely monitored and replaced when needed.

    Persistent uremic toxins may also suppress the bone marrow, although specific compounds have not yet been identified. The enhanced removal of high molecular weight substances by peritoneal dialysis may be a partial explanation of why anemia is less severe in patients treated with this modality; however, the lack of dialysis-associated blood loss is also an important factor.

Blood transfusions in patients with severe anemia produces marrow suppression by increasing tissue oxygenation, which in turn decreases erythropoietin production. Infection is a common complication of dialysis, which diminishes both erythropoiesis, by reticuloendothelial blockade, and the iron supply needed for erythroid synthesis.

While a direct correlation between nutritional status and severity of anemia has not been demonstrated in end-stage renal disease patients, specific nutritional deficiencies can aggravate anemia, for example, folic acid and pyridoxine (vitamin B_6) deficiencies. Histidine has been shown to be essential in renal insufficiency, and an inadequate amount of this amino acid causes a reduction in hemoglobin concentration. An iron-deficient diet will intensify the iron deficiency caused by blood loss. If iron supplements are taken at the same time as phosphate binders, the iron will be bound by the aluminum hydroxide and will not be absorbed.

Finally, it has been reported of both nonuremic and end-stage renal disease patients that hyperparathyroidism may aggravate anemia; however, this abnormality can be mitigated by surgical removal of the excess parathormone-producing tissue. Marrow fibrosis secondary to hyperparathyroidism may also result in compromise of marrow erythropoiesis and may stimulate extramedullary hematopoiesis and splenomegaly.

Shortened erythrocyte survival or increased hemolysis may aggravate the anemia of dialysis patients; the causative factors are listed in Table 5-1. Since most of these factors are avoidable, the clinician must carefully evaluate the dialysis therapy of severely anemic patients, taking every precaution to prevent these occurrences.

Contamination of dialysate by chemicals or metals and abnormal preparation of the dialysate due to accidental overheating or proportioning errors are among the major causes of dialysis-related erythrocyte injury. These forms of injury are now almost totally preventable by appropriate treatment of water used for dialysate and by careful operation and monitoring of dialysate delivery systems, as discussed in Chapter 1.

Various drugs can cause Coombs positive hemolytic anemia in dialyzed patients; hypophosphatemia from overzealous use of binders may also contribute to increased erythrocyte destruction.

It has been shown that splenectomy can effectively treat the increased erythrocyte destruction caused by dialysis-related hypersplenism. Several recent reports have documented that splenomegaly resulted from silicone deposition in macrophages, leading to granuloma formation. It is postulated that the source of silicone may be the tubing used for hemodialysis, because of the shearing stress of blood pumps.

The widespread use of formaldehyde to sterilize hemodialyzers has been implicated in the development of anti-N erythrocyte antibodies. The clinical consequences of this antibody are not clearly defined. Studies by several European centers indicates that reduction of residual dialyzer formaldehyde concentration reduces the incidence of this abnormality.

Clinical Evaluation of Anemia. Patients with anemia of usual severity (hemoglobin concentration, 6–10 g%) usually have minimal or no transfusion requirements and tolerate the anemia without significant symptoms. The routine monitoring of patients with anemia can be simplified as follows:

1. Monthly complete blood count
2. Weekly hematocrit (repeated more often as necessary)
3. Serum ferritin every 4–6 months

It is a simple and routine practice in many dialysis facilities to measure hematocrits with microcapillary tubes that are spun in the dialysis center, thus providing a rapid assessment of anemia. When anemia becomes more severe or transfusions are required, then a more intensive evaluation is required, as outlined in Table 5-2.

Measurement of iron stores is best accomplished by periodic measurement of serum ferritin, a high molecular weight intracellular iron storage compound, which has been shown to correlate best with marrow iron stores in dialysis patients.

Therapy of Anemia. The major therapeutic measures for anemia in dialysis patients are listed in Table 5-3. Provision of adequate dialysis technique, removal of potential hemolytic agents from the dialysis water, and limitation of blood loss associated with dialysis are basic tenets of good therapy; often some improvement in anemia can be observed after 6 months of treatment. Since a majority of patients will have cumulative blood loss that eventually results in iron deficiency, body iron stores must be evaluated on a regular basis and re-

Table 5-2. Clinical Evaluation of Anemia

Adequacy of dialysis therapy
Transfusion frequency (marrow suppression)
Causes of hemolysis
  Drugs
  Chloramine and/or other possible contaminants
  Hypophosphatemia
  Associated leukopenia and thrombocytopenia suggestive of hypersplenism
  Associated disease causing hemolysis
Iron deficiency
  Serum ferritin
  Serum iron/total iron binding capacity
  Erythrocyte indices
Blood loss
  Dialysis-related (clotting of dialyzer, accidental, etc.)
  Occult blood loss (gastrointestinal, vaginal)
Nutritional status
  Dietary deficiency
    Folic acid
    Histidine
    Pyridoxine
  Iron (blood loss or malabsorption of iron due to phosphate binders)

Table 5-3. Therapy of Anemia

Optimize dialysis therapy
Correct/minimize blood loss
Supply good nutrition, including supplemental vitamin therapy
Use arterial pressure monitors
Use treated dialysate water to remove possible chemicals and sub-
    stances injurious to erythrocytes
Replace iron stores as needed
Administer androgen therapy
  Parenteral
     Nandrolone decanoate 2–3 mg/kg/week
     Testosterone enanthate 4 mg/kg/week (males only)
  Oral
     Oxymetholone 1–2 mg/kg/day
     Fluoxymesterone 0.4 mg/kg/day
Provide exercise program as tolerated
Give transfusions, when necessary

pleted as needed. Uremic patients can absorb oral iron normally, the rate of absorption being correlated with body iron stores. When serum ferritin has fallen to the 30–50 µg/L level, iron should be replaced as oral ferrous sulfate or ferrous gluconate, and this therapy should be continued until an adequate response in hematocrit or rise in serum ferritin has been achieved. In those who cannot tolerate, or do not respond to, oral iron therapy, intravenous iron dextran can be given during dialysis (500–1000 mg over 2–3 dialysis treatments) to replace iron stores. The practice of prescribing oral or parenteral iron on a regular basis in all patients should be discouraged, as not all patients need iron in equal quantities or on a continuous basis, and injudicious use of parenteral iron can result in iron overload. Patients who remain significantly anemic, or have symptoms related to anemia despite the above measures, should receive a trial of androgen therapy.

Parenteral androgens (nandrolone decanoate and testosterone enanthate) have proved to be more effective in raising the hematocrit than oral androgens (fluoxymesterone and oxymetholone). While reports of the efficacy of androgens in anephric patients are conflicting, the prevailing experience is that they are usually not effective. Androgens should not be used indefinitely even in patients who respond well to therapy. Often a continued beneficial effect will be present for months after the drug is stopped. Therefore androgens should be administered for 6 months, and then stopped, to determine whether continued administration is necessary.

It has been shown that moderate physical exercise programs for dialysis patients results in improvement of anemia. Those patients who are physically able should be encouraged to perform regular exercise (walking, jogging, bicycling, etc.) to enhance erythrocyte production.

The use of transfusion is unavoidable in some (usually anephric) patients or in older patients with symptomatic coronary artery disease, who require a hematocrit above 30% to avoid tissue hypoxia. In addition, it is now common practice to give routine transfusions (up to 3 units) to all patients waiting for cadaver transplantation, as this practice has been shown to increase graft survival. Since transfusion is always accompanied by the risk of hepatitis, its need should be carefully determined and minimized in each patient, and it should not be employed unless other therapy has proved to be ineffective.

Bleeding Abnormalities

Pathophysiology of Abnormal Bleeding. Patients with untreated advanced uremia often exhibit abnormal bleeding from mucosal surfaces and cutaneous sites; spontaneous intracranial hemorrhage has been observed with increased frequency. While dialytic therapy has been shown to correct the bleeding disorder in some patients, abnormal hemostasis often persists in patients on regular dialysis, possibly as a result of incomplete reversal of uremic platelet abnormalities. The clinical spectrum of bleeding in dialyzed patients varies widely from prolonged oozing at needle puncture sites to serious episodes of gastrointestinal, genitourinary, and intracranial hemorrhage. The regular use of heparin in hemodialysis, along with frequent administration of drugs that can cause platelet dysfunction, make it difficult to identify the exact underlying pathophysiology. Many investigators believe that the chief contributing factor is the intrinsic defects in platelet metabolism.

Abnormal bleeding in uremic patients is probably due to a qualitative platelet defect that is manifested by prolonged bleeding time, decreased platelet adhesion to foreign surfaces, reduced platelet aggregation in response to various agents, and abnormal platelet factor 3 availability (Table 5-4). Recently it has also been shown that an abnormality of platelet arachidonic acid metabolism is present in chronically hemodialyzed patients, which results in reduced thromboxane production, and which may be partially responsible for platelet function abnormalities. Several metabolites present in increased quantities in renal failure, such as guanidinosuccinic acid, urea, and phenols, have been shown to adversely affect platelet function, but not with consistent and reproducible results. A quantitative reduction in platelets has also been reported by several investigators, but the qualitative platelet defect is usually more significant in the pathogenesis of uremic bleeding. Severe anemia can also cause prolongation of bleeding time. Transfusion to a hematocrit above 30% has been shown to shorten abnormal bleeding time and to reduce hemorrhagic complications. This beneficial effect was ascribed to improved rheologic aspects of platelet and vessel wall interaction.

Table 5-4. Pathophysiology of Hematologic
Abnormalities: Coagulation

Platelet function abnormalities
Prolonged bleeding time
Decreased platelet factor 3 availability
Decreased platelet aggregation and adhesion
Decreased platelet thromboxane production
Clotting factors
Normal levels of humoral clotting factors
Decreased multimeric factor VIII:VWF?

Table 5-5. Clinical Evaluation of Bleeding

Exclude underlying disease or other cause of bleeding
Evaluate adequacy of dialysis treatment
Evaluate relationship of bleeding to heparin therapy during dialysis
Discontinue drugs that inhibit platelet function
Perform laboratory studies
  Bleeding time
  Platelet count
  Clotting studies (PT, PTT)

A recent report that prostacyclin-like activity may be present in increased amounts in vascular tissue obtained from patients with renal failure and prolonged bleeding time suggests yet another possible factor that may contribute to abnormal hemostasis in uremia.

Clinical Management of Abnormal Bleeding. An approach to the dialysis patient with a bleeding disorder is outlined in Table 5-5. Underlying disease that can result in bleeding must first be excluded. If none is found, then those factors that are related to dialysis should be considered, including whether the patient may have abnormal platelet function secondary to inadequate dialysis or is bleeding as a result of heparin administration. A careful history for use of the many drugs that can cause abnormal platelet function should be obtained. In addition to well-known drugs such as aspirin and nonsteroidal antiinflammatory agents, there are additional minor agents such as diazepam (Valium), chlordiazepoxide (Librium), and diphenhydramine (Benadryl) that may cause abnormal platelet function. The laboratory test of platelet function that correlates best with abnormal bleeding is the modified Ivy bleeding time (template). While other tests of platelet function, such as aggregation and adhesiveness, may be abnormal, they do not correlate well with clinical bleeding.

Treatment of bleeding secondary to qualitative platelet dysfunction is often difficult and challenging, especially in patients who do not respond to the appropriate measures for treatment of their underlying disease or who require surgical and other invasive diagnostic procedures (see Table 5-6). Fortunately, in the past several years several new therapeutic approaches have been found successful in the treatment of uremic bleeding (see Clotting Factors in Table 5-4). In addition to the use of dialysis and blood transfusion, infusion of cryoprecipitate shortens an abnormal bleeding time and can control major bleeding in a majority of patients. The mechanism for this beneficial effect is not yet understood and has not been shown to alter concentrations of clotting factors. The effect by cryoprecipitate is transient: bleeding time returns to pretreatment

Table 5-6. Treatment Options for Abnormal Bleeding
Secondary to Platelet Dysfunction

Optimize dialysis treatment
Discontinue antiplatelet drugs
Transfuse to hematocrit of 30%
Administer cryoprecipitate (10 units)
Administer 1-deamino-8-D-arginine vasopressin (0.3 µg/kg)

levels by 24 hours after infusion. In addition, 1-deamino-8-D-arginine vasopressin (DDAVP) effectively shortens bleeding time both in normal subjects and in uremic patients with prolonged bleeding times and abnormal hemorrhage. Concomitant with the decrease in bleeding time, this agent produces an increase in circulating multimeric forms of Factor VIII:VWF. This effect is also a transient one, with bleeding times returning to baseline after 4–8 hours. Despite their brief duration of action, these two agents may be extremely helfpul in the temporary correction of bleeding time in patients who have life-threatening bleeding or who need surgical procedures. The effectiveness of cryoprecipitate and 1-deamino-8-D-arginine vasopressin with repeated use remains to be demonstrated.

CARDIOVASCULAR COMPLICATIONS

Cardiovascular disease is the most frequent cause of mortality in chronically dialyzed patients. It contributes significantly to morbidity and to common complications requiring therapy and hospitalization and is a limiting factor in rehabilitation and achievement of satisfactory quality of life for many patients. While the incidence of cardiac disease is high in end-stage renal disease patients, it is possible to prevent or attenuate some of the complications, provided that there is early recognition of the problem, with appropriate therapy. The most common cardiovascular disorders encountered in chronically dialyzed patients are listed in Table 5-7. Hypertension, pericardial disease, and atherosclerosis are the most significant in terms of incidence and therapeutic intervention. Of these, hypertension is probably the most important in terms of its frequency and the high incidence of its sequelae, including heart disease, stroke, and coronary artery disease.

Hypertension

The cause of hypertension in chronic renal disease is still incompletely understood, but at least three major factors have been identified that contribute to the development of this common and serious problem, including volume overload, activation of the renin-angiotensin system, and neurologically mediated factors.

In the well-dialyzed patient, accumulation of salt and water in the interdialytic period commonly results in hypertension, which is then normalized with the next dialysis by removal of fluid. The severity of this form of hypertension

Table 5-7. Cardiovascular Complications

Hypertension
Pericardial disease
Atherosclerosis
Cardiac dysfunction
Arrhythmias
Endocarditis

Table 5-8. Management Strategies of Hypertension

Control of sodium and fluid intake
  2-g sodium diet
  Fluid restriction to limit interdialytic weight gain (1.5–2.0 kg)
Effective ultrafiltration during dialysis
Renin-angiotensin inhibition (where appropriate)
  Beta-blockers (e.g., propranolol)
  Captopril
Neurogenic agents
  Prazosin
  Methyldopa
  Clonidine
Vasodilators
  Hydralazine
  Minoxidil
?Calcium channel blockers (e.g., nifedipine)
(Bilateral nephrectomy)

in the majority of patients (65–75%) is directly related to their understanding of and compliance with dietary sodium and fluid restriction, which, when assiduously applied, can result in only minimal elevation of blood pressure, with the major therapeutic control being provided by dialysis treatment. However, in a significant percentage of dialysis patients (as high as 25–50%) this simple approach to control of blood pressure is unsuccessful due to the contribution of other factors related to the etiology of hypertension, to the inability of the patient to conform to the regimen needed to restrict wide fluctuations in extracellular volume or to a combination of these events.

The clear documentation of renin and other neurogenic factors in the pathophysiology of hypertension in the dialyzed patient is often more difficult than demonstration of the volume component. Multiple factors can alter renin release, including wide fluctuations in extracellular volume, drugs, and abnormalities in renin metabolism secondary to renal damage, as well as alterations in neurogenic stimuli and abnormalities of intrarenal baroreceptors and chemoreceptors. Although measurement of renin levels may be difficult to interpret in many situations, it can be helpful when clearly high in inappropriate situations. Clinical response to renin-angiotensin blocking agents, such as captopril or teprotide, may be useful in documenting the renin-mediated component of hypertension. The lack of reliable indicators for sympathetic activity makes it difficult to quantitate the effect of this system on blood pressure control, but many investigators feel that selective modification of sympathetic tone in hypertensive dialysis patients is helpful in controlling blood pressure. Yet another cause for hypertension may be abnormal prostaglandin production by the diseased kidney with increased vascular resistance.

Treatment of hypertension in dialyzed patients is perhaps the single most important component in the nondialytic therapy of end-stage renal disease. The development of a rational approach to therapy of hypertension is outlined in Table 5-8 and, while not universally applied, is a fairly common regimen used to manage significant interdialytic hypertension. Control of dietary salt and water intake is the cornerstone of antihypertensive therapy. Additionally, failure to achieve full removal of accumulated volume with each dialysis will result in suboptimal control and the need for more pharmacologic agents. Suboptimal fluid removal can also initiate a vicious cycle of drug side effects, that in turn reduces patient tolerance of ultrafiltration during dialysis, which then may reduce compliance with the treatment regimen. The techniques used to achieve ultrafiltration during dialysis are discussed in Chapters 3 and 4 and will not be repeated here.

The selection of antipressor agents varies widely among clinicians, but most use beta-blockers and other renin-angiotensin blocking agents as the next logical step in the therapy of hypertension refractory to ultrafiltration. Extensive experience with propranolol has shown it to be effective; the newer, longer acting preparations with cardiac selectivity can be of additional benefit in achieving better patient compliance. The use of captopril is increasing and may be a better choice in patients with previous cardiac failure. Captopril has a delayed half-life in patients with no renal function, however, and thus requires more careful regulation than the beta-blockers. A variety of neurologically active drugs are also successful, including prazosin, methyldopa, and clonidine. A common practice with the use of these agents is to hold the dose prior to dialysis to prevent hypotension during dialysis. The use of vasodilators has also been very effective in this patient population, with hydralazine being widely used and well tolerated by most patients. The newer, more potent vasodilator, minoxidil, has proven a valuable treatment of patients with severe hypertension. It has nearly eliminated the need for bilateral nephrectomy in the small group (approximately 5% of patients) with refractory hypertension. Vasodilators usually require the concomitant use of a beta-blocker to prevent the reflex increase in heart rate and output.

More recently, calcium channel blocking agents have been found to be effective in controlling hypertension. However, their role and effectiveness in the dialysis population remains to be defined.

Pericardial Disease

Once considered one of the hallmarks of end-stage renal disease in the predialysis era, pericarditis remains a relatively common disease in chronically dialyzed patients. Several reviews indicate that the incidence of pericarditis has remained stable at about 14–17% over the past 15 years. The etiology of pericarditis is still unknown, but the temporal associations in some patients of acute pericarditis with surgical procedures, acute catabolic illness, and inadequate dialysis therapy point to increased production and/or ineffective removal of uremic toxins (probably protein metabolites). The seasonal variation and occasional clustering of cases seen in dialysis facilities also suggest a possible role for infectious agents, although this etiology has not been established with certainty.

The common presenting manifestations of acute pericarditis are listed in Table 5-9. The triad of fever, chest pain, and multicomponent pericardial friction rub occurs in a majority of patients. However, in occasional patients, an atypical presentation of hypotension, especially during dialysis, with clotting of vascular

Table 5-9. Clinical Features of Pericardial Disease

	Acute Pericarditis	Constrictive Pericardial Disease

Presenting manifestations	Chest pain
	Friction rub
	Fever
	Hypotension
	Intolerance of ultrafiltration on
	   dialysis
	Arrhythmias
	Cardiomegaly
	Clotting of vascular access
		Hypotension
		Weight gain
		Fatigue
		Dyspnea
		Ascites
		Normal to increased heart size
		Absence of pulmonary vascular
		   congestion

Complications	Hemorrhagic pericardial effusion Tamponade Arrhythmias Cardiac failure Pleural effusion	Cardiac failure Wasting
Diagnostic procedures	Chest x-ray Electrocardiogram Echocardiography Nuclear magnetic resonance Cardiac catheterization	Chest x-ray Electrocardiogram Cardiac catherization

Management	Optimize dialysis therapy
	   (increased intensity variable)
	Good nutrition
	Control hydration
	Avoid depletion of intravascular
	   volume with dialysis
	Controlled heparinization
	Antiinflammatory drugs
	Intrapericardial steroids
	Surgical drainage of pericardial
	   effusion
		Partial or total pericardiectomy

access may precede the typical clinical symptoms and should always be a signal to evaluate the patient carefully for undiagnosed pericardial disease. Myocarditis with arrhythmias and cardiac failure may also be present.

The major consequence of pericarditis is the development of pericardial effusion, which is variable in quantity, rapidity of formation, and duration. When the effusion is large, or rapidly expands secondary to hemorrhage or to fluid overload, the patient is at serious risk of tamponade and significant compromise of cardiac function. Diagnosis and quantitation of pericardial effusion is easily performed by echocardiography.

The presence of early pericardial tamponade can be evaluated with chest x-ray and measurement of paradoxical pulse. However, right heart catherization should be performed without delay in those patients with clinical evidence of cardiac compromise secondary to tamponade.

The management of pericarditis includes increased intensity and efficiency of dialysis, especially if the patient was underdialyzed prior to onset of pericarditis. The provision of good nutrition is important to provide adequate calories and protein to prevent further tissue catabolism. Volume overload is common secondary to decreased tolerance of ultrafiltration with dialysis; thus, greater dietary sodium restriction may be needed. It is important, however, to avoid intravascular volume depletion during dialysis, since higher filling pressures may be required to maintain cardiac output. Excessively rapid fluid removal can cause a sudden decrease in intramyocardial pressure, which had been resisting compression, and thus result in tamponade. Because uremic pericardial effusions are almost always hemorrhagic, and the pericardium is lined with friable vessels, the avoidance of excessive systemic heparinization is desirable. Low-dose heparin should be used if the patient is hemodialyzed. In those patients with significant symptoms from chest pain and fever, treatment with antiinflammatory drugs is usually beneficial. Indomethacin and other nonsteroidal antiinflammatory agents are most commonly employed. Both systemic steroids and nonabsorbable steroids instilled into the perdicardium through a percutaneous catheter have also been shown to be effective in reducing symptoms. However, it has not been shown convincingly that the use of any of these pharmacologic agents results in shortening illness or in limiting the incidence of other complications.

In over 75% of patients treated with the measures described above, pericarditis will respond satisfactorily, with full resolution over 2–4 weeks. In some patients, however, large effusions result in pericardial tamponade and require surgical intervention to preserve cardiac function. The proper management of pericardial tamponade remains controversial, and while many approaches have been successfully used, the risks associated with each procedure must be carefully evaluated in each individual situation. The risks of pericardiocentesis are high and significant mortality and morbidity can result from vessel and/or myocardial perforation. It is considered safer by many clinicians to use an open procedure for the aspiration of fluid. If pericardial effusion recurs rapidly, either after initial drainage or when loculation prevents full drainage, then an open pericardiactomy should be performed without further delay.

Chronic constrictive pericarditis occurs in a small number of patients within weeks to months following an acute episode of pericarditis. Common presenting manifestations are quite different from those of acute pericarditis: hypotension, fluid overload, fatigue, dyspnea, and ascites. Unless recognized, diagnosed with cardiac catheterization, and treated with surgical pericardial stripping, many of these patients have an unfavorable outcome.

Atherosclerosis

Cardiac disease secondary to atherosclerosis has been estimated to account for over 60% of deaths in long-term dialysis patients. The risk of dying from atherosclerosis has been shown to increase with duration of therapy. Some authors have suggested that atherosclerotic disease is more common in end-stage-renal disease patients than in the nonuremic population. Others, however, have not confirmed a higher incidence of atherosclerotic disease in end-stage renal disease patients when the multiple risk factors present in these patients (Table 5-10) are taken into consideration. There is thus some controversy about the

Table 5-10. Risk Factors for Atherosclerosis

Hypertension
Hyperlipidemia
Abnormal calcium and phosphorus metabolism
Hyperparathyroidism
Abnormal carbohydrate metabolism
Smoking
Sedentery lifestyle

effects of chronic uremia and dialytic therapy on the pathogenesis of atherosclerosis. Survival of chronic dialysis patients with atherosclerotic heart disease is shortened, with a first-year mortality of 25%, compared with 10% in nonaffected patients. As a result of the high incidence of this disease, the clinical problems of angina, peripheral vascular insufficiency, acute myocardial infarction, and cardiac failure are commonly encountered in dialyzed patients. In general, the management of these problems is similar to that for nondialyzed patients; however, the multisystem complications of uremia often make the medical care of these disorders more complex. A common example of this complexity is the superimposition of severe anemia in a patient with symptomatic coronary artery disease. In addition, the stress and attendant risks of dialysis can add to the challenge of controlling the severity of cardiac symptoms and may add to the development of cardiac complications such as arrhythmias, hypotension, and hypokalemia. Some of the special requirements for treatment of atherosclerotic disease in dialysis patients are listed in Table 5-11. More aggressive treatment of anemia to keep the hematocrit $\geq$30% is important in patients who develop tissue hypoxia and allows better tolerance of ultrafiltration with hemodialysis. Control of fluid status is especially important, both to prevent extracellular volume excess, with its resultant strain on cardiac status, and also to avoid to need for ultrafiltration of large volumes, which is often complicated

Table 5-11. Clinical Management of Atherosclerotic Disease

Disorder	Management
Coronary artery disease	
Angina	Maintain hematocrit $\geq$30%
	Control dietary fluid to minimize ultrafiltration requirements
	Conventional pharmacologic agents
Acute myocardial infarction	Delay dialysis 24–48 hours
	Restrict fluid intake
	Transfuse to hematocrit $\geq$30%
	Conventional treatment of pain, arrhythmias, etc.
	Consider peritoneal dialysis if hypotension, arrhythmias are present
Peripheral vascular insufficiency	Avoid hypotension with dialytic therapy
	Control calcium and phosphate levels to avoid soft tissue calcification
	Avoid placement of vascular access in lower extremities
	Transfer to peritoneal dialysis if vascular access is a major problem
Cerebrovascular accident	Avoid heparin with acute bleeding
	Control fluid carefully

by hypotension with aggravation of angina and myocardial ischemia. Patients with severe myocardial dysfunction often walk a very fine line between congestive heart failure secondary to fluid overload, and myocardial ischemia and low output induced by hypotension. Only a few kilograms in either direction can cause symptoms. Thus, dietary management of salt and water, as well as skillful dialysis therapy, is of great importance in these patients.

Patients with peripheral vascular insufficiency are at particular risk of developing hypotension, which significantly aggravates symptoms. Placement of vascular access must also be done with care to avoid both further compromise of distal arterial flow and steal syndromes. The presence of severe vascular compromise and difficulty with vascular access performance may be indications for peritoneal dialysis in this type of patient.

In the patient with established atherosclerotic disease, it may be argued that treatment of the risk factors listed in Table 5-10 may be too late. However, it is possible that progression of the disease may be slowed by treatment or reversal of as many of these abnormalities as is clinically feasible. In particular, control of hypertension, prevention of further vascular calcification by normalization of calcium and phosphorous levels, discontinuation of smoking, and moderate exercise can be achieved in many patients and may lengthen survival.

Cardiac Dysfunction

Abnormal cardiac function leading to cardiac failure is well documented in both acute and chronic renal insufficiency, and occurs in a smaller percentage of chronically dialyzed patients as well. The major clinical manifestations of cardiac dysfunction include left ventricular dysfunction with congestive heart failure and, uncommonly, a clinical picture of cardiomyopathy. Many abnormalities present in chronically dialyzed patients have been implicated in the pathogenesis of these abnormalities, which are listed in Table 5-12. A prominent cause of cardiac failure in dialysis patients is volume overload due to noncompliance with dietary restrictions and/or inadequate removal of excess fluid with dialysis therapy. Hypertension, as a result of increased extracellular volume, may secondarily cause additional cardiac dysfunction by increasing afterload. In patients who present with pulmonary edema due to pure volume overload, prompt ultrafitration to reduce extracellular volume will improve cardiac function; no other therapy is usually required. Anemia can affect cardiac performance by increasing cardiac output and reducing peripheral resistance. Treatment of this factor is achieved by raising the hematocrit to $\geq 30\%$ (Table 5-3). The presence of an arteriovenous fistula, which rarely may have flows of up to 25–30% of cardiac output, creates an additional demand on cardiac performance. Documentation of excessive fistula blood flow can be documented by the presence of bradycardia when the flow through the fistula is acutely compressed (positive Nicoladani-Branham sign).

The role of uremia per se on myocardial function has been debated for many years. Recently, an effect of dialysis therapy on ventricular performance has been

Table 5-12. Pathogenesis of Cardiac Dysfunction

Factor	Possible Effects
Volume overload	Increased peripheral resistance
	Increased end-diastolic volume (preload)
	Increased cardiac output
	Hypertension (afterload)
Anemia	Increased cardiac output
	Low peripheral resistance
Arteriovenous fistula	Increased cardiac output
	Low peripheral resistance
Uremia	Increased pulmonary capillary permeability ("uremic lung")
	"Uremic cardiomyopathy"
	Left ventricular dysfunction (contractility)
	Abnormal baroreceptor response
Electrolyte abnormalities	Decreased myocardial contractility
	Increased vascular resistance
	Soft tissue calcification
	Arrhythmias
Atherosclerosis	Decreased cardiac output and ejection fraction

clearly delineated, separate from volume changes. An increase in left ventricular contractility (as measured by velocity of circumferential fiber shortening) has been documented shortly after completion of regular dialysis therapy. An increase in serum ionized calcium during dialysis correlated with the change in ventricular performance.

Uremia may also indirectly affect cardiac function by a direct effect on capillary permeability, which results in pulmonary interstitial edema in the absence of elevated pressure in the pulmonary vasculature. This syndrome, termed "uremic lung," may have an atypical radiographic appearance, either with fluid unilaterally or localized to certain areas of the lung. This abnormality of capillary permeability usually responds to dialysis therapy with effective removal of uremic toxins rather than fluid.

Significant fluctuations in serum potassium can occur during the interdialytic interval from relatively low normal or subnormal levels immediately following dialysis to elevated levels before the next dialysis. These changes can have an effect on peripheral vascular resistance, as well as on cardiac rhythm and performance. If cardiac glycosides are used, these changes can result in varying myocardial response to the effects of the drug. As discussed in Chapter 3, avoidance of these wide changes in serum potassium concentration can be achieved by a combination of moderate dietary restriction of potassium to 2 g/ day and the prescription of a dialysate potassium concentration to keep potassium levels within the normal range. More constant stabilization of serum potassium levels is achieved with the use of continuous ambulatory peritoneal dialysis.

Fluctuations in ionized calcium and magnesium levels also occur in intermittently dialyzed patients, in part due to removal of anions that complex these cations, and to changes in plasma acid-base composition. As discussed above, changes in calcium concentration may affect myocardial contractility directly and may indirectly affect myocardial function by altering peripheral vessels and hence vascular resistance. Severely elevated calcium and phosphorus concentrations can cause calcification of myocardial tissue and result in conduction disturbances as well as valvular calcification and dysfunction.

Many patients have incomplete correction of metabolic acidosis and develop mild to moderate reduction of serum pH between dialysis treatments. This acidemia is usually not severe enough to cause myocardial depression.

Finally, it must be recognized that the presence of underlying atherosclerotic disease may significantly decrease cardiac function and result in decreased cardiac output and ejection fraction.

The treatment of the patient with chronic severe cardiac disease is very difficult and requires the combination of optimal dialytic maneuvers, to remove volume and control electrolyte shifts, with careful pharmacologic and dietary management in the interdialytic period. Patient education and compliance with the treatment regimen is very important.

Arrhythmias

Significant arrhythmias commonly occur during dialysis. Therapies for this problem include adjustment of the dialysate potassium concentration and the use of antiarrhythmic agents prior to dialysis. In some patients, usually those with underlying atherosclerotic heart disease, arrhythmias may be controlled by continuous drug treatment and careful control of other factors that induce rhythm disturbances, including volume changes, hypotension, hypercalcemia (due to overuse of calcium supplements and vitamin D) and severe anemia. The presence of hyperkalemia and hypocalcemia together significantly increase the incidence of rhythm disturbances. Hypokalemia and hypomagnesemia may precipitate digitalis toxicity.

There is a stable incidence of sudden death in 1–2% of dialysis patients each year. Such deaths often occur in young, healthy patients as well as in individuals with known cardiac disease, and probably result from dietary-induced severe hyperkalemia. These deaths are particularly disturbing because they are potentially preventable, and frustrating because the patients are frequently individuals who resist dietary control of potassium or deny the real and present danger of hyperkalemia. The most common clinical symptoms of such life-threatening hyperkalemia is muscle weakness, often severe enough to prevent ambulation. When these symptoms occur, the patient must be transported immediately to the hospital or dialysis center and dialysis initiated.

Endocarditis

Bacterial endocarditis has been documented as a cause of death in as many as 1–2% of dialysis patients. The true incidence of this complication may be difficult to determine, since sepsis in association with infection of the arteriovenous fistula may be difficult to distinguish from endocardial infection, which itself is introduced by venipunctures of the arteriovenous fistula. Most of these infections are caused by skin organisms, including *Staphylococcus aureus* and *S. epidermidis*. Occasionally streptococci and other bacteria are involved, which suggests other sources of infection than the vascular access site. The diagnosis of endocarditis may be a difficult one, since many patients have flow murmurs, fever may be variable, and mild neurologic symptoms can be attributed to disequilibrium and dialysis-related events. Endovascular graft infection is likewise a difficult diagnosis to make since superficial signs of infection may be minimal or absent. Thus, in many instances, the presence of positive blood cultures with equivocal documentation of endocarditis or graft infection must be treated as presumed endocarditis with 4 to 6 weeks of antibiotic therapy. Careful follow-up of valvular function and cardiac performance and repeat blood cultures are necessary to avoid serious complications and potential mortality.

RENAL OSTEODYSTROPHY

Renal osteodystrophy can be diagnosed histologically in nearly all patients with end-stage-renal disease, although the clinical manifestations are variable in severity and expression. Phosphorus retention and hypocalcemia (sometimes mild and subclinical) are present at some time in most of these patients, who also have elevated serum levels of parathyroid hormone (PTH) and reduced production of calcitriol, $1,25(OH_2)D_3$. In a few patients, progressive skeletal disease is a major cause of physical disability that may limit rehabilitation and even survival. The complex metabolic and structural abnormalities that comprise this disorder include disturbances of mineral metabolism and altered regulation of several hormones, causing pathologically distinct patterns of bone disease.

In addition to these clearly recognizable derangements of skeletal and mineral homeostasis, some features of renal osteodystrophy, particularly the excess production of parathyroid hormone, have also been implicated in the production of uremic symptoms in other organ systems, as summarized in Table 5-13. Parathyroid hormone is considered by some investigators to be an important uremic toxin.

Pathophysiology of Bone Disease

In most patients the onset of renal osteodystrophy probably occurs relatively early in the course of chronic renal insufficiency and is usually well established by the time dialysis is required. The pathogenesis of renal osteodystrophy is complex and incompletely understood; the major factors believed to be causative in this disorder are summarized in Table 5-14.

Two major patterns of bone disease are widely recognized as characteristic of renal osteodystrophy although the pathology of these two types may overlap or coexist in a given patient.

Secondary hyperparathyroidism is the predominant metabolic disturbance of renal osteodystrophy and is manifested in bone by the development of osteitis

Table 5-13. Extraskeletal Disorders
Attributed to Hyperparathyroidism

Proximal myopathy
Anemia
Metabolic disturbances
  Increased catabolism
  Insulin resistance
  Hypertriglyceridemia
  Sexual dysfunction
  Gonadal dysfunction
Neurologic disease
  Peripheral neuropathy
  Abnormal cognitive function
  Electroencephalogram abnormalities
  Personality changes
Dermatologic abnormalities
  Pruritis
  Cutaneous calcification
  Calciphylaxis
Eye disease
  Band keratopathy
  Conjunctival calcification
Cardiovascular disease
  Hypertension
  Cardiac conduction disturbances
  Vascular calcification
Visceral calcification
  Lung
  Heart
  Kidneys

fibrosa cystica. The major pathogenic factor in this disorder is considered to be phosphorus retention, which occurs early in the course of renal failure and leads to progressive, stepwise increases in serum parathyroid hormone levels, which in turn causes skeletal disease. Diminished production of active vitamin D metabolites, as a result of loss of functioning kidney tissue, also plays an important

Table 5-14. Pathogenesis of Renal Osteodystrophy

Hypocalcemia and secondary hyperparathyroidism
  Abnormal vitamin D metabolism
  Hyperphosphatemia
  Increased parathyroid hormone levels and impaired metabolism
  Skeletal resistance to parathyroid hormone
Abnormal skeletal mineralization
  Abnormal collagen synthesis and maturation
  Altered vitamin D metabolism
  Phosphorus depletion
  Abnormal parathyroid hormone levels/response
  Abnormal bone mineral composition
    Magnesium
    Pyrophosphate
    Carbonate
  Toxins
    Aluminum
    Fluoride
    Heparin
    Drugs
  Chronic acidosis

role in hypocalcemia and contributes to the pathogenesis of secondary hyper-parathyroidism. As renal function is progressively lost, hypocalcemia resulting from lack of vitamin D and from phosphorus retention becomes more severe and is associated with rising levels of serum parathyroid hormone. Despite higher levels of circulating parathyroid hormone, mobilization of calcium from bone of patients with renal failure does not occur normally, a state that is referred to as skeletal resistance to parathyroid hormone, which further contributes to hypocalcemia. Parathyroid hormone is metabolized by bone and kidney, with the inactive C-terminal fragment excreted in the urine. Thus, a further consequence of declining renal function is retention of parathyroid hormone metabolites.

Osteomalacia or defective skeletal mineralization is a second major pathologic expression of renal osteodystrophy, which is present in a smaller percentage of patients than secondary hyperparathyroidism. The pathogenesis of this disorder and its relationship to the other skeletal manifestations of renal osteodystrophy remain poorly understood. Present evidence suggests that defective mineralization in dialysis patients does not result primarily from a deficiency of vitamin D as is the case with classic nutritional rickets or osteomalacia. Serum levels of vitamin D_3 and $25(OH)D_3$ have been found to be normal or actually increased in many patients and treatment with multiple forms of vitamin D metabolites has been generally unsuccessful in most patients with osteomalacia. It is possible that several different mechanisms may contribute to the pathogenesis of this disease, but the cause(s) is poorly understood. In a small number of patients, it seems well established that chronic phosphorus depletion resulting from dialysis losses and gastrointestinal malabsorption of phosphorus can lead to osteomalacia; improvement has been noted with phosphorus repletion. There is also a reported relationship of osteomalacia to the use of dialysate prepared with water containing significant amounts of aluminum. Initial reports of clusters of cases from England as well as sporadic reports from other geographic areas has led to documentation that aluminum deposition in bone, specifically along the mineralization front of osteoid, is present more frequently and in greater quantity in patients with defective mineralization of bone. Whether aluminum is a causative factor in this defective bone metabolism remains the subject of intensive investigation. Animal models suggest that aluminum does cause a decrease of total bone and matrix formation, a delay in mineralization and osteoid maturation rate, and increased bone resorption. Because many patients with severe osteomalacia have relatively low or frankly subnormal levels of parathyroid hormone, it has been postulated that the lack of this hormone many contribute to defective mineralization by a reduction in bone turnover. Finally, other factors that have been implicated in the pathogenesis of defective mineralization include abnormal collagen synthesis and abnormal maturation of the osteoid matrix. Impaired nutrition with blunted growth in children may contribute to such abnormalities. Studies of uremic bone composition have revealed that mineral content is abnormal, including increased quantities of magnesium. The presence of chronic acidosis results in gradual loss of bone salts as they are used to buffer the extracellular fluid, a process which would contribute to demineralization of the skeleton.

Clinical Features of Bone Disease

The clinical features of renal osteodystrophy in chronically dialyzed patients can be distinguished for secondary hyperparathyroidism and osteomalacia. There is overlap of some symptoms between the two categories, and both disorders may coexist in some patients. Nevertheless, the contrast between symptoms and other pathophysiologic features in these two disturbances are useful in the clinical diagnosis and management of this challenging complication of end-stage renal disease.

The clinical signs and symptoms of renal osteodystrophy are summarized in Table 5-15. The variety of symptoms that can occur with hyperparathyroidism is much greater than those that usually occur with osteomalacia, but the frequency and severity of skeletal symptoms is significantly higher in patients with osteomalacia. For instance, bone pain can occur in patients with advanced hyperparathyroidism, but is commonly a presenting complaint of osteomalacia, and may progress to severe disabling disease with multiple pathologic fractures, bone deformities, and chronic unremitting pain. Some bone abnormalities seen primarily with hyperparathyroidism and not with osteomalacia include vascular necrosis (especially of the femoral heads), spontaneous tendon ruptures, and occasionally a slipped epiphysis.

Joint symptoms are more common with hyperparathyroidism, including a variety of articular abnormalities, many of which are mediated by abnormal calcification of joint structures. Pseudogout, with deposition of calcium oxalate crystals in the joint fluid, accompanied by acute inflammation, pain, and swelling, is relatively common. Arthrocentesis and microscopic evaluation of the joint fluid is necessary to distinguish this entity from acute gouty arthritis, which symptomatically it resembles closely. Calcification of the joint capsule, tendon sheaths, and other adjacent tissues without abnormality of the joint fluid is known as acute periarthritis and can also mimic acute gout or pseudogout. Synovial tissue biopsy may reveal calcium crystals characteristic of hydroxyapatite, and periarticular calcification may be visible radiographically. Control

Table 5-15. Clinical Signs and Symptoms in Renal Osteodystrophy

Secondary Hyperparathyroidism	Osteomalacia
Musculoskeletal	Bone pain
Bone pain	Proximal muscle weakness
Fractures	Fractures
Slipped epiphyses	Skeletal deformities
Tendon rupture	Dialysis encephalopathy
Avascular necrosis	
Joint disease	
Pseudogout	
Calcific periarthritis	
Tumoral calcification	
Pruritis	
Soft tissue calcification	
Skin	
Calciphylaxis (ischemic ulcers of digits)	
Eye	
Hypertension	

of calcium and phosphorus levels and treatment of hyperparathyroidism will often result in clinical improvement of these entities. In patients with severe hyperparathyroidism and marked elevation of the product of calcium and phosphate concentrations, large masses of amorphous calcium may deposit around the more proximal joints, which is referred to as tumoral calcinosis; this can also be successfully treated by lowering the high serum phosphorus levels and results in resorption of the calcium deposits.

Pruritis is frequently present in dialyzed patients and may be associated with several distinct abnormalities, of which the most common is secondary hyperparathyroidism. In this setting, itching can usually be correlated with elevation of serum phosphorus and hence calcium-phosphate product and may be effectively treated with control of phosphorus levels. It has been suggested that very high parathyroid hormone levels may be causally related to intense unremitting pruritis, and the pruritis can be dramatically improved by parathyroidectomy. However, not all patients are benefited by parathyroid surgery, and clear documentation of the role of parathyroid hormone itself or the deposition of calcium in skin as a cause of pruritis has not been obtained. Skin content of calcium and magnesium have been shown to be elevated in dialysis patients, and occasionally the skin deposition of calcium can be visible as raised lesions that are usually surrounded by excoriations. In patients with very severe disease and associated small vessel calcification, an extremely serious complication can occur marked by ischemic, penetrating ulcers of the digits. This disorder, known as calciphylaxis, can result in loss of digits and, if widespread, in death due to secondary infection. It can be controlled to some extent by maintenance of phosphorus levels in the normal range but may require parathyroidectomy. Another common site of soft tissue calcification associated with hyperparathyroidism is the eye, both in the cornea, in a characteristic distribution known as band keratopathy, and in the conjunctiva, which mimics acute conjunctivitis and has been termed the "red eye syndrome."

Hypercalcemia may be associated with hypertension, or increased severity of hypertension. The pathogenesis of this association is unknown, but the known effects of calcium on vascular smooth muscle and the pharmacologic effects of calcium channel blocking agents suggest that elevated serum calcium levels may have a direct effect on vascular resistance and hence on blood pressure control.

Biochemical, radiographic, and skeletal pathologic features of renal osteodystrophy are summarized in Table 5-16. Secondary hyperparathyroidism is characterized biochemically by variable serum calcium concentration, by an elevated serum phosphorus, and by very high parathyroid hormone levels. Alkaline phosphatase is usually elevated and may be extremely high when bone turnover and formation rates are increased. Spontaneous hypercalcemia may occur when parathyroid gland hyperplasia is marked and may be an indication for subtotal parathyroidectomy. In contrast, patients with predominant osteomalacia on bone biopsy frequently have low or normal calcium concentrations and moderate increases in phosphorus levels. Parathyroid hormone may be normal or only modestly elevated. Alkaline phosphatase is frequently normal as well. When calcium supplements or vitamin D is given, however, serum calcium

Table 5-16. Biochemical, Radiographic, and Pathologic Features of Renal Osteodystrophy

Examination	Secondary Hyperparathyroidism	Osteomalacia

Biochemical	Calcium ↓, N, or ↑
	Phosphorus ↑ ↑
	Magnesium ↑
	Parathyroid hormone ↑ ↑ ↑
	Alkaline phosphatase ↑ ↑
	Vitamin D
	  25(OH)D$_3$ N
	  1,25(OH)$_2$D$_3$ ↓ ↓
	  24,25(OH)$_2$D$_3$ ↓
		Calcium N (or ↑ ↑ with vitamin D)
		Phosphorus N or ↑
		Magnesium ↑
		Parathyroid hormone N or ↑
		Alkaline phosphatase N
		Vitamin D
		  25(OH)d$_3$ N
		  1,25(OH)$_2$D$_3$ ↓ ↓
		  24,25(OH)$_2$D$_3$ ↓

Radiographic	Subperiosteal erosion Cortical striations Cyst formation (brown tumor) "Salt and pepper" skull "Rugger-jersey" spine Periosteal new bone formation Osteonecrosis Osteosclerosis Slipped epiphysis Soft tissue calcification (vascular, joint, visceral)	Diffuse demineralization Pseudofractures (Looser's zones) Skeletal deformities Spontaneous fractures Vertebral collapse

Bone pathology	Osteitis fibrosa cystica
	  Increased bone turnover
	  Marrow fibrosis
	  "Woven bone"
		Increased osteoid seam width and osteoid volume
		Delayed mineralization
		Inactive bone surface increased
		Aluminum deposition at mineralization front

N = normal.

tends to rise sharply, and many patients can tolerate only small doses of each. Vitamin D concentrations are usually depressed in dialysis patients, except for 25(OH)D$_3$, which is normal.

As is the case with the spectrum of clinical symptoms, the radiographic abnormalities that can be seen with secondary hyperparathyroidism are quite numerous and varied in presentation. The classic feature is subperiosteal erosion, best seen along the medical aspect of the middle phalanges, the distal clavicle, and the distal tufts of the phalanges. Cortical striations and cyst formation are frequently present. Increased resorption of the skull causes a mottled "salt and pepper" appearance. Osteosclerosis of the superior and inferior edges, with demineralization of the middle section of the vertebral bodies, causes the typical "rugger-jersey" spine appearance. Osteosclerosis is occasionally seen in patients with long-standing hyperparathyroidism and may represent dense calcification of abnormal quantities of woven bone. Periosteal new bone formation, occurring along the shafts of the long bones can occasionally be seen in hyperparathyroidism, as well as avascular necrosis of the femoral heads.

The radiographic features of osteomalacia are much less striking and may go undetected on routine examination. The major abnormality consists of diffuse demineralization with the occasional appearance of classic Looser's zones, or lucent bands running perpendicular to the cortex of the upper femurs. The other common feature is pathologic fractures occurring in the ribs and weight-bearing areas, especially the pelvis and femurs. Vertebral collapse and marked bone deformity may also occur in severe cases.

The pathologic features of secondary hyperparathyroidism are those of osteitis fibrosa cystica, characterized by increased bone resorption and formation rates, fibrosis of the marrow space, and the presence of abnormal mineralization patterns of irregular bone, called "woven" bone. By contrast, the appearance of the bone in osteomalacia is quite different, with large quantities of unmineralized osteoid, which covers a large portion of the bone surface and appears inactive in that fewer osteoclasts and osteoblasts are evident. Dynamic histomorphometry with tetracycline labeling often shows little or no uptake, indicating markedly reduced mineralization activity. As discussed above under pathogenesis, special stains for aluminum often reveal increased quantities of this mineral along the mineralization front.

Therapy for Bone Disease

The treatment of renal osteodystrophy in the dialyzed patient presents a constant challenge and requires frequent manipulation of diet and pharmacologic agents to achieve acceptable control of serum calcium, phosphorus, and magnesium levels.

Phosphorus. Virtually all patients require therapy to control serum phosphorus. The goal is to prevent hyperphosphatemia, which results in lowering of serum calcium and further stimulation of parathyroid hormone and which places the patient at risk for soft tissue calcification. Target levels for serum phosphorus vary among clinicians, but a predialysis phosphorus level of 4.5–5.0 mg/dl is reasonable and allows some room for removal of phosphorus with dialysis while avoiding severe postdialysis hypophosphatemia. The major therapeutic approaches to control of phosphorus are (1) dietary restriction to 800–1000 mg/day; (2) oral phosphorus binders, of which the most commonly used is aluminum hydroxide; and (3) dialysis therapy. Dietary restriction tends to be underemphasized, but it is important because large unrestricted intake of foods containing phosphorus can exceed the capacity of phosphorus binders and dialysis to control serum phosphorus. Dietary noncompliance often results in escalating doses of binders, which the patient finds unpalatable or which produce constipation. In addition, excessive use of phosphate binders may be harmful, since there is evidence that aluminum deposition in bone may play a role in the pathogenesis of osteomalacia. Serum aluminum levels are correlated with the quantity of aluminum ingested as phosphate binders. The oral route is probably the significant source of this toxin. Thus, dietary phosphorus should be controlled to minimize the need for oral aluminum-containing phosphate binders.

Significant amounts of phosphorus can be removed by dialysis, especially with large surface area, efficient dialyzers, but this alone is usually not adequate to control serum phosphorus in most patients.

Calcium. The next objective is to maintain serum calcium in the normal range to minimize parathyroid hormone stimulation. This can be achieved in several ways. The first is to supplement the diet with calcium in the form of calcium carbonate ($CaCO_3$), since moderate dietary protein and phosphorus restriction obligates a significant reduction of dietary calcium. For instance, a protein intake of 1.0 g protein/kg/day with 800 mg of phosphorus will reduce dietary calcium to only 400 mg daily, ~50% of the recommended intake. Thus, most patients require oral calcium supplements to maintain an intake of 1000–1500 mg/day. Because of variable malabsorption of calcium by the gastrointestinal tract secondary to vitamin D deficiency, higher supplements are required in some patients to maintain a normal serum calcium. If the patient has significant bone demineralization and is avidly repleting calcium in bone, then even larger quantities of calcium (e.g., 5–10 g/day) may be required.

It is now customary to use dialysate containing calcium in a concentration of 3.0–3.5 mEq/L, or 6.0–7.0 mg/dl. Since this is ionized calcium, a favorable gradient for transport of calcium from dialysate to the patient exists. A positive calcium balance of several hundred milligrams occurs with each dialysis. Patients treated with chronic peritoneal dialysis have a less positive gradient and do not obtain significant quantities of calcium by dialysis.

Finally, calcium absorption can be increased by the administration of vitamin D analogs (dihydrotachysterol) or metabolites (calcifediol, calcitriol). Their use is indicated in patients who remain hypocalcemic despite adequate dialysate calcium concentrations and oral calcium supplements.

Magnesium. Since magnesium accumulates in dialysis patients, both in bone and soft tissue, it is important to limit the body load of magnesium by using minimal quantities in dialysate (<1.0 mEq/L) and by avoiding magnesium-containing drugs (laxatives, antacids, etc.)

Dialysate Water Treatment. Current standards established by the Association for Advancement of Medical Instrumentation (AAMI) require that there is appropriate water treatment for preparation of dialysate to remove potentially harmful minerals and substances, as discussed in Chapter 1. Water treatment is especially important in the treatment of renal osteodystrophy because (1) it removes excess calcium and other minerals and allows the use of a controlled and optimal dialysate calcium concentration; (2) it removes aluminum, which can be deposited in bone and may contribute to the development of osteomalacia; (3) it removes fluoride, known to be a cause of osteomalacia in those parts of the world where endemic water supplies contain large quantities of this mineral.

Specific Therapy for Established Renal Osteodystrophy. Despite the careful application of therapy to control calcium and phosphorus levels, many dialysis patients eventually progress to the development of clinically apparent and even symptomatic bone disease. In patients with clinical evidence of hyperparathyroidism (i.e., increased parathyroid hormone and alkaline phosphatase, with radiographic changes) therapy with vitamin D should be given. Many studies in the literature indicate that various forms of vitamin D are equally effective in this situation and thus can be selected by other criteria such as cost and duration of drug action. When any vitamin D preparation is being used, however, it is important to monitor serum calcium at appropriate intervals to adjust the dose until clinical parameters of bone improvement are reached, such as lowering of the alkaline phosphatase into the normal range and healing of bone lesions on x-rays. In some patients with severe disease or in whom control cannot be achieved with vitamin D therapy, subtotal parathyroidectomy may be needed. The usual indications for this procedure are listed in Table 5-17, but must be individualized for each patient. Most patients tolerate parathyroid surgery well, but it does carry the risk of permanent hypoparathyroidism should the remnant gland not be functional and is sometimes unsuccessful if all four glands cannot be located at surgery.

Treatment of osteomalacia is much more difficult. After optimal control of calcium and phosphorus levels and treatment of dialysate water, the disease may continue to progress. Some patients have severe disability due to pain, weakness, and fractures. The use of vitamin D, in particular $25(OH)D_3$, is occasionally helpful in controlling bone pain and symptoms although significant histologic improvement is not often seen. The combination of $24,25(OH)_2D_3$ and $1,25(OH)_2D_3$ has been reported to be effective in a few patients, but more commonly the use of these potent metabolites results in marked hypercalcemia. Since the possible role of aluminum has been documented, attempts to remove excess aluminum with the chelating agent, desferroxamine, have been undertaken with some success. Patients on both hemodialysis and peritoneal dialysis have been administered this drug intravenously; this results in an elevation of serum levels of aluminum bound to the drug, which can then be removed with either form of dialysis. Studies to document histologic as well as clinical improvement of

Table 5-17. Management and Treatment of Renal Osteodystrophy

Secondary Hyperparathyroidism	Osteomalacia
Control phosphate	Normalize calcium and phosphate
Diet	Vitamin D
Binders [$Al(OH)_3$]	$25(OH)D_3$
Dialysis	$24,25(OH)_2D_3$
Normalize serum calcium	Treat water used for dialysis
Calcium carbonate	Desferroxamine to remove aluminum
Dialysis	Avoid parathyroidectomy
Vitamin D	
Dihydrotachysterol	
$25(OH)D_3$	
$1,25(OH)_2D_3$	
Dialysate water treatment	
Parathyroidectomy for	
Persistant ↑ calcium (≥ 11.5 mg/dl)	
Progressive soft tissue calcification	
Calciphylaxis	
Intractable pruritis	
Progressive bone disease unresponsive to	
vitamin D	

Table 5-18. Joint Diseases
Gout
Pseudogout
Calcific periarthritis
Tumoral calcification
Recurrent hemarthrosis
Carpal tunnel syndrome
Septic arthritis
Avascular necrosis

the bone disease with this therapy are currently underway. Because of the potentially adverse effects of low parathyroid hormone levels in patients with osteomalacia, it has been generally advocated that parathyroidectomy not be performed in patients with this form of bone disease. If a patient presents with bone pain but other symptoms and radiographic features are not typical of hyperparathyroidism, a bone biopsy should be performed to look for osteomalacia before proceeding with parathyroidectomy.

Osteomalacia and Dialysis Dementia. Following the initial description of the syndrome known as dialysis dementia or encephalopathy in 1972, this disorder, occurring with bone pain, fractures, and osteomalacia on bone biopsy, began to be reported. A strong relationship between dialysis dementia and osteomalacia has subsequently been demonstrated by several groups of investigators. The presence of aluminum in bone and in the brain tissue of these patients suggests this agent may be the common denominator or perhaps causative factor in the pathogenesis of this disorder.

Joint Abnormalities. Although many of the joint abnormalities listed in Table 5-15 are related to hyperparathyroidism, there are other forms of arthritis and joint disease in end-stage renal disease patients with different causes. A list of joint diseases encountered in dialysis patients is summarized in Table 5-18.

Gout usually occurs in those patients with a history of gout prior to starting dialysis. The diagnosis and management is similar to that for nondialyzed patients. Pseudogout, calcific periarthritis, and tumoral calcification have been described above under joint complications associated with soft tissue calcification.

A pattern of recurrent hemarthrosis, characterized by spontaneous bleeding into the joint in the absence of trauma and progressing to chronic capsulitis, has been described recently. The cause of this syndrome is unclear and does not appear to be related to anticoagulation. It is symptomatically benefited by intraarticular steroid administration.

Carpal tunnel syndrome is relatively common in dialyzed patients and has been reported to occur in 4–6% of patients. The etiology remains uncertain, but a recent report found deposition of amyloid protein in a high percentage of patients. Confirmation of nerve entrapment by electromyogram studies should be followed by surgical treatment.

NUTRITION

Weight loss, muscle wasting, and serum biochemical abnormalities are well-known and frequent complications of patients with progressive chronic renal failure. These derangements are usually ascribed to anorexia and gastrointestinal symptoms of uremia as well as to excessive dietary restriction of protein that is sometimes used to delay the need for dialysis. With the institution of chronic dialytic therapy, uremic symptoms are ameliorated and diet is liberalized, which often results in improved nutrition. However, there has been a growing appreciation (from the National Cooperative Dialysis Study [NCDS] and other studies) that, despite dialysis therapy, many patients have a suboptimal nutritional status.

The nutritional abnormalities listed in Table 5-19, include low-energy intake, changes in body composition, and biochemical derangements. Patients receiving chronic peritoneal dialysis are also known to have special nutritional problems (see Chapter 4) of which decreased serum protein concentration is the most common. Also, in 10–15% of continuous ambulatory peritoneal dialysis patients, excess calorie intake from dialysate glucose results in significant obesity.

Clinical Abnormalities

Decreased Calorie Intake. It has been frequently observed that calorie intake is low in chronic dialysis patients, a factor that may significantly contribute to decreased body weight and compositional abnormalities. There are many possible reasons for this low energy intake, as summarized in Table 5-20. A common cause of inadequate calorie intake is prescribed dietary restriction of various nutrients, which leads to decreased diet palatability or boredom with allowed foods. The frequency of intercurrent illness in dialysis patients also contributes to decreased food intake, either by the production of gastrointestinal symptoms and anorexia, or by the need for procedures and hospitalization.

Anorexia is a common complaint in dialysis patients and may have many causes, such as the requirement for specific medications, including phosphate binders, that must be taken with meals. Depression and the stresses of dealing with chronic illness also contribute to decreased appetite, especially in patients

Table 5-19. Nutritional Abnormalities

Decreased caloric intake
Abnormal body composition
  Decreased fat stores in women
  Decreased muscle mass in men
  Decreased body weight in men and women
Abnormal serum protein concentrations
  Decreased serum albumin in peritoneal dialysis patients
  Decreased transferrin in hemodialysis patients.
  Abnormal plasma amino acids
    Decreased essential/nonessential amino acids
    Decreased branch-chain amino acids
Obesity (in continuous ambulatory peritoneal dialysis patients)

Table 5-20. Causes of Calorie and Protein Deficiencies

Causes of inadequate caloric intake
  Diet restriction (protein, phosphorus, potassium)
  Anorexia
  Depression
  Intercurrent illness, hospitalization, surgery
  Dialysis therapy, scheduling, and related symptoms
Causes of protein deficiency
  Low dietary intake
  Dialysis loss
    Peritoneal dialysis
      CAPD: 9–12 g/day
      IPD: 12–14 g/dialysis
    Hemodialysis: amino acid loss (6–8 g/dialysis)
  Persistant proteinuria
  Inefficient protein utilization secondary to inadequate caloric intake

CAPD, continuous ambulatory peritoneal dialysis; IPD, intermittent peritoneal dialysis.

who may be alone or who lack social support systems necessary to maintain psychological well-being. The increasing numbers of geriatric patients receiving dialysis creates additional problems, as the special nutritional abnormalities of this group become superimposed on those of end-stage renal disease and other chronic illness. It should also be remembered that inadequate therapy of uremia through suboptimal dialysis (see Chapter 3) or other metabolic abnormalities that cannot be corrected by dialysis, such as hypogeusia, may lead to inadequate dietary intake and poor nutrition. Some of these problems are correctable, for instance, by adjusting dialytic therapy or by the use of zinc supplements and multivitamins to optimize taste acuity and appetite.

Dialysis therapy itself may contribute to decreased food intake and increased needs in several ways: (1) mild dialysis symptoms associated with disequilibrium may decrease appetite, delay meals, or cause patients to skip them entirely; (2) eating before or during a dialysis may cause or exacerbate hypotension during dialysis so that most patients do not eat during their treatments; (3) if glucose is not present in the dialysate a small quantity is lost with each dialysis; (4) amino acids are lost with each dialysis, a factor that may contribute to the increased rate of protein catabolism or urea generation which has been demonstrated to occur on dialysis days as compared to nondialysis days; and (5) peritoneal dialysis is regularly accompanied by protein loss, which averages 9–12 g/day in continuous ambulatory peritoneal dialysis patients, and 12–14 g per treatment in intermittent peritoneal dialysis. Finally, if peritonitis occurs in continuous ambulatory peritoneal dialysis patients, protein losses increase and occasionally can reach 50 g/24 hr. Such increased losses may linger for several weeks following treatment of infection, presumably due to persistent alterations in peritoneal membrane permeability.

Body Composition Abnormalities. The National Cooperative Dialysis Study demonstrated several frequent abnormalities in body composition. Both men and women weighed less than their healthy age- and sex-matched controls;

women had a significant reduction in body fat stores; and men had a striking reduction in arm circumference and calculated arm muscle circumference, which are measures of body mass and skeletal muscle mass, respectively. Men tended to have greater abnormalities, while women appeared to achieve better nutritional parameters with age. A relationship between dietary inadequacy and body compositional changes was suggested by positive correlations between urea generation rate (protein intake) and body fat stores as well as with arm muscle circumference. This indicates that patients ingesting more protein, and presumably calories, have better fat and muscle stores.

The significance of these abnormalities is of importance with respect to morbidity and long-term survival. Poor nutrition is known to be associated with impairment of immune function, as evidenced by decreased lymphocyte count and abnormalities of delayed hypersensitivity. Such immune deficiencies may be important in the pathogenesis of infection in end-stage renal disease patients, a major cause of mobidity in this population. It has also been shown through an analysis of many risk factors associated with morbidity in dialysis patients that decreased body mass correlated with poor survival.

Abnormal Serum Protein Concentrations. Unlike assessment of muscle mass and body fat, which are generally thought to reflect long-term nutritional adequacy, the measurement of serum proteins or visceral protein mass is a more dynamic and rapidly changing parameter of nutrition.

Because total serum albumin, as well as serum transferrin and other transport proteins, can be easily and repeatedly measured, they are frequently used along with body weight in a simplified approach to nutritional assessment. These parameters, however, not only are frequently altered by recent changes in dietary intake, but also may be influenced by a variety of acute illnesses and liver dysfunction, thus limiting their specificity for nutritional purposes. Measurement of other transport proteins with shorter turnover time than serum albumin (20 days), such as retinol binding protein and prealbumin, has been advocated as more rapid indicators of change in nutritional therapy. However, these proteins are often elevated in renal insufficiency and thus are probably not appropriate as markers of nutritional status in dialysis patients. Total serum protein and albumin can be normal in chronic hemodialysis patients despite the presence of clearly abnormal body composition. Thus, these measurements can be insensitive for detecting suboptimal nutrition. Serum transferrin was found to be low-normal in the NCDS, although it has been reported to correlate with nutritional status in dialysis patients. However, since transferrin levels may vary with body iron stores, its usefulness in dialysis patients, who have fluctuating iron status, seems uncertain.

A clinical situation in which serum proteins may be more reflective of nutritional status is in peritoneal dialysis patients. Because of the steady dialysate loss of protein, of which about 50–70% is albumin, these is a mild reduction in serum protein concentrations in most chronic peritoneal dialysis patients. With optimal dietary therapy some patients will normalize serum protein concentrations; however, many will have persistantly low values. Protein losses may be exacerbated by recurrent peritonitis or illness, which also results in reduced dietary intake. Monitoring dialysate losses coupled with a concerted effort to maintain dietary protein intake high is an important part of the clinical management of peritoneal dialysis patients.

Abnormal plasma and intracellular muscle amino acid profiles have been noted for years in patients with chronic renal failure. Regular dialysis treatment does not normalize concentrations of all amino acids and may even contribute to persistent abnormalities because there is regular loss of amino acids with dialysis. Other factors that may affect amino acid levels include alterations in lipid and carbohydrate metabolism and chronic elevations in insulin, glucagon, and other peptide hormones. Clinical studies in which specific mixtures of amino acids have been administered to correct amino acid concentrations in plasma have been successful and have improved nutritional status. Such data underscore the point that amino acid abnormalities may result from dietary protein deficiency, even though plasma protein concentrations and other parameters of nutrition may be normal.

Possible causes of protein deficiency in dialysis patients are listed in Table 5-20. In addition to inadequate dietary intake of protein, protein utilization may be inefficient due to poor quality of protein and/or lack of sufficient calories. When energy intake is restricted, nitrogen balance can be negative even when protein intake seems adequate. The number of calories required for optimal incorporation of dietary nitrogen is dependent on many factors, including body energy stores and body protein mass, both of which may be depleted in patients with end-stage renal disease. Thus, a higher ratio of energy/protein in food is needed. Continued losses of protein in continuous ambulatory peritoneal dialysis may contribute significantly to protein deficiency as described above. Despite low glomerular filtration rate, a few patients have persistent proteinuria after starting dialysis, which contributes to protein depletion. Finally, protein requirements may be increased by catabolism due to acute illness and surgical procedures and exceed basal requirements by 30–100%.

Obesity. As discussed in Chapter 4, the high calorie intake (in the form of glucose) and general improvement in the well-being of continuous ambulatory peritoneal dialysis patients has led to obesity in some.

Evaluation

Nutritional assessment is a necessary and inseparable part of chronic dialysis therapy because the two are always linked in any analysis of the adequacy of dialysis treatment as rigorously demonstrated in Chapter 3. The quantity of dietary protein and its attendant rate of urea appearance is a major determinant of the amount of dialysis treatment. Conversely, patients who receive inadequate dialytic treatment often have symptoms of anorexia and decreased dietary intake. While it has been argued that a qualitative, "eyeball," assessment of nutritional

Table 5-21. Assessment of Nutritional Status

Diet history
  Calories
  Protein, carbohydrate, fat
  Minerals (calcium, phosphorus, iron, zinc)
  Vitamins

  Calculated parameters
  Basal energy expenditure (BEE)

  Men   = 66 + (13.7 × W) + (5.0 × H) − (6.8 × A)
  Women = 655 + (9.6 × W) + (1.8 × H) − (4.7 × A)

  W = weight (kg); H = Height (cm); A = age (years)

Anthropometric measurements
  Body weight
  Height (m)
  Skinfold thickness (triceps)
  Midarm circumference (AC)

  Calculated parameters
  Midarm muscle circumference (MAMC) = (triceps skinfold thickness × 3.14) − (arm circumference)
  Body mass index (BMI) = weight/(height)^2. Normal: Men, 20–25 kg/m^2; Women, 19–24 kg/m^2.

Protein measurements
  Serum total protein and albumin
  Serum transferrin
  Assessment of dialysate protein loss in continuous ambulatory peritoneal dialysis

| | | Normal values (ages 35–44) | | | | | | |
| | | Percentiles | | | | | | |
	Mean	5th	10th	25th	50th	75th	90th	95th
Weight (lb)								
Men	172	128	137	152	170	189	211	225
Women	143	104	110	122	137	159	185	203
Triceps skinfold thickness (mm)								
Men	12	5	6	8	12	15	20	23
Women	24	12	14	18	23	29	35	39
Midarm circumference (cm)								
Men	32	26	28	30	32	34	36	37
Women	30	24	25	26	29	32	36	38
Midarm muscle circumference (cm)								
Men	28	24	25	27	28	30	31	33
Women	22	18	19	20	22	24	26	27

status using routine clinical information provides an accurate estimation in a high percentage of hospitalized patients, this method is inadequate in dialysis patients. The results of the NCDS clearly revealed nutritional abnormalities in a group of dialysis patients selected for stability and lack of other serious illness, and in whom other routine clinical evaluation was considered acceptable by current dialysis standards. It is recommended that a group of simple, widely accepted, standardized tests be performed routinely in dialysis patients, along the guidelines given in Table 5-21.

Dietary history. Analysis of dietary intake using recorded diet histories, while subject to known limitations and subjective errors, is nevertheless a valuable tool for evaluating intake of critical nutrients and for monitoring specific dietary prescriptions. Diet histories can be analyzed quickly and thoroughly by the use of interactive computerized systems.

Evaluation of intake of the basic micro- and macronutrients, as well as calculated parameters of basal energy expenditure (BEE), the ratio of calories to BEE, and protein intake are particularly helpful in determining energy needs for dialysis patients. Since these patients have different eating habits on treatment days, diet records should include both dialysis and nondialysis days, as well as weekend days.

Body composition. The quantitative evaluation of body compartments comprising protein and fat reflects protein and calorie nutrient status. Good methods for direct measurement of these parameters are not available for everyday use in clinical medicine, but a variety of indirect assessments can be used which, when combined, can give a reliable profile of nutritional status. Together with dietary analysis, these methods form the basis for identifying those patients with significant nutritional deficiencies who thus need specific therapeutic interventions.

Weight. Longitudinal assessment of body weight as well as static measurements compared with normal reference standards for healthy adults can be a sensitive indicator of malnutrition. Patients who lose more than 5% of body weight in 1 month, or 10% of weight over 6 months, are at risk for developing significant malnutrition. Such weight loss signals a need for careful evaluation of the cause and possible intervention. Rates of growth in stature and weight for children are standard criteria for evaluation of nutritional adequacy. Growth charts should be used routinely in dialyzed patients under the age of 18.

Height. Height measurement, combined with weight, can be used to calculate the body mass index (BMI). This index is the weight (kg) divided by the height^2(m^2), an index of muscle and fat stores. This index has been used extensively in evaluating obesity, but may also be useful to detect severe depletion of body protein and fat stores. However, it can be normal despite evidence for a specific body compartment deficiency, and hence may be of limited use in mild or isolated nutritional deficiency.

Skinfold thickness. Fat stores can be most easily estimated by measurement of skinfold thickness in several body sites. Triceps skinfold thickness measurements have been most widely used. However, measurement of subcutaneous fat in three additional sites (subscapular, biceps, suprailiae) allows for a more accurate estimate of total body fat. The sum of these measurements in four sites has been used to estimate body density and allows a better calculated measurement of total body fat.

Midarm muscle circumference. Measurement of body protein stores is largely an estimate of body muscle mass. A simple and easily performed estimate of body muscle, the midarm muscle circumference can be obtained by multiplying the triceps skinfold thickness by π (3.14) and subtracting this value from the midarm circumference (at the midpoint from the acromion to the olecranon).

Interpretation of data. Interpretation of body composition measurements requires comparison of the individual patient measurement with age- and sex-matched values obtained from healthy controls. The most current and representative standards available for the United States population are those published by the National Center for Health Statistics for data from the National Health and Nutrition Examination Survey, 1971–1974. These data contain reference standards for weight, height, skinfold thickness, arm circumference, and midarm muscle circumference for healthy adults, which are grouped into population percentiles by age and sex. Patients who fall below the 15% percentile of the normal population are felt to be at risk for development of significant nutritional deficiency reflected by those parameters, and below the 5% percentile as having significant depletion. A summary of these data is given in Table 5-21.

Therapy

Specific recommendations for diet and supplemental nutrition therapy in dialysis patients is outlined in Table 5-22.

Table 5-22. Recommendations for Nutritional Therapy
Energy   35 kcal/kg/day
Protein   1.0–1.2 g/kg/day (hemodialysis)
1.2–1.5 g/kg/day (peritoneal dialysis)
Distribution of calories
Carbohydrate   55% of total calories
Fat   30% of total calories
Protein   15% of total calories
Electrolyte intake
Sodium   80–100 mEq (individualized)
Potassium   40–80 mEq (individualized)
Phosphorus   800–1000 mg/day
Multivitamins   B, C, folate, niacin, biotin, but without A and D
Calcium carbonate supplement   1000–1500 mg/day
Optional dietary supplements
Additional calories
Dialysate glucose
Oral carbohydrate concentrate
Liquid protein-calorie supplements
Protein
Liquid protein-calorie supplements
Hyperalimentation during hemodialysis
Oral amino acid capsules
Zinc sulfate   67 mg (15 mg elemental zinc/day)
Ferrous sulfate   (320–960 mg/day)

Energy. Energy needs are difficult to predict in individual patients, but a general recommendation of 35 kcal/kg body weight daily has been found to be adequate for most dialysis patients without associated stress or concurrent illness. Another method for estimation of energy requirement is based on calculation of basal energy expenditure (BEE) (Table 5-21) adjusted for usual activity level, with an increase of 30, 50, and 75% for light, moderate, and heavy activity, respectively. For instance, the BEE of a 30-year-old man weighing 78 kg who is 68 inches (150 cm) in height is

$$BEE = 66 + (13.7 \times weight) + (5.0 \times height) - (6.8 \times age)$$
$$= 66 + 1069 + 750 - 204$$
$$= 1681 \text{ kcal/day}$$

BEE adjusted for light activity:

$$BEE = BEE \times 130\%$$
$$= 1681 \times 130\%$$
$$= 2185 \text{ kcal/day}$$

Protein. The minimum daily dietary protein requirement recommended for healthy adults consuming a standard American diet is 0.8 g/kg/day. Patients on chronic dialysis are subject to additional stress associated with chronic illness, as well as regular losses of protein into the dialysate. Protein requirements are therefore increased to 1.0–1.2 g/kg/day in hemodialysis patients. Chronic peritoneal dialysis is associated with greater loss of dialysate protein and thus requires an intake of 1.2–1.5 g/kg/day to maintain adequate serum protein concentrations. Most stable dialysis patients do not have difficulty ingesting this amount of protein, since it closely approximates the standard American diet.

In patients whose protein intake is marginal, efficiency of protein utilization can be achieved by increasing energy intake and also by moderate exercise. Recent studies of exercise programs in dialysis patients show not only a beneficial effect on nutrition with weight gain, but also other clinical benefits including improved cardiac function, lower blood pressure, and improved anemia.

If these conservative measures are not possible or effective, and evidence for protein deficiency persists, then dietary supplements should be tried. There are numerous commercial formulations of protein-calorie supplements that provide a wide range of choice regarding nutrient content and palatibility. Since these preparations are all relatively expensive, use of specific table foods and homemade preparations, such as "milk shakes" using nondairy cream substitutes, may be more acceptable and equally effective in many patients. An oral amino acid preparation in capsule form is available but is expensive and requires the ingestion of numerous capsules to achieve a significant quantity of protein.

It is also possible to provide parenteral protein supplementation during hemodialysis which results in significant positive protein balance. Negative aspects of this therapy include expense, occasional technical problems associated with infusion into the venous side of the dialyzer where pressures may be elevated, and associated symptoms of nausea and vomiting, which may due to the rapid infusion of the mixture.

Distribution of Calories. The Committee on Dietary Allowances of the National Academy of Sciences suggests that the distribution of calories between carbohydrate, protein, and fat be 58, 12, and 30%, respectively. Because the increased need for protein in dialysis patients, this percentage has been increased to 15%, which is close to the actual intake of 16% noted in the NCDS study population. Thus, intake of 55% carbohydrate, and 30% fat would be close to the recommended levels.

Electrolyte Intake. Sodium intake in dialyzed patients must be individualized somewhat but generally should range between 80 and 100 mEq/day to prevent interdialytic volume overload and hypertension. Potassium should be mildly restricted to allow a reasonably normal diet but to prevent severe hyperkalemia between dialysis. The practice of using a very low potassium dialysate to allow greater freedom with diet may be associated with hypotension or arrhythmias on dialysis. Patients on continuous peritoneal dialysis seem to tolerate higher levels of dietary potassium because of better removal.

Phosphorus should be restricted to 800–1000 mg/day to limit the quantity of phosphate binders that must be taken and thus avoid potential toxicity from aluminum absorption, and to reduce the risk of soft tissue calcification and worsening hyperparathyroidism due to hyperphosphatemia.

Multivitamins. It is customary to provide dialysis patients with a multivitamin preparation to replace dialysis losses of soluble vitamins and to correct any dietary deficiencies. This vitamin should not include either vitamin A, which is elevated in dialysis patients, or vitamin D, which should be prescribed separately and individually as specific therapy for renal osteodystrophy.

Calcium Carbonate Supplement. The restriction of phosphorus will limit the use of dairy products and hence the ingestion of calcium. Thus, most patients should receive supplemental calcium carbonate at the level of 1000–1500 mg/day. This may need to be increased for patients who remain hypocalcemic or who are repleting demineralized bone.

Optional Dietary Supplements. Zinc is often prescribed to dialysis patients for treatment of sexual dysfunction or for anorexia. The recommended level of zinc supplement is 15 mg elemental zinc per day. Iron therapy should not be uniformly prescribed for all patients, but should be given based on individual needs determined from serum ferritin levels.

ENDOCRINE-METABOLIC ABNORMALITIES

Chronic renal failure is associated with disturbances of many hormones, due to abnormal renal metabolism and excretion. However, the presence of renal insufficiency can also affect hormone production and metabolism at extrarenal sites, as well as affect target organs. Table 5-23 summarizes the major mechanisms that can result in abnormal hormonal function in renal failure, and lists examples of those hormones thought to be influenced by each mechanism.

The clinical manifestation of these endocrine disturbances are variable in the frequency and severity with which they result in specific functional abnormalities. Some endocrine disturbances such as thyroid are associated with numerous biochemical abnormalities but only occasionally result in impaired thyroid function of clinical significance. However, many of the hormone disturbances described in Table 5-23 result in significant clinical abnormalities although our understanding of the specific pathophysiology in many cases remains incomplete. Since regular dialysis treatment does not correct these disturbances, patients on dialysis have persistent hormonal abnormalities. Abnormal gonadal function and associated sexual dysfunction can result in markedly impaired quality of life for many patients. As discussed previously, the numerous skeletal and metabolic disturbances resulting from abnormal parathyroid hormone and vitamin D metabolism can cause serious physical limitations and chronic pain, which may limit rehabilitation and survival. The complex disturbances associated with carbohydrate metabolism, pancreatic hormones, and their interrelated effects on lipid abnormalities may contribute to atherogenesis, which is the major disease limiting survival in dialysis patients.

Thyroid Dysfunction

There are many biochemical abnormalities of thyroid function in patients with renal failure, summarized in Table 5-24. Iodide accumulates secondary to decreased renal excretion. Thyroid hormones are either normal or decreased. Despite the frequent documentation of reduced T_4 and T_3 levels, most dialysis

Table 5-23. Pathogenesis of Endocrine-Metabolic Abnormalities

Mechanisms	Examples
Increased hormone levels	
Impaired degradation	
Decreased renal catabolism	Insulin, proinsulin, glucagon, C-peptide of parathyroid hormone, calcitonin, growth hormone, prolactin, gastrin, secretin, cholecystikinin
Heterogeneous hormone immunoreactivity	Glucagon, parathyroid hormone, calcitonin
Impaired extrarenal hormone degradation	Insulin, parathyroid hormone
Increased production	
Increased secretion as adaptation	Parathyroid hormone, aldosterone
Increased secretion resulting from abnormal feedback control	Luteinizing hormone, follicle-stimulating hormone
Decreased hormone levels	
Decreased secretion	
Impaired renal production	Erythropoietin, vitamin D
Dysfunction of other glands	Testosterone, progesterone, estrogen
Impaired conversion of prohormones to active components	$25(OH)D_3$, thyroxine
Altered organ responsiveness to hormone	Glucagon, insulin, parathyroid hormone

Table 5-24. Thyroid Hormone Abnormalities

Plasma iodide and iodide pool increased
Thyroxine binding to serum proteins decreased
T_4 levels normal or decreased
T_3 levels low
Conversion of T_4 to T_3 impaired
Reverse T_3 normal
Thyrotropin normal
^{131}I uptake depressed

patients are clinically euthyroid and do not benefit from therapy to increase these levels. Rather, the converse may be true: an increase in free thryoxine may occur during dialysis due to heparin-induced changes in protein binding. Despite the impaired conversation of T_4 to T_3, the levels of reverse T_3 are usually normal and thus different from what occurs in other types of chronic illness. Thyrotropin is usually normal, rises slowly after administration of thyrotropin-releasing hormone, and has a delayed rate of disappearance.

Several studies of serial thyroid function in dialyzed patients demonstrate wide variation in the incidence of goiter and in other clinical manifestations of thyroid abnormalities. The diagnosis of primary hypothyroidism may be difficult in end-stage renal disease patients, but thyrotropin levels are probably the most reliable index for evaluating this disorder.

Pituitary-Gonadal Dysfunction

Pituitary-gonadal hormone concentrations are abnormal in many chronic dialysis patients and account in part for the symptoms of sexual dysfunction that are so disturbing to these patients.

Table 5-25 lists the primary alterations in gonadotropin and gonadal hormones that occur in male and female dialysis patients. Luteinizing hormone has been found to be consistently elevated by most investigators while follicle-stim-

Table 5-25. Pituitary-Gonadal Abnormalities

	Men	Women
Hormonal abnormalities	Increased LH Normal to increased FSH Elevated LH and FSH response to LH-RH Increased prolactin Normal or decreased testosterone	Increased LH Increased prolactin Low or normal estrogen, progesterone, testosterone Loss of normal pulsatile release of gonadotropins
Clinical disorders	Decreased libido Decreased potency Reduced testicular size and azoospermia Gynecomastia	Amenorrhea Infertility Decreased libido Menorrhagia Abnormal lactation
Therapy	Zinc supplements Testosterone (if low) Optimize dialysis therapy Bromocriptine	Bromocriptine

LH, luteinizing hormone; FSH, follicle-stimulating hormone; LH-RH, luteinizing hormone releasing hormone.

ulating hormone is more variable and has been reported to be either normal or elevated. Even when elevated, however, these levels are felt to be inappropriately low for the degree of end-organ dysfunction. There is therefore a double defect, one at the hypothalamic level as well as the end-organ or gonadal level. This abnormal feedback control system is documented by an abnormal follicle-stimulating hormone response to luteinizing hormone releasing hormone in men and impaired positive estradiol-associated cyclic release of luteinizing hormone in women. High prolactin levels are observed in both men and women but are more common in women. In some patients elevated prolactin levels may be further aggravated by a methyldopa antihypertensive therapy. Very high levels are sometimes associated with galactorrhea in women, but are not consistently improved by the use of the dopamine receptor agonist, bromocriptine. Increased prolactin in men has been linked with impotence. However, these correlations are often weak, and the therapeutic efficacy of bromocriptine again is equivocal.

Testosterone levels are often, but not consistently, low in male dialysis patients. Institution or optimization of dialysis can sometimes result in improved sexual function but may not help in other patients. This is suggestive that a circulating toxin may suppress testosterone production. Several reports have found that low plasma zinc levels correlated with low serum testosterone and luteinizing hormone levels. Both zinc and testosterone levels could be normalized by the use of supplemental zinc acetate (50 mg daily) for 6 months. Sperm counts were also normalized, follicle-stimulating hormone levels were persistantly abnormal in some patients. Sexual function was subjectively improved in many but not all patients.

Zinc therapy is currently recommended as relatively benign and potentially beneficial for sexual dysfunction in men when zinc levels are depressed. In addition, if serum testosterone is low, testosterone supplements may be used. If not successful, bromocriptine may be used but this drug produces hypotension in a large percentage of patients. Estrogen and progesterone levels are often reduced in women.

The primary clinical symptoms of gonadal dysfunction encountered in men and women on chronic dialysis are listed in Table 5-25. Complaints of decreased libido and potency occur in as many as 50–70% of men. These symptoms are always difficult to evaluate, since they may be related to uremic abnormalities or to antihypertensive therapy. Psychological factors also play a role. Management of sexual dysfunction in men varies considerably, but a reasonable approach to evaluation and treatment is as follows:

1. Measure serum zinc and testosterone.
2. If zinc level is low, treat with oral zinc supplement for 6 months and reevaluate.
3. If testosterone level is low, give parenteral testosterone injections (which may also be efficacious for treatment of anemia).
4. Evaluate adequacy of dialysis therapy.
5. If symptoms persist and/or zinc and testosterone levels are normal, a trial of bromocriptine therapy may be warranted.

6. Bromocriptine has been used with some success in women with disorders of gonadal function. Fertility is, however, markedly reduced in all women undergoing dialysis.

Carbohydrate Metabolism

Abnormal glucose metabolism, known historically as "uremic pseudo-diabetes," has been recognized in connection with advanced renal failure for many years. Conversely, patients with diabetes mellitus with renal failure often have diminished insulin requirements and improved glucose control. Clinically, fasting hyperglycemia is rarely seen in patients with end-stage renal disease, but the converse situation, hypoglycemia, is occasionally seen in patients who have prolonged fasting or have very poor dietary intake of calories. Mild hypoglycemia may occur in poorly nourished patients who are dialyzed against a bath free of glucose.

The metabolic abnormalities that cause these clinical disturbances include alterations in insulin and glucagon metabolism and perhaps uremic toxins, which are presently unidentified.

Documented disturbances in insulin metabolism are summarized in Table 5-26. Since the renal proximal tubule is an important site of catabolism of both insulin and proinsulin, it is not surprising that these hormones are elevated in patients with renal insufficiency. Proinsulin, the metabolically inactive precursor of insulin, is elevated to a greater extent than insulin. Insulin resistance is well described, although the mechanism is controversial.

Dialysis therapy partially corrects the abnormal response of plasma glucose and insulin levels to glucose infusion. However, hyperinsulinemia persists in many patients on dialysis.

Glucagon is universally elevated in patients with advanced renal insufficiency and remains elevated in chronic dialysis patients. A major fraction of this elevation, however, represents a large inactive molecular form of glucagon, so the clinical effects of such elevated glucagon levels in these patients is uncertain. Hyperglucogonemia may increase mobilization of muscle amino acids utilized

---

Table 5-26. Abnormalities of Carbohydrate Metabolism

Insulin metabolism
  Increased insulin levels
  Increased ratio of proinsulin to insulin
  Peripheral insulin resistance
  Circulating insulin antagonists
  Decreased insulin catabolism secondary to decreased renal mass
Glucagon metabolism
  Increased plasma levels secondary to decreased renal function
  Increased ratio of inactive to active hormone
Glucose
  Fasting hyperglycemia rare
  Fasting hypoglycemia can occur in response to prolonged fasting
  Abnormal glucose tolerance curves

for gluconeogenesis, hence may be a cause of increased catabolism in uremic patients.

Impaired glucose metabolism usually does not require specific therapy in dialyzed patients. The use of dialysate containing glucose is preferred in hemodialysis patients, because it avoids the small loss of calories associated with glucose removal in the dialysate and it prevents a mild decrease in plasma glucose during dialysis. In diabetic patients, insulin requirements and prolonged half-life of administered insulin are reflected in decreased insulin needed. In diabetics dialysate should always contain glucose to prevent insulin-induced hypoglycemia during dialysis.

Adrenal Steroid Metabolism

Glucocorticoids. Plasma cortisol is normal in end-stage renal disease patients. However, cortisol metabolites, the 17-hydroxycorticosteroids, are primarily excreted by the kidney and thus accumulate in the plasma of patients with renal failure. Cortisol production and response to adrenocorticotropic hormone (ACTH) is normal, but plasma disappearance of administered cortisol is somewhat delayed. Cortisol levels are not affected by hemodialysis therapy, since only small amounts (<1 mg) are removed with each dialysis.

Adrenal insufficiency is occasionally seen in the dialyzed patient, the most frequent cause being prolonged treatment and then discontinuation of prednisone for renal transplantation. Clinical manifestations are weakness, hyperkalemia, and pigmentation. Diagnosis can be made in the usual manner by lack of stimulation of cortisol by ACTH infusion.

Aldosterone. Reported abnormalities in aldosterone metabolism associated with renal disease appear to be inconsistant, and perhaps relate to the stage of renal failure and amount of functional residual renal mass. Before the start of dialysis treatment, plasma aldosterone levels have been generally reported to be elevated, but respond normally to stimulatory and inhibitory factors. Such increased aldosterone concentrations may be an adaptation to higher serum potassium levels and the increased production of renin in response to intrarenal disease and ischemia. However, patients receiving regular dialysis have plasma levels that are usually normal, but the response to volume depletion is blunted. Anephric patients have a loss of renin activity and frequently very low levels of aldosterone, and are also unresponsive to decreased extracellular volume. In dialysis patients, especially those who are anephric, serum potassium is usually the primary factor regulating aldosterone. The quantity of aldosterone removed by dialysis is small, so that changes in plasma levels represent changes in production. Hemodialysis does not significantly affect the plasma levels of other adrenal hormones (corticosterone, deoxycorticosterone, or 18-hydroxycorticosterone).

Metabolism of Other Hormones

Growth Hormone. Plasma levels of growth hormone are usually elevated in patients with renal failure, since this hormone is cleared by the kidney. Elevated levels may persist after institution of hemodialysis and may increase even further in patients on chronic peritoneal dialysis. Secretion of growth hormone may also be abnormal in renal failure, since plasma levels do not fall (and may even rise) with glucose administration. This paradoxical response may be due to protein-calorie malnutrition.

Somatomedin. Somatomedin levels are depressed in children with uremia and may be a contributing factor to abnormal growth in these patients. Hemodialysis can result in improvement in somatomedin levels, but it is uncertain if this change contributes to improved growth. Somatomedin levels in adult hemodialysis patients have been reported to be elevated.

Gastrointestinal Hormones. Gastrin, secretin, cholecystikinin and gastric inhibitory polypeptide are elevated in renal insufficiency, largely because of their dependence on renal tissue for metabolism and excretion. No definite correlation between gastrin levels and gastrointestinal disease has been made as yet. The effects of hemodialysis therapy on these hormones is inconsistent, with conflicting data on whether there is lowering of gastrin. There is no apparent effect on cholecystikinin when gastric inhibitory polypeptide is lowered.

Catecholamines. Catecholamines, primarily norepinephrine levels, have been reported to be elevated in dialysis patients, but detailed studies of the effects of hemodialysis on catecholamine metabolism are not available.

Lipid Metabolism

Abnormal lipid levels are present in the majority of patients with chronic renal failure, and these abnormalities persist or may even be worsened with the institution of chronic dialysis. Some of the features of abnormal metabolism of lipids in these patients are summarized in Table 5-27.

An absolute increase in total plasma triglyceride concentration is present in about a third of patients on chronic hemodialysis and perhaps two thirds on chronic peritoneal dialysis. The degree of elevation is variable and ranges from mild increases to severely elevated levels in the 1000–2000 mg/dl range in some

Table 5-27. Abnormalities of Lipid Metabolism

Increased total triglyceride level
Low normal total plasma cholesterol
Decreased high density lipoprotein cholesterol fraction (HDL)
Increased low density lipoprotein fraction (LDL) and increased LDL/HDL ratio
Increased HDL, LDL, and very low density lipoprotein (VLDL) triglyceride

patients. Triglyceride is increased in all three major lipoprotein groups: low density lipoprotein (LDL), high density lipoprotein (HDL), and very low density lipoprotein (VLDL). There is accumulation of incompletely metabolized remnant VLDL particles as well.

Of perhaps greater significance in regard to atherosclerosis is the frequent observation that HDL is depressed while LDL cholesterol and the LDL/HDL ratio is elevated in a high percentage of dialysis patients. Racial differences in the lipoprotein abnormalities have been reported, with white males having higher levels of total triglyceride and lower levels of HDL cholesterol and apoprotein fractions than black men. These differences may account for the higher mortality from atherosclerosis in white men compared with black men, despite the latter group's higher incidence of nephrosclerosis.

The mechanism underlying these abnormalities remains incompletely understood, but several mechanisms related to decreased triglyceride removal and perhaps abnormal HDL metabolism have been identified as outlined in Table 5-28. Triglyceride production is not elevated in uremia, but there is impaired triglyceride removal from the plasma. One reason for this impaired removal is decreased basal adipose tissue lipoprotein lipase (LPL) activity, which fails to increase postprandially. A circulating lipoprotein lipase inhibitor has also been proposed as another mechanism, as well as abnormalities in apolipoprotein cofactors carried on high density lipoprotein, which normally stimulate lipoprotein lipase.

Other possible factors that may contribute to abnormal lipid levels in end-stage renal disease include carnitine deficiency, especially in those treated with peritoneal dialysis. This amino acid mediates the intracellular transport of fatty acids and thus oxidative metabolism. Studies to evaluate the effects of carnitine replacement therapy and its possible effect on lipid metabolism are currently being conducted. Certain drugs increase triglyceride levels, including high-dose anabolic steroids and propanolol.

It has been suggested that chronic acidosis might adversely affect triglyceride transport, but further data are needed. Concern that acetate or glucose in the dialysate may contribute to increased lipid production has not been substantiated.

Treatment of hyperlipidemia in end-stage renal disease patients is presently controversial because the relative importance of this factor in the development of atherosclerosis remains uncertain and because the therapeutic modalities available for lowering serum triglycerides and increasing high density lipoprotein are not always effective or without risk. Dietary therapy with a reduction in

Table 5-28. Pathogenesis of Hyperlipidemia

Decreased metabolism of triglycerides
  Decreased lipoprotein lipase
  Lipoprotein lipase inhibitor
    Abnormal apolipoprotein cofactors in high density lipoprotein
Carnitine deficiency
Drug therapy
? Chronic acidosis

carbohydrate and an increase in polyunsaturated/saturated fat ratio has been demonstrated to be effective in reducing triglyceride levels. However, this type of diet may be difficult with regard to compliance and may be deleterious to overall nutrition, since suboptimal carbohydrate intake is already present in many dialysis patients. The use of a diet relatively rich in complex carbohydrates and low in saturated fats is probably a reasonable compromise, although further studies are required to document an effect on lipid metabolism.

The use of clofibrate has been successful in lowering triglycerides, raising high density lipoprotein and increasing adipose tissue lipoprotein lipase. However, this drug has potentially serious side effects, including hyperkalemia from muscle toxicity, elevated muscle enzymes and skeletal muscle pathology, and a possible increased incidence of gastrointestinal neoplasms. Increased triglyceride levels noted with peritoneal dialysis therapy is thought to be mediated by the intraperitoneal absorption of large quantities of glucose from the dialysate. However, the administration of insulin in the dialysate in sufficient quantities to lower blood glucose levels has not resulted in significant changes in plasma lipids in nondiabetic patients. Dietary restriction of carbohydrate to compensate for glucose received from the dialysate may be necessary to control severe elevations of serum triglycerides.

NEUROLOGIC COMPLICATIONS

Abnormalities of the nervous system are unique among all the other organ system complications in that most of the complications seen in chronically dialyzed patients are distinctly different from those that classically occur in patients with advanced renal failure. Dialysis therapy effectively reverses the many manifestations of uremic encephalopathy and even results in improvement in peripheral neuropathic symptoms. However, dialysis therapy itself commonly results in a series of mild neurologic disturbances known as dialysis disequilibrium and, rarely, can cause a progressive fatal disorder called dialysis encephalopathy. Other common disturbances of the nervous system in dialysis patients result not from dialysis therapy directly, but may be indirect consequences of disease complications that occur as a result of prolonged survival on dialysis.

Disturbances of the Central Nervous System

Uremic Encephalopathy. The nervous system is said to have the greatest sensitivity to uremic toxins, and it is thus one of the earliest organ systems to manifest clinical signs and symptoms of advancing renal failure. The type of metabolic encephalopathy known as uremic encephalopathy presents as a continuum of central nervous system dysfunction, ranging from mild symptoms of altered concentration and sleep disturbances to changes in alertness, orientation, and sensorium, which interfere with the ability to perform routine daily activities. If allowed to progress, motor disturbances, including tremulousness, asterixis, myoclonus, and seizures, may occur in association with further deterioration of level of consciousness, including obtundation, stupor, and coma. The severity of symptoms often waxes and wanes as renal failure progresses. The psychological stress resulting from these symptoms is often very disturbing to patients and may result in further worsening of the patient's status because of associated depression, anger, fear, and occasional psychotic symptoms. The institution of dialysis produces marked improvement in these symptoms after only a few treatments.

In regularly dialyzed patients, signs or symptoms of uremic encephalopathy should not recur, and if a clinical picture of metabolic encephalopathy is seen, another cause must be actively sought.

Dialysis Disequilibrium. Dialysis disequilibrium is a prominent and common abnormality that occurs in connection with dialysis therapy, and, if severe, may occasionally persist into the interdialytic interval. The common features of dialysis disequilibrium are listed in Table 5-29, and include mild symptoms frequently encountered in perhaps as many as 50–60% of chronic hemodialysis patients. The more severe symptoms listed in the table are usually seen only in severely azotemic patients treated with efficient dialysis that results in a rapid and large fall in BUN. This disorder is preventable by the use of decreased dialysis rate and amount with frequent, shorter dialysis sessions until good biochemical control has been achieved, as discussed in Chapter 3.

The pathogenesis of dialysis disequilibrium is not fully understood, but several abnormalities have been identified. Rapid removal of solute from the extracellular fluid compartment results in an osmolar gradient between brain and blood, which results in cerebral edema. A fall in the pH of spinal fluid has also been noted to occur.

Prevention of symptoms of disequilibrium can best be achieved by limiting the amount and rate of dialysis in the setting of a high BUN and pharmacologic maneuvers. Use of high dialysate sodium levels, bicarbonate dialysate buffer, and intravenous infusion of hypertonic dextrose, sodium, or mannitol to maintain plasma osmolality at a higher level are often helpful. Treatment of symptoms after they occur is more difficult, but muscle cramps and some of the other mild

Table 5-29. Clinical Manifestations of
Dialysis Disequilibrium

Mild	Headache
	Fatigue
	Nausea
	Vomiting
	Muscle cramps
	Restlessness
Severe	Hypertension
	Agitation
	Confusion
	Seizures
	Stupor
	Coma

Table 5-30. Clinical Approach to Dialysis Encephalopathy

Clinical signs and symptoms	Dysarthria and speech apraxia Personality changes Myoclonus Seizures Progressive dementia

Diagnostic studies	Electroencephalogram
	Lumbar puncture
	Computed tomography scan
	Skeletal evaluation for osteomalacia
	    Bone x-rays
	    Bone biopsy with stains for aluminum
	Aluminum concentration in dialysate water supply

Therapy	Dialysis water treatment to remove aluminum
	Desferroxamine treatment to remove body aluminum
	Symptomatic treatment
	    Diazepam
	    Clonazepam

features may be helped by injection of the above hypertonic solutes during dialysis.

Dialysis Encephalopathy. Dialysis encephalopathy is characterized by the features listed in Table 5-30. This is a devastating complication, which usually occurs after a number of years of dialysis, and progresses relentlessly in most patients, resulting in death 9–12 months after onset.

The presenting symptoms are most frequently those of speech disturbances that initially seem worse with or after a dialysis and tend to be intermittent and of varying severity. Changes in personality eventually emerge with progressive decline of intellectual function. A variety of motor disturbances, including twitching, jerks, and hemiballismus, as well as focal or grand mal seizures are often present.

Many patients ultimately succumb to progressive inanition, malnutrition, and infection, though discontinuation of treatment has been elected in some cases as the diagnosis and poor prognosis is appreciated.

The pathogenesis of this disorder remained poorly understood until recently. Patients with dialysis encephalopathy have been found to have very high levels of aluminum in brain gray matter, compared with other dialysis patients. Occurrence of several epidemics of dialysis encephalopathy in European centers, associated with severe osteomalacia and multiple fractures, led to the identification of increased aluminum deposition in bone as well. The water used for preparation of dialysate in these centers had high concentrations of aluminum. When water treatment to remove aluminum was instituted, the incidence of new cases of dialysis encephalopathy decreased dramatically. Better treatment of dialysate water has resulted in fewer epidemic occurrences of this disorder. However, sporadic cases continue to be seen throughout the world in patients who have been dialyzed with low dialysate aluminum. In these cases the implication of oral aluminum hydroxide (phosphorus binders) in the pathogenesis of both bone disease and encephalopathy is likely.

Diagnostic evaluation of patients with dialysis encephalopathy includes the usual studies to evaluate dementia and other neurologic disease that can produce a picture of metabolic encephalopathy. Electroencephalographic changes are often present early, with distinctive patterns of episodic bursts of spikes against a background of slow wave activity. The lumbar puncture is usually negative, as is the computed tomography (CT) scan.

Because of the documented association with bone disease, it is appropriate to evaluate patients with dialysis encephalopathy for osteomalacia. The dialysate water should be checked for increased aluminum levels (>15 μg/L).

Treatment of this disorder has been very discouraging. Changes in dialysis therapy as well as successful transplantation have not been effective. Symptomatic treatment of neurologic symptoms with diazepam is helpful, but does not alter the course of the disease. Beneficial results have been achieved by removal of aluminum from the water, (deionization and reverse osmosis) and by chelation and removal of body aluminum using desferroxamine.

Toxic Encephalopathy. Dialysis encephalopathy has a very characteristic clinical appearance and is fairly readily distinguished from other types of metabolic encephalopathies. However, uremic encephalopathy may be mimicked by toxic (drug) or metabolic encephalopathies, which occasionally occur in dialysis patients. A list of some of the common causes of altered mental status and other neurologic symptoms that can be confused with uremic encephalopathy are listed in Table 5-31.

There are many drugs that can cause neurologic side effects in chronic renal failure, including penicillin, metabolites of meperidine, procainamide, aminophylline, and others. Long-acting barbiturates and other sedatives may result in altered sensorium. Hypercalcemia due to vitamin D therapy can frequently cause symptoms if the serum calcium rises above 13–14 mg/dl. Hypoglycemia in the

Table 5-31. Differential Diagnosis of Altered
    Mental States in the Dialyzed Patient

Drug toxicity
   Penicillin
   Meperidine
   Procainamide
   Aminophylline
   Cimetidine
Hypercalcemia
Hypoglycemia
Sepsis
Intracranial bleeding
   Subdural hematoma
   Intracranial hemorrhage
Psychological disturbances
   Depression
Dementia
   Dialysis dementia
   Multiple infarcts secondary to hypertension
   Presenile (Alzheimer's type)

malnourished patient or occult sepsis can each present with an alteration in mental status. Intracranial bleeding (described below), psychological disturbances, and other causes of dementia occur with sufficient frequency that they must be considered in the differential diagnosis of altered mental status in the dialyzed patient.

Peripheral Neuropathy

Peripheral neuropathy is one of the classic features of chronic renal failure, which occurs rather frequently but is subclinical or subtle in presentation in most cases. With adequate dialysis, it is rather uncommon for patients to present with severe disease.

The clinical presentation of peripheral neuropathy begins with mild sensory symptoms of the lower extremities. The restless leg syndrome, a nocturnal sensation of ill-defined discomfort in the feet and legs, relieved by continuous movement of the legs, is often an early presentation. Subsequently, there are typical symptoms of sensory neuropathy, such as paresthesia and numbness, especially in the lower extremities. Sensory symptoms tend to be followed by motor impairment, such as weakness of the feet and calf muscles. Rapid progression to widespread weakness and quadriplegia has been reported rarely.

The diagnosis of peripheral neuropathy can usually be made on clinical evaluation. In many clinically unaffected patients, motor nerve conduction studies will reveal slowing, which is consistent with early disease, and which may remain abnormal indefinitely, despite regular dialysis treatment. However, regular measurement of motor nerve conduction velocity is not recommended, since it will not change therapy in patients with mild subclinical abnormalities, is uncomfortable, and has a large intrinsic degree of variation.

The observation that peripheral neuropathy is improved by dialysis and transplantation is strongly suggestive that uremic toxin(s) are responsible for its pathogenesis. Many substances and possible deficiencies, listed in Table 5-32, have been proposed as causes of nerve toxicity. The pathogenic role of each of these factors remains unproven.

Peripheral neuropathy in the undialyzed patient without predisposing factors for neuropathy (diabetes mellitus, drugs, etc.), is an indication to begin dialysis therapy. The appearance or progression of neuropathy in the previously dialyzed patient requires evaluation of the adequacy of dialysis. Transplantation should be considered in those patients who have severe or disabling disease. Drugs that can exacerbate or cause peripheral neuropathy should obviously be avoided.

The combination of severe diabetic neuropathy and uremia can sometimes result in a synergistic worsening of neuropathic symptoms. These patients should receive optimal dialysis therapy and careful attention to nutritional management. Diabetic patients with loss of sensation may have pressure-induced ischemic nerve damage during surgery if their extremities are not adequately protected.

Table 5-32. Possible Etiologic Factors of Uremic
Polyneuropathy

Primary factors
  Uremic neurotoxins
    Guanidine compounds
    Phenols
    Myoinositol
  Nutritional
    Protein malnutrition
    Vitamin deficiency
  Endocrine disorders
    Parathyroid hormone
    Abnormal calcium and phosphate metabolism
    Disordered carbohydrate metabolism
  Fluid, electrolyte, osmotic shifts
  Disease of the vasa nervorum
    Accelerated atherosclerosis
    Vascular calcification
Aggravating factors
  Drugs
  Systemic disease
    Diabetes mellitus
  Local nerve damage secondary to vascular access procedure

Cerebrovascular Disease

Intracranial hemorrhage and stroke are common because of the high incidence of long-standing hypertension and common occurrence of atherosclerotic vascular disease in the dialysis patient. The regular use of systemic anticoagulation in hemodialysis patients may also contribute to the increased incidence of spontaneous subdural hematoma that occurs in dialyzed patients.

Intracerebral Hemorrhage. The presence of hypertension and intermittent heparin for dialysis are major factors in the production of this serious complication. Clinically, the patient represents with an abrupt onset of neurologic symptoms which rapidly progress. Confirmation of diagnosis and localization can be made with CT scan. Conservative management is the rule, except in large cerebellar hemorrhage where surgical evacuation may be indicated.

Subdural Hematomas. These may occur either following head trauma or spontaneously and appear most commonly after a routine dialysis treatment. Because the initial presentation may include alterations in sensorium, confusion, and even dementia, the diagnosis is not always immediately apparent. However, a suspected diagnosis can be easily confirmed with CT scan, and usually requires surgical treatment. Dialysis with as low systemic heparinization as possible (preferably with peritoneal dialysis or hemodialysis using prostacycline or EDTA-calcium anticoagulation) should be employed for 7–10 days following this type of hemorrhage to avoid rebleeding. Since platelet function may be impaired, bleeding time should be measured and, if prolonged, corrected with those measures listed in Table 5-6.

Dementia Secondary to Lacunar Infarcts (Multiinfarct Dementia). In addition to acute hemorrhagic disease, hypertension can produce a chronic progressive form of central nervous system disease due to multiple small infarcts localized around arterioles. This lesion results in progressive deterioration in intellectual function and neurologic abnormalities, including pseudobulbar palsy and other pyramidal signs, dysarthria and dysphagia.

Stroke. Stroke secondary to atherosclerotic disease may occur due to thrombosis emboli from thrombus in the heart or carotid plaque. Standard treatment is used.

GASTROINTESTINAL COMPLICATIONS

See Table 5-33 for outline of gastrointestinal complications.

Nonspecific Manifestations

Nausea and Vomiting. These symptoms are among the most common in patients with advanced renal failure and are often correlated with severity of azotemia. Chronic dialysis therapy usually results in improvement in such symptoms. However, they may occur in dialyzed patients in association with dialysis disequilibrium, as a result of drugs prescribed for other complications, and often as a manifestation of gastrointestinal or liver diseases.

Constipation. Constipation is present in a majority of dialysis patients who take aluminum hydroxide regularly. Constipation should be treated with any of the usual preparations that increase stool bulk to encourage compliance with phosphate binder therapy. Chronic use of laxatives, especially those containing magnesium, should be avoided if possible.

Singultus. Singultus (hiccups) is a long-recognized complication of uremia of unknown pathogenesis. It is a symptom of uremia, and hence when it occurs repeatedly in a dialysis patient, is suggestive of underdialysis. However, singultus

---

Table 5-33. Gastrointestinal Complications

Nonspecific manifestations
  Nausea and vomiting
  Constipation
  Singultus (hiccup)
Diseases of the gastrointestinal tract
  Bleeding
  Mucosal abnormalities
  Peptic ulcer disease
  Diverticulosis (in patients with polycystic kidney disease)
Ascites
Hepatitis

can occur with many unrelated disorders, such as central nervous system diseases, esophagitis, phrenic nerve irritation, and infectious diseases. Treatment measures of variable effectiveness have included sedatives, tranquilizers, antacids, and antispasmodics.

Major Enteric Syndromes

Bleeding. Subclinical. Small but continuous blood loss from the gastrointestinal tract is fairly common in dialysis patients, and may reflect undetected disease or mild, chronic irritation that is aggravated by intermittent anticoagulation for hemodialysis. The magnitude of such blood loss has been documented using chromium-labeled red cells to be 6 ml blood/day lost by dialyzed patients, compared with 3 ml/day by undialyzed azotemic patients and with <1 ml/day by normal controls. Elective evaluation by radiographic and endoscopic techniques in these patients revealed a very high incidence of previously unrecognized pathology including inflammation of esophagus, stomach, and duodenum; hiatus hernia; and peptic ulcer disease. This chronic blood loss adds to that already incurred from dialysis therapy and blood sampling. Gastrointestinal bleeding may be aggravated by ingestion of irritants, including alcohol, nonsteroidal antiinflammatory agents, and aspirin, as well as by the presence of an incompletely corrected qualitative platelet defect.

Clinically significant. Clinically apparent bleeding is also quite common in dialysis patients and may occur from any portion of the gastrointestinal tract. Causes are similar to those seen in other patients, and include reflux esophagitis, gastritis, Mallory-Weiss tears from prolonged vomiting, and peptic ulcer disease of the stomach and duodenum. Diverticular disease of the colon is common in older patients, and there is an increased frequency (up to 85%) in patients with polycystic kidney disease.

Mallory-Weiss syndrome. Standard diagnostic and therapeutic strategies are employed. Anticoagulation during hemodialysis is minimized to avoid aggravating the bleeding. Increased dialysis therapy may be necessary because of the increased rate of protein catabolism from blood in the gastrointestinal tract, and the stress of acute illness, and from lack of caloric intake.

Mucosal Abnormalities. Enlarged gastric (12% of dialysis patients) and duodenal (42% of patients) rugae are frequently noted on radiographic examination. Biopsy proven gastritis is present in as many as 46% of patients. Duodenitis has been found in 60% and esophagitis in 13% of patients by radiography or endoscopy and often correlate with symptoms of nausea, vomiting, pain, and heartburn. Several mechanisms have been proposed to explain increased gastrointestinal tract bleeding in dialysis patients: (1) increased ammonia production in the gastrointestinal tract from bacterial degradation of urea, which may irritate the mucosa; (2) frequent prescription of irritative drugs; (3) increased levels of gastric polypeptides, though correlation of gastrin levels with mucosal abnormalities and peptic disease has been poor; and (4) stress secondary to chronic disease and dialysis treatment.

Peptic Ulcer Disease. Ulcers were previously thought to be increased in chronic renal disease. However, the current incidence is about 10%, which probably does not exceed that of the general population.

Diverticulosis. Patients with polycystic kidney disease have a very high incidence of diverticulosis, approaching 83%, compared with 32% of other patients on chronic hemodialysis and with 38% of normal age and sex matched controls. Of patients with diverticular disease, 40% present with colonic perforation secondary to diverticulitis. In patients on continuous ambulatory peritoneal dialysis, patients with diverticulosis have an increased incidence of perforation and fecal peritonitis.

Ascites

Refractory ascites can occur in patients on chronic hemodialysis therapy, which in most cases cannot be attributed to underlying cardiac, liver, abdominal, or identifiable infectious diseases. The ascitic protein concentration is usually high, and many patients have hypoalbuminemia, which effectively limits the mobilization of ascitic fluid with dialysis or ultrafiltration.

The pathogenesis of this abnormality remains undetermined, but the frequent association with prior peritoneal dialysis therapy in a majority of patients suggests an alteration in peritoneal membrane capillary permeability, secondary to the use of hypertonic dialysate, that persists after peritoneal dialysis has been discontinued.

Treatment of this serious complication has often been unsuccessful, despite the use of rigid fluid control, intensive dialysis, ultrafiltration, albumin infusion, and high protein diets. However, despite the poor prognosis for this disorder, some success has been recorded with the following therapies: (1) transplantation; (2) reinfusion of fluid with the LaVeen shunt (which has been left in place for several years in some patients); and (3) drainage of all ascitic fluid, followed by instillation of a nonreabsorbable steroid, with repetition of this maneuver if ascites recurs.

Hepatitis

Hepatitis B. Incidence. Hepatitis is the most significant infectious problem occurring in hemodialysis facilities; staff may be infected as well as patients.

An increased incidence of hepatitis B became evident in the early days of chronic hemodialysis as a result of frequent transfusion to treat anemia and the need to prime older large volume dialysis circuits. The subsequent development of serologic tests to identify and to isolate patients with acute hepatitis and those individuals with chronic carrier state controlled the spread of infection. Widespread screening of blood donors has also decreased risk of transmission of hepatitis B virus. For the past 10 years, the use of guidelines established by the Center for Disease Control led to a steady decline in hepatitis incidence, from 7.8% to 2.7% positive for HBsAg between 1976 and 1982.

In 1982, an effective vaccine against hepatitis B was released, and testing in dialysis centers showed that it was protective for 94% and 60% of staff and patients, respectively. With widespread immunization of patients and staff on entry to the dialysis centers, the incidence of hepatitis should be very low in the future.

Clinical presentation. Acute hepatitis in the dialyzed patient is usually a mild disease, with no symptoms or only fatigue, pruritis, and anorexia. The disease is almost always anicteric with small rises in transaminases to levels 3–5 times normal. Serum enzyme abnormalities usually return to normal within 3–8 weeks. Persistent elevation may be seen in patients who remain chronic carriers for HBsAg and may be indicative of chronic persistent or chronic active hepatitis. Unlike patients, dialysis staff who develop acute hepatitis are more acutely ill with typical symptoms.

Etiology and laboratory testing. The majority of hepatitis in dialysis patients during the past 20 years has been due to hepatitis B virus. This virus, which as an incubation period of 6 weeks to 6 months, is probably initially introduced to a center via contaminated blood but may be subsequently transmitted to other patients and staff by blood contamination of hands, objects, and equipment, and by accidental needle stick. The major route of entry into the body is through small skin breaks or mucous membranes, but there may also be spread via the oral route.

HBsAg and Anti-HBsAg. HBsAg appears during the late incubation or early clinical illness phases and is followed weeks to months later by the appearance of Anti-HBsAg. Persistence of HBsAg in dialysis patients is quite high, with perhaps 50% of patients becoming asymptomatic chronic carriers. The carrier state can persist for years. The presence of Anti-HBsAg without HBsAg indicates healing and the presence of immunity.

HBcAg and Anti-HBcAg. HBcAg is in the viral core but is not found in the circulation. Anti-HBcAg occurs in response to virus replication in liver cells during the acute phase of hepatitis when HBsAg is present, and may persist long after recovery from the acute disease. Persistant anti-HBcAg without HBsAg may represent continued viral replication in the liver and therefore infectivity, although the risk is low.

HBeAg and Anti-HBeAg. HBeAg may be an integral part of the virus core or may develop from the host response and is most useful as an indicator of infectivity. HBeAg is found more often in chronic hepatitis and anti-HBeAg in chronic HBsAg carriers with normal liver histology.

Table 5-34. Schedule for Screening Hepatitis B

	Frequency
Patients	
HBsAg negative	Every 1–2 months
HBsAg positive	Biannual
Anti-HBsAg negative	Screen new patients and patients with known prior acute hepatitis; then every 12 months
Anti-HBsAg positive	No further testing needed
Anti-HBc	Biannual, especially in HBsAg positive carriers
Staff	
HBsAg negative	Quarterly
Anti-HBsAg negative	Quarterly
HBsAg positive	Biannual
Anti-HBsAg positive	No further testing needed

Control and prevention. The guidelines published by the Center for Disease Control regarding precautions for hepatitis in dialysis centers provide a practical and effective approach to control of this problem. It is also important to be constantly vigilant regarding good hygiene, with strict adherence to proscription of eating, drinking, and smoking in the dialysis center, and adequate cleaning of dialysis equipment.

Physical isolation of chronic HBsAg carriers is desirable, but not absolutely necessary. Reuse of dialyzers should be avoided in all patients with acute hepatitis or chronic HBsAg carriers.

Recommendations for hepatitis testing in chronic dialysis centers vary widely. A limited schedule for hepatitis B screening (for HBsAg and anti-HBsAg) in patients and staff is given in Table 5-34. Of considerable concern is that about 25–50% of these cases will progress to chronic hepatitis.

Non-A Non-B Hepatitis. Unfortunately, as the incidence and prevalence of hepatitis B has declined steadily in dialysis units, the number of cases of sporadic non-A, non-B hepatitis appears to be increasing. In Europe recently, 24% of reported cases of hepatitis was non-A, non-B in patients, and 8% in staff.

Transfusion is the major source of infection, although nonparenteral spread may occur. Clinical disease is of similar severity and manifestations as hepatitis B among patients, but staff do not contract disease. The incubation period is shorter, 2 weeks to 3 months. Progression to chronic disease may occur in as many as 50% of afflicted patients. Control will not be possible until reliable serologic testing for this virus becomes available.

MISCELLANEOUS COMPLICATIONS

Metabolic Acidosis

Despite regular dialysis treatment, many patients have persistent metabolic acidosis on predialysis blood testing which varies in severity. Mean blood gas values of patients evaluated in the National Cooperative Dialysis Study were: pH 7.37; Pco_2 33 mm Hg; Po_2 95 mm Hg; bicarbonate 18 mEq/L. The anion gap was 19 mEq/L. The most important cause of the acidosis was insufficient base delivery on dialysis to match the rate of endogenous acid production. Patients ingesting higher levels of protein or who become catabolic secondary to illness or stress have higher rates of endogenous acid production. Another minor factor is interdialytic extracellular volume expansion and dilution of the plasma bicarbonate concentration. It is also likely that bone buffers do not defend against acidosis normally in dialysis patients, since skeletal demineralization has progressed over many years.

Treatment of acidosis in dialyzed patients should be undertaken. It is now common to use dialysate acetate concentrations of 39–41 mEq/L and bicarbonate dialysate of 36–39 mEq/L to provide a significant base to correct acidosis. If this is inadequate, then evaluation of dietary protein intake may be indicated. Supplemental sodium bicarbonate in a dose of 1 mEq/kg/day can be used to titrate endogenous acid production.

Hyperkalemia

During the interdialytic interval serum potassium rises slowly from the usual low normal postdialysis levels to concentrations in the upper normal range predialysis. This control is achieved by moderate restriction of dietary potassium intake to ~50–80 mEq/day and through stool losses of potassium, which may account for up to 50% of dietary intake. Stool potassium and transport of potassium from plasma to intracellular space is significantly influenced by plasma aldosterone concentration. If renin production is impaired, decreased aldosterone production will result in higher serum potassium levels. Persistent metabolic acidosis may also contribute to hyperkalemia.

However, the major factor affecting predialysis potassium levels is dietary intake, and patients who ingest larger amounts of potassium though dietary indiscretion may chronically have predialysis potassium concentrations of 5–7 mEq/L and occasionally 8–9 mEq/L. As mentioned previously, when a dialysis patient complains of acute muscle weakness, this must be considered severe hyperkalemia until proven otherwise. Suspected hyperkalemia can be confirmed with an EKG and then followed by immediate hemodialysis using a zero or low dialysate potassium as described in Chapter 3. Intravenous glucose and bicarbonate may also be helpful acutely but should not be used in place of dialysis, which should begin as soon as possible.

Skin Abnormalities

Dry Skin. Many patients complain of dry skin of varying degree, which is often associated with decreased sweating as well. This is best managed with liberal use of lanolin-based creams for lubrication, avoidance of drying soaps, and less frequent bathing.

Pruritis. Chronic itching is a complaint in many patients; it can be very severe and limit tolerance of hemodialysis. In the majority of patients, this symptom is more troublesome after the start of hemodialysis, than during advanced renal failure, possibly due to sensitivity to heparin or other chemicals leached from the dialyzer circuit. In addition, pruritis is commonly associated with other uremic complications, including dry skin, elevated calcium-phosphorus product, and secondary hyperparathyroidism. Control of serum phosphorus with diet and binders usually results in some improvement in pruritus but some patients require parathyroidectomy. Finally, pruritis may be a prominent symptom in patients with acute or chronic hepatitis.

Treatment for dialysis-associated pruritis is not very successful but some patients will respond favorably to the following maneuvers.

Ultraviolet light therapy. Gradually increasing doses of ultraviolet light therapy administered in a treatment cabinet has been associated with reduction in symptoms in about 80–90% of patients. Improvement occurs after 2–3 weeks of treatment and persists for 6–7 months after discontinuation. A comparable response in placebo-treated patients has also been reported, thus making the effects of this treatment difficult to assess.

Parenteral lidocaine. Intravenous administration of lidocaine (100 mg in saline over 15 min) has been found to be effective in about 60% of patients with severe pruritis during dialysis. Relatively few side effects have been reported if the dose is limited and the infusion rate does not exceed 7 mg/min. Its mechanism of action is unknown.

Topical agents. Itching is often temporarily relieved by the topical creams and lotions available for this purpose. An effective and pleasant preparation, which is well-liked by our patients, is CME cream (1% camphor, $\frac{1}{4}$% menthol in eucerin) which can be easily mixed by the pharmacist.

Antihistamines. The antihistamines are frequently used for itching and may be helpful at night, but they often produce drowsiness and only partial relief of pruritis.

OUTCOME OF CHRONIC DIALYSIS THERAPY

The management of patients during hemodialysis is appropriately focused on technical concerns and optimal performance of dialysis, including prevention and treatment of dialysis-associated symptoms and complications. During the interdialytic interval, patients are usually seen for other complications and sequelae of dialysis therapy. However, it is important from time to time to step back from these more immediate concerns and direct attention to the overall care of the patient, to reassess the success or failures of current treatment, and to reestablish long term goals and best options for attaining them. The success of therapy should be evaluated not only in terms of survival but also of the quality of life experienced by dialysis patients.

Morbidity

Hospitalization has been reported to be necessary in as many as half of stable chronic hemodialysis patients during a 12 month period. Vascular access revision was the most common reason for inpatient care, followed by cardio-vascular disease and infection. While comparable data for patients on chronic peritoneal dialysis are not available, general experience indicates that peritoneal access problems are not as frequent as in hemodialysis and probably account for a smaller percentage of morbidity. However, because of the high rates of peritonitis at least in the early experience with continuous ambulatory peritoneal dialysis, this complication is probably the most common cause of morbidity and hospitalization.

Medical Results: Hemodialysis versus Continuous Ambulatory Peritoneal Dialysis

The review in this chapter of complications which persist or can occur as a result of dialysis therapy is a sobering testimony to the continuing challenges of renal replacement therapy. But it is both misleading and unfair to concentrate only on the failures of dialysis without commenting on the fact that many patients do well, have relatively few medical complications, and may have 10–15 years of effective life that would not have been possible a generation ago. The availability of dialysis technology and a wider range of dialysis therapy options than existed even 5–10 years ago now make it possible to choose the technique that best meets each individual's needs and to change modality when indicated. The rapid growth and development of peritoneal dialysis over the past 5 years has compelled the nephrology community to look closely at this new trend and to compare the results thus far with hemodialysis.

Long-term randomized comparisons of patients on chronic peritoneal di-alysis and hemodialysis are not yet available. Such comparisons are also limited by the deliberate selection of patients with specific medical complications (e.g., diabetes mellitus and cardiovascular disease) for chronic peritoneal dialysis, which creates significant bias regarding morbidity and survival. However, a growing collective experience with intermittent peritoneal dialysis and contin-uous ambulatory peritoneal dialysis during the past 5 years allows some general observations on the medical results obtained with these types of therapy com-pared with hemodialysis.

Anemia. Patients on continuous ambulatory peritoneal dialysis are usually less anemic than those on hemodialysis, at least partially due to the lack of blood loss that is obligatory with hemodialysis. This is an important advantage for patients with cardiac disease and those who refuse blood transfusion. It is also probably one of several factors that contribute to the increased sense of well-being in patients on continuous ambulatory peritoneal dialysis and may promote better rehabilitation.

Hypertension and Volume Overload. Sustained extracellular volume control is significantly better with CAPD therapy because of continuous ultrafiltration and results in better blood pressure control in a majority of patients. In the Toronto experience, 68% of patients starting continuous ambulatory peritoneal dialysis became normotensive without medication and 26% were better controlled with lower medication requirements than they required while on hemodialysis. Since persistent hypertension is an important risk factor in the development of atherosclerosis and coronary artery disease, this therapeutic advantage may be beneficial in long-term survival. The frequency of atherosclerosis in patients on continuous ambulatory peritoneal dialysis remains high, however, in part due to patient selection bias, but also due to other factors associated with chronic peritoneal dialysis (e.g., hyperlipidemia).

Renal Osteodystrophy. Reports of the effects of continuous ambulatory peritoneal dialysis treatment on the skeletal complications of end-stage renal disease are conflicting, and indicate that longer periods of observation with histologic studies are needed. Both improvement and worsening of bone disease on CAPD have been reported in short term studies. It has been suggested that beneficial changes in bone mineralization on CAPD may result from reduced aluminum exposure, either in dialysate or from binders, due to better control of serum phosphorus.

Nutrition. Nutritional assessment data comparable to those obtained in the NCDS are not available for large numbers of patients on continuous ambulatory peritoneal dialysis. However, based on general experience thus far, it would seem that caloric intake is better for these patients, due to dialysate glucose, but visceral protein stores may be reduced, compared with hemodialysis patients.

Endocrine-Metabolic. Significant differences between continuous ambulatory peritoneal dialysis and hemodialysis regarding thyroid, gonadal, and adrenal hormone function have not yet been identified. However, abnormalities of carbohydrate and lipid metabolism may be more severe in continuous ambulatory peritoneal dialysis. Elevations of total triglycerides are present in a greater percentage of patients on continuous ambulatory peritoneal dialysis, while abnormalities of high density lipoprotein and low density lipoprotein cholesterol appear to be similar to that found in hemodialyzed patients.

Diabetics on continuous ambulatory peritoneal dialysis appear to achieve better control of blood glucose with lower quantities of insulin. The long-term benefits remain to be determined.

Gastrointestinal Disease. Few differences in the incidence of gastrointestinal complications between continuous ambulatory peritoneal dialysis and hemodialysis patients have been reported. There may be decreased incidence and prevalence of hepatitis in continuous ambulatory peritoneal dialysis because of the lesser need for transfusions, and because it is performed at home, placing patients at reduced risk of cross-contamination.

Neurologic. Significant differences exist between hemodialysis and continuous ambulatory peritoneal dialysis regarding neurologic disease. Symptoms of dialysis disequilibrium are almost totally eliminated in CAPD therapy. Also, while dialysis dementia has been reported in patients on peritoneal dialysis, it is largely a disease of chronic hemodialysis therapy. Finally, patients treated with chronic peritoneal dialysis appear to have a decreased incidence of peripheral neuropathy.

Serum Electrolytes. More normal levels of serum potassium are present in patients on continuous ambulatory peritoneal dialysis compared with those on hemodialysis. This occurs in the face of more liberal dietary potassium intake in many patients. Control of systemic acidosis has also been found to be better than in hemodialysis patients, especially with the use of dialysate solutions with higher lactate concentrations.

Rehabilitation

The ability of dialysis to sustain life for long periods of time has been well demonstrated. However, there is growing concern that the maintenance of life without rehabilitation or without restoration of the capacity to perform activities required for a satisfactory quality of life is not an acceptable outcome. Current sentiment is that renal replacement therapy should be both cost-effective and capable of returning most patients to productive life. Data on the rehabilitation of patients available from the European Dialysis and Transplantation registry indicate that about 70% of all dialyzed male patients are classified as able to work, while 85–90% of patients with a functioning transplant can work. Work rehabilitation is better for home patients (81%) than for center hemodialysis (65%). Occupational rehabilitation was lower in women on dialysis (26–33%). Comparable statistics are unfortunately not available in the United States. However, one report on rehabilitation from a multicenter study was quite discouraging and revealed a low rate of rehabilitation, especially in diabetic patients. However, these data may not be representative of the general experience in this country.

Survival

A recent report of survival rates following dialysis and transplantation for the years 1977–1980 in the United States revealed 1 and 3 year survival rates for dialysis therapy of 81% and 56%, respectively; comparable survival figures for cadaver transplantation were 86% and 78% and for living-related transplantation were 95% and 91%. Comparison of these data to European results is made difficult by the fact that rates of entry on dialysis and of transplantations are three times higher in the United States than in Europe, which may reflect not only greater population but also different criteria for admission to these programs. However, when the data are compared, the survival for transplantation is somewhat higher in the United States, but survival with center dialysis is slightly lower than in Europe. Data on survival rates for hemodialysis compared with peritoneal dialysis will be of great interest but are not yet available. Preliminary reports suggest survival on continuous ambulatory peritoneal dialysis is equivalent to hemodialysis.

OUTCOME IN CHILDREN
(Donald E. Potter)

Acute hemodialysis has been performed in premature infants and chronic hemodialysis has been performed in infants as small as 4 kg. The first child was started on chronic dialysis in 1962 and several pediatric dialysis centers have accumulated experience extending more than 17 years. Most children, at least in North America, receive renal transplants after relatively short periods of dialysis; therefore, there is little experience with long-term dialysis in children.

Figures from Europe indicate that the actuarial 4-year survival of children is 66% with center dialysis and 85% with home dialysis. These figures are similar to those in young adults and even better survival has been reported from individual centers. The most frequent causes of death are cerebrovascular accidents, hypertensive heart failure, hyperkalemia, and infections.

Although the survival of children undergoing dialysis is good, children are subject to the same complications of hypertension, heart failure, osteodystrophy, anemia, and failure of vascular access as adults. Most children also have retarded growth and sexual development, the former related to calorie deficiency, vitamin D resistance, and other less well understood factors. In addition, it is apparent that chronic dialysis imposes stresses on children that interfere with normal emotional development and psychosocial functioning. Children are invariably dialyzed in a center, usually during the day, and are unable to participate fully in school and social activities. Feelings of isolation are common, and adaptation is especially difficult in adolescents who are trying to achieve independence but are dependent on a machine and medical personnel for their existence.

For these reasons pediatric nephrologists have considered transplantation, rather than hemodialysis, to be the optimum form of treatment for children with end-stage renal disease. Continuous ambulatory peritoneal dialysis has also become an important alternative to chronic hemodialysis for may children.

REFERENCES

Alpers DH, Clouse RE, Stenson WF: Manual of nutritional therapeutics. Little, Brown, Boston, 1983

Arismendi GS, Izard MW, Hampton WR, Maher JF: The clinical spectrum of ascites associated with maintenance dialysis. Am J Med 60:46, 1976

Bagdade JD: Hyperlipidemia and atherosclerosis in chronic dialysis patients. p. 588. In Drukker W, Parsons FM, Maher J (eds): Replacement of Renal Function by Dialysis. Martinus Nijhoff, Boston, 1983

Bagdade JD: Chronic renal failure and atherogenesis: Serum factors stimulate the poliferation of human arterial smooth muscle cells. Atherosclerosis 34:243, 1979

Bailey GL, Hampers CL, Merrill JP: Reversible cardiomyopathy in uremia. Trans Am Soc Artif Intern Organs 13:263, 1967

Beallo R, Dallman PR, Schoenfeld PY, et al: Serum ferritin and iron deficiency in patients on chronic hemodialysis. Trans Ann Soc Artif Intern Organs 22:73, 1976

Berl T, Berns AS, Huffer WE, et al: 1,25-Dihydroxycholecalciferol effects in chronic dialysis. Ann Intern Med 88:774, 1978

Berl T, Katz FH, Henrich WL, et al: Role of aldosterone in the control of sodium excretion in patients with advanced renal failure. Kidney Int 14:228, 1978

Bischel MD, Neiman RS, Berne TV, et al: Hyperplenism in the uremic hemodialyzed patient. Nephron 9:146, 1972

Bishop CW, Bowen PE, Ritchey SJ: Norms for nutritional assessment of American adults by upper arm anthropometries. Am J Clin Nutr 34:2530, 1981

Blumberg A, Jarti HR: Red cell metabolism and hemodialysis in patients on dialysis. Proc Eur Dial Transplant Assoc 9:91, 1972

Brunzell JD, Albers JJ, Hass LB, et al: Prevalence of serum lipid abnormalities in chronic hemodialysis, metabolism 26:903, 1977

Cannata JB, Briggs JD, Junor BJR: Aluminium hydroxide intake: Real risk of aluminium toxicity. Br Med J 286:1937, 1983

Coburn JW, Llach F: Renal osteodystrophy and maintenance dialysis. p. 679. In Drukker W, Parsons FM, Maher J (eds): Replacement of renal function with dialysis. Martinus Nijhoff, Boston, 1983

Committee on Dietary Allowances, Food and Nutrition Board, National Research Council: Recommended Dietary Allowances. 9th Ed. National Academy of Science, Washington, DC, 1980

Comty CM, Shapiro FL: Cardiac complications of regular dialysis therapy. p. 595. In Drukker W, Parsons FM, Maher J (eds): Replacement of renal functions by dialysis. Martinus Nijhoff, Boston, 1983

Comty CM, Cohen SL, Shapiro FL: Pericarditis in chronic uremia and its sequelae. Ann Intern Med 75:173, 1971

Costaldi PA, Rosenberg MC, Stewart JH: The bleeding disorder of uremia. A qualitative platelet defect. Lancet 2:66, 1966

Durnin JVGA, Womersby J: Body fat assessed from total body density and its estimation for skinfold thickness: Measurements in 481 men and women aged from 16–72 years. Br J Nutr 32:77, 1974

Eastwood JB, Bordier J, DeWardener HE: Some biochemical, histological, radiological and clinical features of renal osteodystrophy. Kidney Int 4:128, 1973

Emmanouel DS, Lindhemier MD, Katz AI: Metabolic and endocrine abnormalities in chronic renal failure. p. 46. In Brenner BM, Stein JH, (eds): Contemporary Issues in Nephrology: Chronic Renal Failure. Churchill Livingstone, New York, 1981

Emmanouel DS, Lindhemier MD, Katz AI: Pathogenesis of endocrine abnormalities in uremia. Endocrine Rev 1:28, 1980

Epstein M: Peritoneovenous shunt in the management of ascites and the hepato-renal syndrome. Gastroenterology 82:790, 1982

Eschbach, JW: Hematologic problems of dialysis patients. p. 630 In Drukker W, Parsons FM, Maher JF (eds): Replacement of Renal Function by Dialysis. Martinus Nijhoff, Boston, 1983

Eschbach JW, Cook JD, Scribner BH, et al: Iron balance in hemodialysis patients. Ann Intern Med 87:710, 1977

Feldman HA, Singer I: Endocrinology and metabolism in uremia and dialysis: A clinical review. Medicine 54:345, 1974

Fisher JW: Prostaglandins and kidney erythropoietin production. Nephron 25:53, 1980

Forst DH, O'Rourke RA: Cardiovascular complications of chronic renal failure. p. 84. In Brenner BM, Stein JH (eds): Contemporary Issues in Nephrology. Chronic Renal Failure. Churchill Livingstone, New York, 1981

Fournier A, Bordier P, Gueris J, et al: Comparison of 1-hydroxycholecalciferol and 25-hydroxycholecalciferol in the treatment of renal osteodystrophy: Greater effect of 25-hydroxycholecalciferol on bone mineralization. Kidney Int 15:196, 1979

Gilchrest BA, Rowe JW, Brown RS, et al: Relief of uremic pruritus with ultraviolet light phototherapy. N Engl J Med 297:136, 1977

Goldberg AP, Harter HR, Patsch W, et al: Racial differences in plasma high density lipoproteins in patients receiving hemodialysis. N Engl J Med 308:1246, 1983

Goldberg A, Sherrard DJ, Brunzell JD: Adipose tissue lipoprotein lipase in chronic hemodialysis: Role in plasma triglyceride metabolism. J Clin Endocrinol Metab 47:1173, 1978

Gipstein RM, Coburn JW, Adams DA, et al: Calciphylaxis in man. Arch Intern Med 136:1273, 1976

Graber SE, Krantz SB: Erythropoietin and the control of red cell production. Annu Rev Med 29:51, 1978

Hampers CL, Katz AI, Wilson RE, Merrill JP: Disappearance of uremic itching after subtotal parathyroidectomy. N Engl J Med 279:695, 1968

Harter HR: Review of significant findings from the National Cooperative Dialysis Study and recommendations. Kidney Int 23, Suppl 13:S107, 1983

Henrich WL, Hunt JM, Nixon JV: Increased ionized calcium and left ventricular contractility during hemodialysis. N Engl J Med 310:19, 1984

Hodsman AB, Sherrard DJ, Wong EGC, et al: Vitamin-D-resistant osteomalacia in hemodialysis patients lacking secondary hyperparathyroidism. Ann Intern Med 94:629, 1981

Hung J, Harris PJ, Uren RF, et al: Uremic cardiomyopathy: Effect of hemodialysis on left ventricular function in end-stage renal failure. N Engl J Med 302:547, 1980

Janson PA, Jubelier SJ, Weinstein MJ, et al: Treatment of the bleeding tendency in uremia with cryoprecipitate. N Engl J Med 303:1318, 1980

Jennekens FGI, Jennekens-Schinkel A: Neurological aspects of dialysis patients. p. 724. In Drukker W, Parsons EM, Maher J, (eds): Replacement of Renal Function by Dialysis. Martinus Nijhoff, Boston, 1983

Kim KE, Onesti G, Del Guercio ET, et al: Sequential hemodynamic changes in end-stage renal disease and the anephric state during volume expansion. Hypertension 2:102, 1980

Knochel JP: Endocrine changes in patients on chronic dialysis. p. 712. In Drukker W, Parsons FM, Maher J (eds): Replacement of Renal Function by Dialysis. Martinus Nijhoff, Boston, 1983

Krakauer H, Grauman JS, McMullan MR, Creede CC: The recent U.S. experience in the treatment of end stage renal disease by dialysis and transplantation. N Engl J Med 308:1558, 1983

Lindner A, Charra B, Sherrard DJ, Scribner BH: Accelerated atherosclerosis in prolonged maintenance hemodialysis. N Engl J Med 290:697, 1974

Lindsay RM, Burton JA, Dangie HJ, et al: Dialyzer blood loss. Clin Nephrol 1:24, 1973

Mahajan SK, Abbasi AA, Prasad AS, et al: Effects of oral zinc therapy on gonadal function in hemodialysis patients. Ann Intern Med 97:357, 1982

Mahoney CA, Arieff AI: Uremic encephalopathies: Clinical, biochemical, and experimental features. Am J Kidney Dis 2:324, 1982

Mannuci PM, Remuzzi G, Pusineri F, et al: Deamino-8-D-arginine vasopressin shortens the bleeding time in uremia. N Engl J Med 308:8, 1983

Margolis DM, Saylor JL, Geisse G, et al: Upper gastrointestinal disease in chronic renal failure. Arch Intern Med 138:1214, 1978

Massry SG, Coburn JW, Lee DB, et al: Skeletal resistance to parathyroid hormone in renal failure. Ann Intern Med 78:357, 1973

Mooradian AD, Morley JE: Endocrine dysfunction in chronic renal failure. Arch Intern Med 144:351, 1984

Morrison G, Michelson EL, Brown ST, Morganroth J: Mechanism and prevention of cardiac arrhythmias in chronic hemodialysis patients. Kidney Int 17:811, 1980

National Center for Health Statistics: Basic data on anthropometric measurements and angular measurements of the hip and knee joints for selected age groups 1–74 years of age, United States, 1971–1975 (Vital and Health Statistics: Series II, No 219) DHHS publication, No (PHS) 81–1669, 1981

National Center for Health Statistics: Weight by height and age for adults 18–74 years. United States, 1971–1974: (Vital and health statistics: Series II, No 208) DHHS publication, No (PHS) 79–1656, 1979

Neff MS, Goldberg J, Slifkin RF, et al: A comparison of androgens for anemia in patients on hemodialysis. N Engl J Med 304:871, 1981

Nestel PJ, Fidge NH, Tan MH: Increased lipoprotein-remnant formation in chronic renal failure. N Engl J Med 307:329, 1982

Nixon JV, Mitchell JH, McPhaul JJ, Henrich WL: Effect of hemodialysis on left ventricular function. J Clin Invest 71:377, 1983

Ott SM, Maloney NA, Coburn JW, et al: The prevalence of bone aluminum deposition in renal osteodystrophy and its relation to the response to calcitrol therapy. N Engl J Med 307:709, 1982

Parkinson IS, Ward MK, Feest TG, et al: Fracturing dialysis osteodystrophy and dialysis encephalopathy. Lancet 1:406, 1979

Polakoff S: Dialysis associated hepatitis. p. 659. In Drukker W, Parsons FM, Maher J (eds): Replacement of Renal Function by Dialysis. Martinus Nijhoff, Boston, 1983

Raskin NH, Fishman RA: Neurological disorders in renal failure (two parts). N Engl J Med 294:143; 204, 1976

Renfrew R, Buselmeier TJ, Kjellstrand CM: Pericarditis and renal failure. Annu Rev Med 31:345, 1980

Rosenblatt SG, Drake S, Fadem S, et al: Gastrointestinal blood loss in patients with chronic renal failure. Am J Kidney Dis 1:232, 1982

Rostand SG, Greter JC, Kirk KA, et al: Ischemic heart disease in patients with uremia undergoing maintenance hemodialysis. Kidney Int 16:600, 1979

Sargent J, Gotch FA, Borah M, et al: Urea Kinetics: A guide to nutritional management of renal failure. Am J Clin Nutr 31:1696, 1978

Savazzi GM, Buzio C, Migone L: Lights and shadows on the pathogenesis of uremic polyneuropathy. Clin Nephrol 18:219, 1982

Scheff RT, Zuckerman G, Harter HR, et al: Diverticular disease in patients with chronic renal failure due to polycystic kidney disease. Ann Intern Med 92:202, 1980

Schoenfeld, PY, Henry RF, Laird NM, Roxe DM: Assessment of nutritional status of the National Cooperative Dialysis Study population. Kidney Int 23, Suppl 13:P S-80, 1980

Steiner RW, Coggins C, Carvalho ACA: Bleeding time in uremia: A useful test to assess clinical bleeding. Am J Hematol 7:107, 1979

Strickland ID, Choputde Saintonge DM, Boulton FE, et al: The therapeutic equivalance of oral and intravenous iron in renal dialysis patients. Clin Nephrol 7:55, 1977

Tapia L, Cheigh JS, David DS, et al: Pruritis in dialysis patients treated with parenteral lidocaine. N Engl J Med 296:261, 1977

Teehan BP, Laird NM, Harter HR: Influences of dialysis prescription on electrolyte and acid-base metabolism. Kidney Int 23, Suppl 13:S66, 1983

Thunberg BJ, Swamy AP, Cestero RUM: Cross-sectional and longitudinal nutritional measurements in maintenance hemodialysis patients. Am J Clin Nutr 34:2005, 1981

Van Ypersele de Strihou, C: Potassium Homeostasis in renal failure. Kidney Int 11:491, 1977

Vertes V, Cangiano JL, Berman LB, Gould A: Hypertension in end-stage renal disease. N Engl J Med 280:978, 1971

Vollmer WM, Wahl PW, Blagg CR: Survival with dialysis and transplantation in patients with end stage renal disease. N Engl J Med 308:1553, 1983

Weideman P, Maxwell MH, Lupu AN, et al: Plasma renin activity and blood pressure in terminal renal failure. N Engl J Med 285:757, 1971

White RP, Rubin AL: Blood pressure control in chronic dialysis patients. p. 575. In Drukker, W, Parsons FM, Maher J (eds): Replacement of Renal Function by Dialysis. Martinus Nijhoff, Boston, 1983

Wing AJ, Brunner FP, Brynger HOA, et al: Comparative review between dialysis and transplantation. p. 850. In Drukker W, Parsons FM, Maher J (eds): Replacement of Renal Function by Dialysis. Martinus Nijhoff, Boston, 1983

Yawata Y, Howe R, Jacob HS: Abnormal red cell metabolism causing hemolysis in uremia. A defect potentiated by tap water hemodialysis. Ann Intern Med 79:362, 1973

6

DRUG OVERDOSE AND PHARMACOLOGIC CONSIDERATIONS IN DIALYSIS

Donald P. Alexander   John G. Gambertoglio

Various forms of dialysis are used in the treatment of acute and chronic renal disease. Although the primary purpose of dialysis is to remove accumulated toxic waste products from the body, it also has the effect of removing drugs as well. Recently, it has been shown that chronic dialysis patients receive an average of eight drugs for a variety of medical indications. Thus, it is important to know the extent to which drugs are removed, as it may alter the patient's response to therapy. Supplemental doses or revised dosage regimens may be required under these circumstances. Dialysis procedures, including hemoperfusion, have also been used in treating drug overdoses as a means of eliminating a drug or its metabolites from the body. It is essential to know how effective these procedures are and whether they offer substantial advantages, as compared with conventional or conservative approaches to treating drug overdoses.

The objectives of this chapter are threefold: (1) to review basic concepts of extracorporeal removal of drugs in renal failure patients and in the overdose setting; (2) to critically evaluate the various methods used to calculate the dialysis clearance and fractional removal of a drug; and (3) to provide the skills that will help predict and interpret the extent of drug removal by dialysis.

BASIC CONCEPTS

The optimal therapy for the use of extracorporeal dialysis in the treatment of renal failure and in the overdose situation is unknown. Appropriate data collection and analysis of the role of dialysis in drug overdose is difficult to accomplish. The evidence demonstrating the effectiveness of this intervention as a treatment modality in the overdosed patient is insufficient. Since plasma drug concentrations often reflect total body burden of a drug, this measurement is frequently used as a means of assessing the degree of drug removal. Furthermore, for many drugs plasma concentrations correlate with clinical effect and are used as a guide in monitoring therapy. Appropriate interpretation of plasma drug concentrations necessitates recognition of certain limitations, such as delayed gastrointestinal absorption, active metabolites, altered distributional characteristics, and saturable elimination pathways. In addition, the use of any extracorporeal procedure for drug removal from the body is limited by access for drug removal from the blood or central compartment. That is, drugs having large distribution volumes are not greatly eliminated by these procedures. The use of pharmacokinetic information can be especially useful for drugs whose exact dialyzability has not been determined. Applying these pharmacokinetic principles can be useful in both the therapeutic situation and overdose setting, but they should be used in conjunction with clinical information, which can aid in the decision as to whether dialysis should be used in the treatment of drug overdose.

In the use of extracorporeal intervention, many reports in the literature are primarily qualitative and commonly anecdotal, especially in the overdose setting. Often the effectiveness of dialysis in drug removal is assumed by changes in the patient's clinical response alone. For example, a comatose patient awakens during or shortly after dialysis, and it is assumed that dialysis removed the drug and accounted for the improved clinical status of the patient. In the absence of measured drug levels in blood or dialysate, a proper assessment of drug removal cannot be made. Commonly, the type of dialysis system is unspecified; there are insufficient patient data, such as weight, hemotocrit, and renal or hepatic function, that are useful in determining the patient's ability to eliminate drugs. Furthermore, the methods used for calculation of drug dialysis clearance are frequently unspecified.

Most pharmacokinetic data used in predicting a drug's dialyzability are obtained from normal, healthy subjects or from renal failure patients receiving dialysis. Obviously this information may not directly apply to the overdosed individual being considered for dialysis. Furthermore, advances in dialysis technology have outdated many previous studies determining drug dialyzability in the renal failure patient.

In determining a drug's dialyzability, both dialysis-related factors and drug-related factors must be considered. Dialysis-related factors include dialyzer membrane characteristics and surface area, blood flow to the dialyzer, degree of ultrafiltration, and duration of dialysis. Drug-related factors include availability of the drug for dialysis and specific drug characteristics. As shown in Figure 1-6 in Chapter 1, drugs with a low molecular weight (<500) cross dialyzer membranes more readily, the degree of transfer being dependent upon blood flow, dialysate flow, and effective membrane surface area. The dialyzability of larger molecules is more dependent upon membrane surface area and less on effective blood flow (see Fig. 1-7, Chapter 1). Large molecules, such as amphotericin B (mol wt 924), vancomycin (mol wt 3300), and heparin (mol wt 6,000–20,000), cross membranes with difficulty, and their removal is thus limited during hemodialysis or even peritoneal dialysis. Drugs with greater water solubility are more readily removed by the aqueous dialysate. Lipid-soluble compounds such as glutethimide are dialyzed with difficulty. Moreover, lipid-soluble drugs generally have larger distribution volumes and are less concentrated in the blood from which the dialysis procedure has access. Drugs with large distribution volumes (e.g., digoxin, 600 L) are not substantially dialyzed, since the majority of drug is not in the blood compartment but, rather, in tissue storage sites, and is not readily accessible for removal. Furthermore, some drugs exhibit a rebound in plasma concentration at the completion of dialysis due to the relatively slow transfer of drug from tissue to blood (e.g., lithium, ethchlorvynol). Another important factor in predicting drug dialyzability is plasma protein binding, since only the free (unbound) drug can cross dialysis membranes. Drugs that are normally highly protein-bound (e.g., warfarin, 98–99%, and propranolol, 90–94%) are not significantly removed by dialysis, since the drug-protein complex is too large to effectively cross the dialysis membrane.

PHARMACOKINETIC CONSIDERATIONS IN THE OVERDOSED PATIENT

In the overdosed patient, collection and interpretation of adequate data to assess drug removal by dialysis is often difficult. Frequently, the amount of drug and time of ingestion are unknown, making quantitative estimates of the fractional drug loss by dialysis impossible. In the overdosed setting, there can be prolonged gastrointestinal absorption (e.g., tricyclic antidepressants, narcotics) due to the formation of concretions or by depressed gastrointestinal motility. This may provide a constant input of drug into the systemic circulation. Furthermore, the first-pass metabolism of some drugs (e.g., propranolol, propoxyphene) becomes saturated with large ingestions, causing increased systemic availability. For many drugs there is a lack of correlation between plasma concentration and clinical response in the overdose situation. The presence of active metabolites may contribute to this poor correlation. Saturation of plasma protein binding with increased unbound drug may result in increased volume of distribution and drug clearance. In the presence of a saturated metabolic pathway for drug elimination, the contribution of extracorporeal drug removal may increase. Furthermore, changes in plasma concentration may be disproportionate to the amount of drug in the body. It should also be recognized that certain drug overdoses may result in pathologic damage to organs of elimination (e.g., acetaminophen, mercury), causing decreased drug clearance. Other factors, such as hypotension, hypothermia, cardiac failure, and hepatic congestion, may also diminish the body's capability of removing toxic substances.

METHODS USED TO CALCULATE DIALYSIS CLEARANCE

There are several methods of calculating dialysis clearance of solutes and drugs, as discussed in Chapter 1. Dialysis clearance (K) of a substance is defined as the volume of fluid that is cleared by the dialyzer per unit time, and is used as an index of the efficiency of solute removal. Simply, clearance of a solute or drug is dependent on the efficiency (ER, extraction ratio) of the dialyzer and the blood flow rate entering the dialyzer (Q_{Bi}) when convective flux is low, as shown in Equation (1-13) from Chapter 1:

$$K = Q_{Bi}ER \tag{6-1}$$

Since

$$ER = \frac{C_{Bi} - C_{Bo}}{C_{Bi}} \tag{6-2}$$

Then

$$K = Q_{Bi} \times \frac{C_{Bi} - C_{Bo}}{C_{Bi}} \tag{6-3}$$

Clearance is sometimes calculated from plasma flow [blood flow multiplied by 1 minus the hematocrit (H)] and/or from plasma water (P) drug concentrations:

$$K = Q_{Bi}(1 - H) \times \frac{C_{Pi} - C_{Po}}{C_{Pi}} \tag{6-4}$$

It is important to point out that the dialysis clearance and dialysance of a drug are the same when a single-pass dialysate system is used, because the concentration of a drug in the entering dialysate is zero. Many dialysis systems in the past have used a recirculating dialysate bath, which decreases the drug concentration gradient between blood and dialysate with time.

There are several problems with using these equations for drug clearance. Since a value for blood flow is available from the dialysis machine, and it is usually plasma drug concentrations that are measured, this method treats the blood as a simple solution and ignores any differences between whole blood and plasma drug concentrations. Over- or underestimation of dialysis clearance may result. Furthermore, if plasma flow is used and the drug is distributed to more than just the plasma, dialysis clearance will be underestimated.

The relationship between blood and plasma concentrations can be estimated in Equation (6-5):

$$C_B = C_P(1 - H) + C_{RBC}H \tag{6-5}$$

where C_B, C_P, and C_{RBC} are the concentrations in blood, plasma, and red blood cell, respectively, and H is the hematocrit.

When drug is present in the red blood cell, Equation (6-6) represents the dialysis clearance, utilizing the combined contribution of the plasma and red blood cell flow:

$$K = Q_{Bi}[(1 - H) + ZH] \times ER_P \qquad (6\text{-}6)$$

where $Z = C_{RBC}/C_P$.

If the drug partitions into the red blood cell extensively, then Equation (6-4) will underestimate the true dialysis clearance. At present few data are available regarding the red blood cell : plasma ratio of drugs.

The use of these equations also assumes that rapid equilibration of the drug occurs between plasma and the red blood cell. If rapid equilibration of the drug does not occur, then the calculations of dialysis clearance will be inaccurate.

Most importantly, the use of these methods for determining dialysis clearance requires that accurate measurements of blood flow, hematocrit, and extraction ratio can be made and remain constant over the dialysis interval measured. The blood flow rates determined from dialysis machine pump dials have been shown to vary as much as $\pm 30\%$ of the actual blood flow. Furthermore, ultrafiltration may falsely decrease the arteriovenous difference across the dialyzer, thereby underestimating dialysis clearance. The variability in drug analysis may also contribute to an inaccurate calculation of clearance. If one is unable to collect and measure the amount of drug recovered in dialysate, measuring drug concentrations in plasma and whole blood will provide the best estimate of true dialysis clearance.

The most accurate and reliable manner of determining dialysis clearance is to use the method utilizing the total amount of drug recovered in the dialysate:

$$K = \left[\frac{Q_{Do} \times C_{Do}}{\overline{C}_B} \right]_o^t \qquad (6\text{-}7)$$

where $Q_{Do} \times C_{Do}$ is the amount of drug recovered in the dialysate during the measured interval of dialysis (t), divided by average blood drug concentration during that period $(\overline{C}_B)$ or the area under the blood concentration-time curve for the measured interval (t). When one measures only plasma concentrations and substitutes average plasma drug concentration or the area under the plasma concentration-time curve for the interval (t) for $\overline{C}_B$, the calculation of K may be inaccurate.

Accurate measurements of dialysate flow and concentration are practical problems in the use of this method. The collection of large volumes of dialysate, and the ability to measure the drug in very dilute solutions, have hindered the more widespread use of this method. However, this is a direct and reliable method of determining dialysis clearance that is not influenced by ultrafiltration or the ability to accurately measure blood flow.

Other methods used to assess the effectiveness of extracorporeal removal are by comparison of the drug's half-life, or area under the plasma concentration time curve, on- and off-dialysis; by the reduction of plasma concentrations before and after the intervention; or by calculation of the fraction removed by dialysis. There are several problems that make these methods of determining effectiveness of extracorporeal removal less than ideal. The calculation of half-life is determined from the drug's elimination rate constant. This rate constant is a composite of the volume of distribution (V) and body clearance; it must be assumed that V does not change with concentration or the dialysis procedure and that the elimination rate constant reflects clearance of the drug. Little information is presently available regarding the volume changes that may occur during dialysis. The interpretation of clearance by this method requires a second study off-dialysis or comparison to population values in the literature. The accuracy of the values for half-life are dependent upon the number of samples taken, length of sampling time, and sensitivity of the assay used to determine drug concentrations. Area under the plasma concentration-time curve during a dialysis period reflects the combination of normal body clearance plus clearance by dialysis and requires the knowledge of the total body burden at the time of dialysis and usual values of normal body clearance. Unfortunately, the amount of drug in the body at the start of dialysis is not usually known, especially in the case of the overdosed patient.

Reduction in plasma concentration is a very insensitive and inaccurate method of assessing drug removal by dialysis. Plasma concentrations are subject to influences from distribution, hemoconcentration, and redistribution of the drug. In the overdose situation, the slopes of the plasma concentration-time curve may be confounded by delayed absorption of the drug, therefore not representing accurately the extracorporeal removal of the drug. If one uses the change in plasma concentration before and after dialysis, one must know the V and/or the amount of drug in the body and assume that V does not change during the procedure. In the overdose situation, the amount of drug in the body is rarely known and the normal population values of V may not apply because of possible concentration-dependent pharmacokinetics.

EXAMPLES OF DRUG REMOVAL BY HEMODIALYSIS

The extraction efficiency and dialysis clearance parameters do not quantitate the effectiveness of extracorporeal removal of drug. The best method to evaluate the effectiveness of extracorporeal removal is by the fractional drug removal (f) of the procedure. For drugs described by a one-compartment body model, or drugs with multicompartmental characteristics, f may be determined by appropriate modeling equations. However, technical problems of obtaining information for such drug pharmacokinetics may be different in an overdose situation, and the use of these equations to determine fractional drug removal may not be appropriate.

When attempting to predict the dialyzability of a drug, the dialysis clearance of the drug must be compared to the clearance of the drug by the body. Clearance terms are additive:

$$K_{\text{body}} + K_{\text{dialysis}} = K_{\text{total}} \tag{6-8}$$

Thus, the clearance (renal, hepatic, etc.) by the body (K_{body}) and by dialysis

(K_{dialysis}) can be added together to give a total combined clearance K_{total}. If dialysis clearance adds substantially to body clearance, forming a much larger total clearance, elimination will be that much faster. Thus, Equation (6-9) shows that the fraction of drug in the body that is lost during a dialysis period f can be calculated as follows:

$$f = \text{Fraction lost during a dialysis period} \qquad (6\text{-}9)$$
$$= 1 - e^{-(K_{\text{body}} + K_{\text{dialysis}}) \frac{t}{V}}$$

where t is the duration of the dialysis. This equation allows calculation of the fraction of drug in the body that is lost during a dialysis period by all routes of elimination (i.e., renal excretion, metabolism, and dialysis). From literature sources it is possible to obtain values for distribution volume, plasma clearance, and dialysis clearance. Again, it should be emphasized that the clearance and volume terms may change under different conditions, such as in renal failure and drug overdose, to name only two.

Discussion of some examples will illustrate the use of the above concepts in predicting the effect of hemodialysis on drug removal. The parameter estimates for several drugs are listed in Table 6-1.

In a patient with normal renal function overdosed on digoxin, using a distribution volume of 560 liters, with a body clearance of 150 ml/min and a dialysis clearance of 20 ml/min, there would be a drug half-life off dialysis of ~43 hours, but on the half-life on dialysis would decrease to only 38 hours. The fraction of drug lost from the body during 4 hours of dialysis would be only 7%. Thus, hemodialysis would not be very useful in treating digoxin overdose, primarily because of its large volume of distribution. If the same patient were anephric, the values for volume and clearance would be decreased (Table 6-1), and the drug half-life both off and on dialysis would change from 86 hours to 58 hours. Although this is a larger change than in the previous example, it would mean that the patient would require 58 hours of dialysis in order to remove half the drug from the body, with only 5% being lost in a 4-hour period.

For a patient overdosed with phenobarbital, since dialysis clearance adds substantially to the body clearance, the decrease in half-life is large, declining

Table 6-1. Parameter Estimates of Representative Drugs for Determining Utility of Hemodialysis

Drug	Total Body Clearance (ml/min)	Dialysis Clearance (ml/min)	Volume of Distribution (L)	Half-life off Dialysis (h)	Half-life on Dialysis (h)	FL*
Digoxin						
Normal[†]	150	20	560	43	38	0.07
Anephric[††]	40	20	300	86	58	0.05
Phenobarbital	5	70	50	115	8	0.30
Ethchlorvynol	35	60	300	100	36	0.07
Phenytoin	5	10	100	231	77	0.04
Salicylates	20	100	40	23	4	0.51

* FL: fraction lost during a 4-hour period of hemodialysis.
† Normal: Parameters for a patient with normal renal function.
†† Anephric: Parameters for a patient with no renal function.

from 115 hours to 8 hours with dialysis. During a 4-hour dialysis, 30% of the drug is eliminated from the body.

The next three drugs, ethchlorvynol, phenytoin, and salicylates, have been shown to exhibit concentration-dependent pharmacokinetics. Therefore, estimates of distribution volume and clearance would be expected to be altered in the overdose situation. Ethchlorvynol has a half-life of 26 hours after usual therapeutic doses, but during an overdose its half-life may increase to 100 hours or more. This is probably due to a decreased metabolic clearance at high drug concentrations. Although the dialysis clearance is 60 ml/min, greater than the expected body clearance, only 7% of the drug would be eliminated from the body during 4 hours of dialysis. Again, the limiting factor of its removal by dialysis is the large distribution volume of this drug. Furthermore, ethchlorvynol appears to show a postdialysis rebound in plasma concentrations because of redistribution of drug back into the systemic circulation from tissue storage sites.

The half-life of phenytoin is 18–36 hours in the therapeutic concentration range, whereas in the overdose setting it may be greatly prolonged due to a decrease in the body clearance from the usual rate of 15–30 ml/min. The usual volume of distribution of ~50 L and plasma protein binding of 90% would increase and decrease, respectively, at high plasma concentrations. Thus, in an overdosed patient with parameter estimates of those shown in Table 6-1, there would be a tremendous change in drug half-life, from 231 to 77 hours, with dialysis. However, with this still very long half-life on dialysis, it appears that dialysis would contribute little to the detoxification of overdosed patients.

In patients with aspirin overdose with plasma salicylate concentrations of ~100 mg/dl, the estimated pharmacokinetic parameters for salicylates are shown in Table 6-1. The dialysis clearance of salicylate is 100 ml/min and adds substantially to the body clearance, so that the half-life on-dialysis is about 4 hours. Thus, an 8-hour period of hemodialysis could possibly remove 75% of the drug from the body.

USE OF HEMOPERFUSION

In the treatment of drug overdose, the use of resin or activated charcoal hemoperfusion techniques exist as a means of drug removal from the body. These act by adsorbing or binding drugs present in the patient's blood. Resin hemoperfusion is advocated primarily for lipid-soluble drugs and drugs whose removal by conventional dialysis (peritoneal or hemodialysis) is limited. Commonly, drug concentrations in the blood demonstrate a dramatic decrease over the hemoperfusion period, and values for drug clearance and extraction ratio are usually much greater than those seen with hemodialysis. However, because lipid-soluble drugs frequently have large distribution volumes in the body, their removal by hemoperfusion is limited, since the majority of drug resides in peripheral tissues, which serve as a depot from which the drug returns to the blood once hemoperfusion is discontinued. The degree of drug protein binding is not a limitation of hemoperfusion because the drug is removed from plasma proteins as it passes the adsorbent material. Furthermore, molecular weight is not a limitation for hemoperfusion techniques, as the drug is adsorbed onto a high-surface-area material. The efficiency of hemoperfusion has been shown to diminish over time as the adsorbent material becomes saturated with accumulated drug. Overall, the use of hemoperfusion in drug overdose should be restricted to more severe cases, and its risks, primarily bleeding due to thrombocytopenia secondary to platelet adhesion to the hemoperfusion substrate, must be compared to its proposed benefits in enhancing drug removal. Table 6-2 provides specific information on the hemoperfusion removal of several drugs.

USE OF PERITONEAL DIALYSIS

Peritoneal dialysis is not generally considered an efficient means of drug removal in the overdose setting. This is due to the low peritoneal clearances for drugs in relation to the body's clearance of the drug. In the therapeutic situation, chronic peritoneal dialysis usually causes only a slight increase in drug removal, which may necessitate some drug dosage alteration. However, very little quantitative data are available describing drug elimination by peritoneal dialysis. Basically, the same principles as discussed under hemodialysis apply to the peritoneal dialysis situation. Refer to Table 6-2 for information regarding available data on the peritoneal removal of drugs.

REFERENCES

Anderson RJ, Bennett WM, Gambertoglio JG, Schrier RW: Fate of drugs in renal failure. p. 2659. Brenner BM, Rector Jr, FC (ed): The Kidney. Saunders, Philadelphia, 1981

Anderson RJ, Melikian DM, Gambertoglio JG, et al: Prescribing medication in long term dialysis units. Arch Intern Med 142:1305, 1982

Anderson RJ, Schrier RW (eds): Clinical Use of Drugs in Patients with Kidney and Liver Disease. Saunders, Philadelphia, 1981

Benet LZ, Massoud N, Gambertoglio JG (eds): The Pharmacokinetic Basis of Drug Therapeutics. Raven Press, New York, 1983

Benet LZ, Sheiner LB: Design and optimization of dosage regimens: Pharmacokinetic data (Appendix II). p. 1675. Gilman AG, Goodman LS, Gilman A (eds): The Pharmacological Basis of Therapeutics. Macmillan, New York, 1980

Bennet WM, Aronoff GR, Morrison G, et al: Drug prescribing in renal failure: Dosing guidelines for adults. Am J Kidney Dis 3:155–193, 1983

Bennett WM, Muther RS, Parker RA, et al: Drug therapy in renal failure: Dosing guidelines for adults. Ann Intern Med 93:62, 286, 1980

Gibson TP, Matusik E, Nelson LD, et al: Artificial kidneys and clearance calculations. Clin Pharmacol Ther 20:720, 1976

Gibson TP, Nelson HA: Drug kinetics and artificial kidneys. Clin Pharmacokinet 2:403, 1977

Gwilt PR: General equation for assessing drug removal by extracorporeal devices. J Pharm Sci 70:345, 1981

Gwilt PR, Perrier D: Plasma protein binding and distribution characteristics of drugs as indices of their hemodialyzability. Clin Pharmacol Ther 24:154, 1978

Lee CS: The assessment of fractional drug removal by extracorporeal dialysis. Biopharm Drug Dispos 3:165, 1982

Lee CS, Marbury TC, Benet LZ: Clearance calculations in hemodialysis: Application to blood, plasma, and dialysate measurements for ethambutol. J Pharmacokinet Biopharm 8:69, 1980

Pond, S, Rosenberg J, Benowitz NL, et al: Pharmacokinetics of haemoperfusion for drug overdose. Clin Pharmacokinet 4:329, 1979

Rosenberg J, Benowitz NL, Pond S: Pharmacokinetics of drug overdose. Clin Pharmacokinet 6:161, 1981

Takki S, Gambertoglio JG, Honda DH, et al: Pharmacokinetic evaluation of hemodialysis in acute overdose. J Pharmacokinet Biopharm 6:427, 1978

Tilstone WJ, Winchester JF, Reavey PC: The use of pharmacokinetic principles in determining the effectiveness of removal of toxins from blood. Clin Pharmacokinet 4:23, 1979

Table 6-2. DRUG DIALYSIS REFERENCE DATA

Table 6-2 on the following pages lists information on the effect of hemodialysis (HD), peritoneal dialysis (PD), and hemoperfusion (HP) on the removal of commonly used drugs. For each drug, we have attempted to critically evaluate the literature and have provided a qualitative statement to describe the extent of removal by the three techniques using the standard procedure time.

The following abbreviations are used:

ND = not dialyzed (0–5% removed)
SD = slightly dialyzed (5–20% removed)
MD = moderately dialyzed (20–50% removed)
D   = dialyzed (50–100% removed)
MW = molecular weight
S   = water solubility (base)
  S   = soluble
  IS = insoluble
  SS = slightly soluble
  *   = Data reporting the removal of the drug by a dialysis procedure was less than optimal for evaluation

We define a standard dialysis procedure to include a blood flow rate of 200–300 ml/min; a dialysate flow rate of 500 ml/min; a duration of hemodialysis or hemoperfusion of 3–4 hours (e.g., $Kt/V \simeq 1.0$–1.2).

A list of general and selected references is provided after the end of the table so that further details on specific drugs may be obtained.

ANTIBACTERIAL AGENTS

DRUG	MW	S	HD	PD	HP	COMMENTS	REFERENCES
Aminoglycosides							
Amikacin	781	S	D	SD–MD		50–75% of the loading dose postdialysis; use plasma levels as a guide to dosing	1
Gentamicin	543	S	D	SD–MD		See amikacin	2–5
Kanamycin	582	S	D	SD–MD		See amikacin	2, 6
Neomycin	614	S	D*			See amikacin	7
Netilmicin		S	D			See amikacin	8
Streptomycin	581	S	MD–D*			See amikacin	9
Tobramycin	467	S	D (64 ml/min)	MD		See amikacin	10–14
Penicillins							
Amdinocillin	325	S	MD*			Usual dose post-HD	15
Amoxicillin	364	S	MD*	SD		1-g dose post-HD	16, 17
Ampicillin	349	S	MD*	ND*		1-g dose post-HD	18, 19
Azlocillin	461	S	MD (26–44 ml/min)			1–2-g dose post-HD	20, 21
Carbenicillin	399	S	MD	SD*		0.75–1.5-g dose post-HD	22, 23
Cloxacillin	453	S	ND*				24

Drug					Recommendation	Ref.
Dicloxacillin	487	S	ND*			25, 26
Methicillin	397	S	ND*			27
Mezlocillin	557	S	MD (29 ± 9 ml/min)	SD	0.5–1.0-g dose post-HD	28, 29
Nafcillin	432	S	ND*			30, 31
Oxacillin	418	S	ND*	ND*		19, 27
Penicillin G	334	S	MD (46 ± 12 ml/min)		500,000-U dose post-HD	32
Piperacillin	517	S	MD		1-g dose post-HD	33, 34
Ticarcillin	405	S	MD*	ND–SD*	0.75–1.5-g dose post-HD	35
Cephalosporins						
Cefaclor	386	S	MD		Usual dose post-HD	36, 37
Cefamandole	463	S	MD	SD* (24 ± 12 ml/min)	One-half usual dose post-HD	38, 39
Cefazolin	454	S	MD	SD*	25–50% usual dose post-HD	40–42
Cefoperazone	644	S			No data	
Cefotaxime	454	S	SD*	ND	Active (1/8) desacetyl metabolite; half-usual dose post-HD	43, 44
Desacetyl metabolite	395		MD*	SD		
Cefonicid	586	S	ND–SD		No supplemental dose	45
Cefoxitin	426	S	MD*	SD*	One-half usual dose post-HD	46, 47

ANTIBACTERIAL AGENTS (Continued)

DRUG	MW	S	HD	PD	HP	COMMENTS	REFERENCES
Cephalexin	365	S	MD*	SD*		Usual dose post-HD	42, 48
Cephalothin	395	S	MD*			Active (1/2) desacetyl metabolite; half-usual dose post-HD	49
Cephapirin	422	S	MD*			See cephalothin	50
Cephradine	349	S	MD*			Usual dose post-HD	51
Moxalactam	518	S	D	SD*		One-half usual dose post-HD	52, 53
Miscellaneous							
Chloramphenicol	323	SS	SD*	ND		No supplemental dose required	54–56
						Increased dialysis removal in hepatic failure	
Chloroquine	320	SS	ND*	ND*		HD data derived from dogs	57, 58
Cinoxacin	262	IS				No data	
Clindamycin	423	SS	ND*	ND			13, 59
Doxycycline	463	SS	ND*	ND–SD*			60, 61
Erythromycin	734	SS	ND				62
Metronidazole	171	SS	D	SD*		500 mg after each HD	63, 64
Minocycline	457	SS	ND*	ND*			65
Nalidixic acid	232	IS				No data	

DRUG	MW	S	HD	PD	HP	COMMENTS	REFERENCES
Nitrofurantoin	238	SS				No data	
Sulfamethoxazole	253	SS	SD–MD*	ND		Give daily dose after dialysis	66, 67
Sulfisoxazole	267	SS				No data	56
Tetracycline	444	SS		SD			
Trimethoprim	290	SS	SD–MD*	ND		Give daily dose after dialysis	66, 67
Vancomycin	3300		ND*	SD–MD			68–71

ANTIFUNGAL AGENTS

DRUG	MW	S	HD	PD	HP	COMMENTS	REFERENCES
Amphotericin B	924	IS	ND				72
Flucytosine	129	S	D	MD*		20 mg/kg after HD	72–74
Ketoconazole	531	S	ND*				75
Miconazole	416	SS	ND*				76

ANTIVIRAL AGENTS

DRUG	MW	S	HD	PD	HP	COMMENTS	REFERENCES
Acyclovir	225	S	D (113 ± 22 ml/min)			One-half usual dose post-HD	77, 78
Amantadine	151	S	ND–SD	SD*			79–81

ANTIVIRAL AGENTS (*Continued*)

DRUG	MW	S	HD	PD	HP	COMMENTS	REFERENCES
Vidarabine	285	S				No data	

ANTITUBERCULAR AGENTS

DRUG	MW	S	HD	PD	HP	COMMENTS	REFERENCES
Ethambutol	208	S	SD (85 ml/min)			No supplemental doses needed after HD	82
Isoniazid	137	S	D	MD		Dose post-HD	83, 84
Rifampin	823	SS				Not dialyzed due to large distribution volume and molecular size	

SEDATIVES–HYPNOTICS

DRUG	MW	S	HD	PD	HP	COMMENTS	REFERENCES
Chloral hydrate	165	S	MD–D (117 ± 9 ml/min)			Data are for the trichloroethanol active metabolite	85
Chlordiazepoxide	300		ND*			Active metabolites	86
Diazepam	285		ND*			Active metabolites	
Ethchlorvynol	145	IS	ND–SD	ND	SD–MD	Concentration-dependent kinetics; rebound blood level after HP	87–90

	MW	S	HD	PD	HP	Active metabolites	REFERENCES
Flurazepam	388	S	ND*	ND*	SD–MD	Active metabolite	91, 92
Glutethimide	217	IS	ND–SD*	ND–SD*	SD	Active metabolite	93–97
Meprobamate	218	S	SD	ND–SD*	SD		91, 98, 99
Methaqualone	250	IS	SD*	SD*	SD*		100
Oxazepam	287	IS	ND				
Pentobarbital	225	S	SD*	ND–SD*	SD–MD		91, 101–104
Secobarbital	237	S	SD*	ND–SD*	SD–MD		91, 101, 102, 104

ANTIEPILEPTICS AND PSYCHOTROPICS

DRUG	MW	S	HD	PD	HP	COMMENTS	REFERENCES
Carbamazepine	236	IS		ND*	See comments	Active epoxide metabolite. One case report using HP, insufficient data	105, 106
Ethosuximide	141	S	MD–D (143 ± 15 ml/min)			Give dose after dialysis	107
Haloperidol	376	IS				Probably insignificant removal due to large distribution volume	
Lithium	7		MD–D*	MD*		Rebound rise in plasma levels postdialysis. Case reports suggest 300–600 mg lithium carbonate after each HD in renal failure patients	108–112

ANTIEPILEPTICS AND PSYCHOTROPICS (*Continued*)

DRUG	MW	S	HD	PD	HP	COMMENTS	REFERENCES
Phenobarbital	232	S	MD–D*	SD–MD*	D	Give dose after dialysis	91, 101, 104, 113–117
Phenothiazines (e.g., chlorpromazine)	319		ND*			Numerous metabolites; toxicity and dialyzability unknown	118
Phenytoin	252	IS	ND (12 ± 3 ml/min)	ND	SD–MD	Concentration-dependent kinetics	119–124
Primidone	218	S	MD (98 ± 14 ml/min)			Partly metabolized to phenobarbital	125
Tricyclic antidepressants (e.g., nortriptyline)	263		ND	ND	ND	Multiple metabolites	91, 126–131
Valproic acid	144	SS	SD	ND			132, 133

ANALGESICS

DRUG	MW	S	HD	PD	HP	COMMENTS	REFERENCES
Acetaminophen	151	SS	SD (138 ± 27 ml/min)	ND*	SD*	Concentration-dependent kinetics, increased dialysis removal in overdose. HD or HP has not been shown to prevent hepatic or renal toxicity	134–137

278

	MW	S	HD	PD	HP	COMMENTS	REFERENCES
Acetylsalicylic	300	IS	D*	MD*	D*	Concentration-dependent kinetics; HD preferred over HP for overdose	91, 116, 138–142
Codeine	397	S				No data	
Dextropropoxy-phene	339	S	ND			Active metabolite poorly dialyzed	143
Meperidine	217	S				Active metabolite accumulates in renal failure	
Methadone	346	S				No data	
Morphine	669	S				No data	
Pentazocine	285	IS				No data	

ANTIINFLAMMATORY AGENTS

DRUG	MW	S	HD	PD	HP	COMMENTS	REFERENCES
Allopurinol	136	SS				Active metabolite; oxypurinol dialyzed similar to creatinine	144
Fenoprofen	242					No data	
Ibuprofen	206	IS				No data	
Indomethacin	358	IS				No data	
Methylpredniso-lone	374	SS	SD*				145
Naproxen	230					No data	

ANTIINFLAMMATORY AGENTS (Continued)

DRUG	MW	S	HD	PD	HP	COMMENTS	REFERENCES
Penicillamine	149	S				No data	
Phenylbutazone	308	S			SD*		146
Prednisone (prednisolone, active moiety)	360	SS	SD				147
Probenicid	285	IS				No data	

CARDIAC AGENTS

DRUG	MW	S	HD	PD	HP	COMMENTS	REFERENCES
Atenolol	266		MD*				148
Bretylium	237		MD*				149
Digitoxin	765	SS	ND*	ND*			150
Digoxin	781		ND	ND	ND	Post-HD and -HP rebound in serum levels	91, 151–155
Diltiazem	415					No data	
Disopyramide	339		ND			Concentration-dependent kinetics	156
Lidocaine	234	IS	ND (27 ml/min)			Active metabolites	157
Metoprolol	267					No data	

DRUG	MW	S	HD	PD	HP	COMMENTS	REFERENCES
N-Acetylprocain-amide	261		MD*	ND			158–161
Nadolol	309		SD*				162
Nifedipine	346	IS				No data	
Procainamide	236		MD*	ND*			158, 159, 161
Propranolol	259		ND*				163, 164
Quinidine	324	SS	ND–SD*	ND			165–167
Tocainide			SD–MD*				168
Verapamil	455	IS				Probably poorly dialyzed due to large body distribution	

ANTIHYPERTENSIVES

DRUG	MW	S	HD	PD	HP	COMMENTS	REFERENCES
Captopril	218		MD*				169
Clonidine	230		ND*				170
Guanethidine	198					No data	
Hydralazine	160					No data	
Methyldopa	211		SD–MD*	SD*		Parent drug and metabolite data	171
Minoxidil						No data	
Nitroprusside	252					No data	
Prazosin	382					No data	

DIURETICS

DRUG	MW	S	HD	PD	HP	COMMENTS	REFERENCES
Acetazolamide	222	SS	MD				172
Ethacrynic acid	303	SS				No data	
Furosemide	331	SS	ND*				173, 174
Hydrochlorothia-zide	298	IS				No data	
Metolazone	366					No data	
Spironolactone	417	IS				No data	
Triamterene	253					No data	

ANTINEOPLASTIC AGENTS

DRUG	MW	S	HD	PD	HP	COMMENTS	REFERENCES
Azathioprine (6-mercaptopurine)	152	SS	SD–MD*			Data for azathioprine and metabolites using nonspecific assay	175
Bleomycin	>1400	S				No data; probably poorly dialyzed due to large size	
Cis-platinum	195					No data	
Cyclophospha-mide	261	S	MD (104 ± 15 ml/min)				176

DRUG	MW	S	HD	PD	HP	COMMENTS	REFERENCES
Cytarabine	243					No data	
5-Fluorouracil	130					No data	
Melphalan	305	IS				No data	
Methotrexate	454		ND*	ND*	ND–SD*		177–179
Mithramycin	1085	SS				No data; probably poorly dialyzed due to large size	
Vinblastine	811	IS				No data; probably poorly dialyzes due to large body distribution	
Vincristine	825	IS				No data; probably poorly dialyzed due to large body distribution	

HYPOGLYCEMIC AGENTS

DRUG	MW	S	HD	PD	HP	COMMENTS	REFERENCES
Acetohexamide	324			ND*		Active metabolite	180
Chlorpropamide	277	IS		ND*		Active metabolite	181
Insulin	>6000					No data; probably poorly dialyzed due to large size	
Tolazamide	311					Active metabolites	
Tolbutamide	270		ND*			Inactive and less active metabolites	182

MISCELLANEOUS AGENTS

DRUG	MW	S	HD	PD	HP	COMMENTS	REFERENCES
Cimetidine	252	S	SD	ND	SD–MD*	Supplemental doses post-dialysis unnecessary; coincide doses around dialysis	183–189
Diphenhydramine	255	S				No data	
Ethanol	46	S	D				116, 190
Ethylene glycol	62	S	D*			Toxic metabolites formed	116
Heparin	6,000–20,000	S				No data; probably poorly dialyzed due to large size	
Isopropanol	60	S	D*			Major toxic metabolite is acetone	116, 191
Levodopa	197	S				No data	
Methanol	32	S	D	SD–MD*		Major toxic metabolites are formaldehyde and formic acid	116, 190, 192
Ranitidine						No data	
Theophylline	180	SS	D (88 ± 6 ml/min)	SD–MD*	D	Nonlinear disposition; supplemental doses needed following dialysis	91, 193–196
Warfarin	308	IS				Probably poorly dialyzed due to high protein binding	

REFERENCES FOR TABLE 6-2

1. Madhavan T, Yaremchuk K, Levin N, et al: Effect of renal failure and dialysis on the serum concentration of the aminoglycoside amikacin. Antimicrob Agents Chemother 10:464, 1976
2. Danish M, Schultz R, Jusko WJ: Pharmacokinetics of gentamicin and kanamycin during hemodialysis. Antimicrob Agents Chemother 6:841, 1974
3. Jusko WJ, Baliah T, Kim KH, et al: Pharmacokinetics of gentamicin during peritoneal dialysis in children. Kidney Int 9:430, 1976
4. Gary NE: Peritoneal clearance and removal of gentamicin. J Infect Dis Suppl 124:S96, 1971
5. Somani P, Shapiro RS, Stockard H, et al: Unidirectional absorption of gentamicin from the peritoneum during continuous ambulatory peritoneal dialysis. Clin Pharmacol Ther 32:113, 1982
6. Atkins RC, Mion C, Despaux E, et al: Peritoneal transfer of kanamycin and its use in peritoneal dialysis. Kidney Int 3:391, 1973
7. Krumlovsky FA, Emmerman J, Parker RH, et al: Dialysis treatment of neomycin overdosage. Ann Intern Med 76:443, 1976
8. Humbert G, Leroy A, Fillastre JP, et al: Pharmacokinetics of netilmicin in the presence of normal or impaired renal function. Antimicrob Agents Chemother 14:40, 1978
9. Langer T, de Bercovich C, Barousse AP: Extraccion de estreptimicina por hemodialisis extracorporea. Medicina (B Aires) 29:105, 1969
10. Bunke CM, Aronoff GR, Brier ME, et al: Tobramycin kinetics during continuous ambulatory peritoneal dialysis. Clin Pharmacol Ther 34:110, 1983
11. Firsov AA, Bogomolova NS, Treskina OS, et al: Comparative characteristics of procedures for estimation of aminoglycoside extraction with "artificial kidney" apparatus: Clearance and dialyzing of tobramycin. Antibiotiki 26:290, 1981
12. Lockwood WR, Bower JD: Tobramycin and gentamicin concentrations in the serum of normal and anephric patients. Antimicrob Agents Chemother 3:125, 1973
13. Jaffe G, Meyers BR, Hirschman SZ: Pharmacokinetics of tobramycin in patients with stable renal impairment, patients undergoing peritoneal dialysis, and patients on chronic hemodialysis. Antimicrob Agents Chemother 5:611, 1974
14. Malacoff RF, Finkelstein FO, Andriole VT: Effect of peritoneal dialysis on serum levels of tobramycin and clindamycin. Antimicrob Agents Chemother 8:574, 1975
15. Bailey K, Cruickshank JG, Bisson PG, et al: Mecillinam in patients on hemodialysis. Br J Clin Pharmacol 10:177, 1980
16. Francke EL, Appel GB, Neu HC: Kinetics of amoxicillin in patients on long-term dialysis. Clin Pharmacol Ther 26:31, 1979
17. Jones RH, Cundy T, Bullock R, et al: Concentrations of amoxycillin in serum and dialysate of uraemic patients undergoing peritoneal dialysis. J Infect 1:235, 1979
18. Jusko WJ, Lewis GP, Schmitt GW: Ampicillin and hetacillin. Clin Pharmacol Ther 14:90, 1972
19. Ruedy J: The effects of peritoneal dialysis on the physiological disposition of oxacillin, ampicillin and tetracycline in patients with renal disease. Can Med Assoc J 94:257, 1966
20. Schurig VR, Kampf D, Becker H, et al: Pharmacokinetik von Azlocillin bei Niereninsuffizienz und Hämodialyse. Arzenim Forsch 29:1944, 1979
21. Aletta JM, Francke EF, Neu HC: Intravenous azlocillin kinetics in patients on long-term hemodialysis. Clin Pharmacol Ther 27:563, 1980
22. Latos DL, Bryan CS, Stone WJ: Carbenicillin therapy with normal and impaired renal function. Clin Pharmacol Ther 17:692, 1975
23. Eastwood JB, Curtis JR: Carbenicillin administration in patients with severe renal failure. Br Med J 1:486, 1968
24. Nauta EH, Mattie H, Gosling WRO: Pharmacokinetics of cloxacillin in patients on chronic intermittent haemodialysis and in healthy subjects. Chemotherapy 19:261, 1973
25. McCloskey RV, Hayes Jr CP: Plasma levels of dicloxacillin in oliguric patients and the effects of hemodialysis. Antimicrob Agents Chemother 7:770, 1967
26. Williams Jr TW, Lawson SA, Brook MI, et al: Effect of hemodialysis on dicloxacillin concentration in plasma. Antimicrob Agents Chemother 7:767, 1967

27. Bulger RJ, Lindholm DP, Murray JS, et al: Effect of uremia on methicillin and oxacillin blood levels. JAMA 187:319, 1964

28. Janicke DM, Mangione A, Schultz RW, et al, Mezlocillin disposition in chronic hemodialysis patients. Antimicrob Agents Chemother 20:590, 1981

29. Kampf D, Schurig R, Weihermuller K, et al: Effects of impaired renal function, hemodialysis, and peritoneal dialysis on the pharmacokinetics of mezlocillin. Antimicrob Agents Chemother 18:81, 1980

30. Rudnick M, Morrison G, Walker B, et al: Renal failure, hemodialysis and nafcillin kinetics. Clin Pharmacol Ther 20:413, 1976

31. Diaz CR, Kane JG, Parker RH, et al: Pharmacokinetics in patients with renal failure. Antimicrob Agents Chemother 12:98 1977

32. Bryan CS, Stone WJ: "Comparably massive" pencillin G therapy in renal failure. Ann Intern Med 82:189, 1975

33. Francke EL, Appel GB, Neu HC: Pharmacokinetics of intravenous piperacillin in patients undergoing chronic hemodialysis. Antimicrob Agents Chemother 16:788, 1979

34. Alexander DP, Ethridge S, Kaysen G: Unusual pharmacokinetics of piperacellin in a patient with liver and renal dysfunction. In preparation, 1984.

35. Parry MF, Neu HC: Pharmacokinetics of ticarcillin in patients with abnormal renal function. J Infect Dis 133:46, 1976

36. Berman SJ, Boughton WH, Sugihara JG, et al: Pharmacokinetics of cefaclor in patients with end-stage renal disease and during hemodialysis. Antimicrob Agents Chemother 14:281, 1978

37. Fillastre JP, Leroy A, Humbert G, et al: Cefaclor pharmacokinetics and renal impairment. J Antimicrob Chemother 6:155, 1980

38. Gambertoglio JG, Aziz NS, Lin ET, et al: Cefamandole kinetics in uremic patients undergoing hemodialysis. Clin Pharmacol Ther 26:592, 1979

39. Ahern MJ, Finkelstein O, Andriole VT: Pharmacokinetics of cefamandole in patients undergoing hemodialysis and peritoneal dialysis. Antimicrob Agents Chemother 10:457, 1976

40. McCloskey RV, Forland MF, Sweeney MJ, et al: Hemodialysis of cefazolin. J Infect Dis Suppl 128:S358, 1973

41. Madhavan T, Yaremchuk K, Levin N, et al: Effects of renal failure and dialysis on cefazolin pharmacokinetics. Antimicrob Agents Chemother 8:63, 1975

42. Bunke CM, Aronoff GR, Brier ME, et al: Cefazolin and cephalexin in continuous ambulatory peritoneal dialysis. Clin Pharmacol Ther 33:66, 1983

43. Alexander DP, Gambertoglio JG, Barriere SL, et al: Cefotaxime in continuous ambulatory peritoneal dialysis. In preparation, 1984.

44. Chodos J, Francke EL, Saltzman M, et al: Pharmacokinetics of intravenous cefotaxime in patients undergoing chronic hemodialysis. Ther Drug Monit 3:71, 1981

45. Barrier S, Gambertoglio JG. Alexander DP, et al: Pharmacokinetic disposition of cefonicid in patients with renal failure and on hemodialysis. Rev Infect Dis. In press, 1984.

46. Garcia MJ, Dominguez-Gil A, Tabernero JM, et al: Pharmacokinetics of cefoxitin in patients undergoing hemodialysis. Int J Clin Pharmacol 17:366, 1979

47. Greaves WL, Kreeft JH, Ogilvie RI, et al: Cefoxitin disposition during peritoneal dialysis. Antimicrob Agents Chemother 19:253, 1981

48. Reisberg BE, Mandelbaum JM: Cephalexin: Absorption and excretion as related to renal function and hemodialysis. Infect Immun. 3:540, 1971

49. Venuto RC, Plaut NE: Cephalothin handling in patients with undergoing hemodialysis. Antimicrob Agents Chemother 10:50, 1971

50. McCloskey RV, Terry EE, McCracken AW et al: Effect of hemodialysis and renal failure on serum and urine concentrations of cephapirin sodium. Antimicrob Agents Chemother 1:90, 1972

51. Solomon AE, Briggs JD, McGeachy et al: The administration of cephradine to patients in renal failure. Br J Clin Pharmacol 2:443, 1975

52. Aronoff GR, Sloan RS, Mong SA, et al: Moxalactam pharmacokinetics during hemodialysis. Antimicrob Agents Chemother 19:575, 1981

53. Wright N, Wills PJ, Wise R: The pharmacokinetics of moxalactam in renal failure. J Antimicrob Chemother 8:395, 1981
54. Slaughter RL, Cerra FB, Koup JR: Effect of hemodialysis on total body clearance of chloramphenicol. Am J Hosp Pharm 37:1083, 1980
55. Blouin RA, Erwin WG, Dutro MP, et al: Chloramphenicol hemodialysis clearance. Ther Drug Monit 2:351, 1980
56. Greenberg PA, Sanford JP: Removal and absorption of antibiotics in patients with renal failure undergoing peritoneal dialysis; tetracycline, chloramphenicol, kanamycin and colistimethate. Ann Intern Med 66:465, 1967
57. Van Stone JC: Hemodialysis and chloroquine poisoning. J Lab Clin Med 88:87, 1976
58. McCann WP, Permisohn R, Palmisano PA: Fatal chloroquine poisoning in a child: Experience with peritoneal dialysis. Pediatrics 55:536, 1975
59. Roberts AP, Eastwood JB, Gower PE, et al: Serum and plasma concentrations of clindamycin following a single intramuscular injection of clindamycin phosphate in maintenance haemodialysis patients and normal subjects. Eur J Clin Pharmacol 14:435, 1978
60. Whelton A, von Wittenau MS, Twomey TM, et al: Doxycycline pharmacokinetics in the absence of renal function. Kidney Int 5:365, 1974
61. Letteri JM, Miraflor F, Tablante V, et al: Doxycycline (vibramycin) in chronic renal failure. Nephron 11:318, 1973
62. Iliopoulou A, Downey K, de Saintonge C., et al: Should erythromycin dose be altered in haemodialysis patients? Eur J Clin Pharmacol 23:435, 1982
63. Gabriel R, Page M, Weller IVD, et al: The pharmacokinetics of metronidazole in patients with chronic renal failure. p. 49. In Finegold SM (ed): Proceedings of the 2nd International Symposium on Anaerobic Infections. Series 18. Royal Society of Medicine, Geneva, Switzerland, 1979
64. Holten E, Smith-Ericksen N: Concentration of metronidazole in serum during peritoneal dialysis. Chemotherapy 27:414, 1981
65. Carney S, Butcher RA, Dawborn JK et al: Minocycline excretion and distribution in relation to renal function in man. Clin Exp Pharmacol Physiol 1:299, 1974
66. Craig WA, Kunin CM: Trimethoprim-sulfamethoxazole: Pharmacokinetic effects of urinary pH and impaired renal function; studies in humans. Ann Intern Med 78:491, 1973
67. Singlas E, Colin JN, Rottenbourg J, et al: Pharmacokinetics of sulfamethoxazole-trimethoprim combination during chronic peritoneal dialysis: Effect of peritonitis. Eur J Clin Pharmacol 21:409, 1982
68. Mollering RC, Krogstad DJ, Greenblatt DJ: Vancomycin therapy in patients with impaired renal function: A nomogram for dosage. Ann Intern Med 94:343, 1981
69. Lindholm DD, Murray JS: Persistence of vancomycin in the blood during renal failure and its treatment by hemodialysis. N Engl J Med 274:1047, 1966
70. Nielson HE, Sorensen I, Hansen HE: Peritoneal transport of vancomycin during peritoneal dialysis. Nephron 24:274, 1979
71. Ayus JC, Eneas JF, Tong TG, et al: Peritoneal clearance and total body elimination of vancomycin during chronic intermittent peritoneal dialysis. Clin Nephrol 11:129, 1979
72. Block ER, Bennett JE, Livoti ZG, et al: Flucytosine and amphotericin B: Hemodialysis effects on the plasma concentration and clearance; studies in man. Ann Intern Med 80:613, 1974
73. Cutler RE, Blair AD, Kelly MR: Flucytosine kinetics in subjects with normal and impaired renal function. Clin Pharmacol Ther 24:333, 1978
74. Polak A: Pharmacokinetics of amphotericin B and flucytosine. Postgrad Med J 55:667, 1979
75. Ken CM, Perfect JR, Craven PC, et al: Fungal peritonitis in patients on continuous ambulatory peritoneal dialysis. Ann Intern Med 99:334, 1983
76. Lewi PJ, Boelaert J, Daneels R, et al: Pharmacokinetic profile of intravenous miconazole in man: Comparison of normal subjects and patients in renal insufficiency. Eur J Clin Pharmacol 10:49, 1976
77. Krasny HC, Liao SH, de Miranda P, et al: Influence of hemodialysis on acyclovir pharmacokinetics in patients with chronic renal failure. Am J Med Suppl 73:202, 1982

78. Laskin OL, Longstreth JA, Whelton A, et al: Acyclovir kinetics in end-stage renal disease. Clin Pharmacol Ther 31:594, 1982

79. Horadam VW, Sharp JG, Smilack JD, et al: Pharmacokinetics of amantadine hydrochloride in subjects with normal and impaired renal function. Ann Intern Med 94(Part 1):454, 1981

80. Ing TS, Mahurkar SD, Dunea G, et al: Removal of amantadine hydrochloride by dialysis in patients with renal insufficiency. Can Med Assoc J 115:515, 1976

81. Soung L-S, Ing TS, Daugirdas JT, et al: Amantadine hydrochloride pharmacokinetics in hemodialysis patients. Ann Intern Med 93(Part 1):46, 1980

82. Lee CS, Marbury TS, Benet LZ: Clearance calculations in hemodialysis: Application to blood, plasma, and dialysate measurements for ethambutol. J Pharmacokinet Biopharm 8:69, 1980

83. Gold CH, Buchanan N, Tringham, V, et al: Isoniazid pharmacokinetics in patients in chronic renal failure. Clin Nephrol 6:365, 1976

84. Cocco AE, Pazoureh LJ: Acute isoniazid intoxication: Management by peritoneal dialysis. N Engl J Med 269:852, 1963

85. Stalker NE, Gambertoglio JG, Fukumitsu CJ, et al: Acute massive chloral hydrate intoxication treated with hemodialysis: A clinical pharmacokinetic analysis. Clin Pharmacol 18:136, 1978

86. Cruz IA, Cramer NC, Parrish AE: Hemodialysis in chlordiazepoxide toxicity. JAMA 202:136, 1967

87. Tozer TN, Witt LD, Gee L, et al: Evaluation of hemodialysis for ethchlorvynol (Placidyl) overdose. Am J Hosp Pharm 31:986, 1974

88. Hedley-Whyte J, Laasberg LH: Ethchlorvynol poisoning: Gas liquid chromatography in management. Anesthesiology 30:107, 1969

89. Lynn RI, Honig CL, Jatlow PI, et al: Resin hemoperfusion for treatment of ethchlorvynol overdose. Ann Intern Med 91:549, 1979

90. Benowitz N, Abolin C, Tozer T, et al: Resin hemoperfusion in ethchlorvynol overdose. Clin Pharmacol Ther 27:236, 1980

91. Pond S, Rosenberg J, Benowitz NL, et al: Pharmacokinetics of haemoperfusion for drug overdose. Clin Pharmacokinet 4:329, 1974

92. Ozdemir AI, Tannenberg AM: Peritoneal and hemodialysis for acute glutethimide overdosage. NY State J Med 72:2076, 1972

93. Lobo PI, Spyker D, Surratt P, et al: Use of hemodialysis in meprobamate overdosage. Clin Nephrol 7:73, 1977

94. Hagstam K-R, Lindholm T, Treatment of exogenous poisoning with special regard to the need for artificial kidney in severe complicated cases. Acta Med Scand 175:507, 1964

95. Castell DO, Sode J: Meprobamate intoxication treated with peritoneal dialysis. Ill Med J 131:298, 1967

96. Mouston DE, Cohen RJ, Barrett Jr O: Meprobamate poisoning: Successful treatment with peritoneal dialysis. Am J Med Sci 253:706, 1967

97. Hoy WE, Rieveo A, Marin MG, et al: Resin hemoperfusion for treatment of a massive meprobamate overdose. Ann Intern Med 93:455, 1980

98. Proudfoot AT, Noble J, Nimmo SS, et al: Peritoneal dialysis and haemodialysis in methaqualone (Mandrax) poisoning. Scott Med J 13:232, 1968

99. Chang TMS, Coffey JF, Barre P, et al: Microcapsule artificial kidney: Treatment of patients with acute drug intoxication. Can Med Assoc J 108:429, 1973

100. Murray TG, Chiang ST, Koepke HH, et al: Renal disease, age and oxazepam kinetics. Clin Pharmacol Ther 30:805, 1981

101. Berman LB, Jeghers HJ, Schreiner GE, et al: Hemodialysis, an effective therapy for acute barbiturate poisoning. JAMA 161:820, 1956

102. Setter JG, Freeman RB, Maher JF, et al: Factors influencing the dialysis of barbiturates. Trans Am Soc Artif Intern Organs 10, 340, 1964

103. Bloomer HA: Limited usefulness of alkaline diuresis and peritoneal dialysis in pentobarbital intoxication. N Engl J Med 272:1309, 1965

104. Berman LB, Vogelsang P: Removal rates for barbiturates using two types of peritoneal dialysis. N Engl Med 270:77, 1964

105. Gary NE, Byra WM, Eisinger RP: Carbamazepine poisoning: Treatment by hemoperfusion. Nephron 27:202, 1981
106. Gruska H, Beyer KH, Kubicki ST, et al: Klinik, Toxikologie und Therapie einer schweren Carbamazepin-Vergiftung. Arch Toxicol 27:193, 1971
107. Marbury TC, Lee CC, Perchalski RJ, et al: Hemodialysis clearance of ethosuximide in patients with chronic renal disease. Am J Hosp Pharm 38:1757, 1981
108. Hawkins JB, Dorken PR: Lithium. Lancet 1:839, 1969
109. Amdisen A, Skjoldborg H: Haemodialysis for lithium poisoning. Lancet 2:213, 1969
110. Wilson HP, Donker AJM, Van der Hem K, et al: Peritoneal dialysis for lithium poisoning. Br Med J 2:749, 1971
111. Procci WR: Mania during maintenance hemodialysis successfully treated with oral lithium carbonate. J Nerv Ment Dis 164:355, 1977
112. Port FK, Kroll PD, Rosenzweig J: Lithium therapy during maintenance hemodialysis. Psychosomatics 20:130, 1979
113. Lee HA: The Role of peritoneal and hemodialysis treatment. p. 205. In Matthew H (ed): Acute Barbiturate Poisoning. Excerpta Medica, Amsterdam, 1971
114. Whiting EG, Barrett Jr ON, Immon TW: Treatment of barbiturate poisoning: The use of peritoneal dialysis. Calif Med 102:367, 1965
115. Kennedy AC, Briggs JD, Young N, et al: Successful treatment of three cases of very severe barbiturate poisoning. Lancet 1:995, 1969
116. Winchester JF, Gelfand MC, Knepshield JH, et al: Dialysis and hemoperfusion of poisons and drugs: Update. Trans Am Soc Artif Intern Organs 23:762, 1977
117. Chow-Tung E, Lau AH, Vidyasagar D, et al: Clearance of phenobarbital by peritoneal dialysis in a neonate. Clin Pharm 1:266, 1982
118. Avram MM, McGinn JT: Extracorporeal hemodialysis in phenothiazine overdosage. JAMA 197:182, 1966
119. Martin E, Gambertoglio JG, Adler DS, et al: Removal of phenytoin by hemodialysis in uremic patients. JAMA 238:1750, 1977
120. Rubinger D, Levy M, Roll D, et al: Inefficiency of haemodialysis in acute phenytoin intoxication. Br J Clin Pharmacol 7:405, 1979
121. Dodson WE, Loney LC: Hemodialysis reduces the unbound phenytoin in plasma. J Pediatr 101:465, 1982
122. Tenckhoff H, Sherrard DJ, Hickman RO, et al: Acute diphenylhydantoin intoxication. Am J Dis Child 116:422, 1968
123. Blair AAD, Hallpike JF, Lascelles PT, et al: Acute diphenylhydantoin and primadone poisoning treated by peritoneal dialysis. J Neurol Neurosurg Psychiatry 31:520, 1968
124. Czajka PA, Anderson WH, Christoph RA, et al: A pharmacokinetic evaluation of peritoneal dialysis for phenytoin intoxication. J Clin Pharmacol 20:565, 1980
125. Lee CC, Marbury TC, Perchalohi RT, et al: Pharmacokinetics of primadone elimination by uremic patients. J Clin Pharmacol 22:301, 1982
126. Bailey RR, Sharman JR, O'Rourke J, et al: Haemodialysis and forced diuresis for tricyclic antidepressant poisoning. Br Med J 4:230, 1974
127. Oreopoulos DG, Lal S: Recovery from massive amitriptyline overdosage. Lancet 2:221, 1968
128. Halle MA, Collipp PJ: Amitriptyline hydrochloride poisoning: Unsuccessful treatment by peritoneal dialysis. NY State J Med 69:1434, 1969
129. Sunshine P, Yaffe S: Amitriptyline poisoning: Clinical and pathological findings in a fatal case. Am J Dis Child 106:501, 1963
130. Dawling S, Lynn K, Rosser R, et al: Nortriptyline metabolism in chronic failure: Metabolite elimination. Clin Pharmacol Ther 32:322, 1982
131. Comstock TJ, Watson WA, Jennison TA: Severe amitriptyline intoxication and the use of charcoal hemoperfusion. Clin Pharm 2:85, 1983
132. Marbury TC, Lee CS, Bruni J, et al: Hemodialysis of valproic acid in uremic patients. Dial Transplant 9:961, 1980
133. Orr JM, Farrell K, Abbott FS, et al: The effects of peritoneal dialysis on the single dose and

steady state pharmacokinetics of valproic acid in a uremic epileptic child. Eur J Clin Pharmacol 24:387, 1983

134. Marbury TC, Wang LH, Lee CS: Hemodialysis of acetaminophen in uremic patients. Int J Artif Organs 3:263, 1980

135. Øie, S, Lowenthal DT, Briggs WA, et al: Effect of hemodialysis on kinetics of acetaminophen elimination by anephric patients. Clin Pharmacol Ther 18:680, 1975

136. Maclean D, Peters TJ, Brown RAG, et al: Treatment of acute paracetamol poisoning. Lancet 2:849, 1968

137. Gazzard BG, Willson RA, Weston MJ, et al: Charcoal haemoperfusion for paracetamol overdose. Br J Clin Pharmacol 1:271, 1974

138. Doolan PD, Walsh WP, Kyle LH, et al: Acetylsalicylic acid intoxication: A proposed method of treatment, JAMA 146:105, 1951

139. Kallen RJ, Zaltzman S, Coe FL, et al: Hemodialysis in children: Technique, kinetic aspects related to varying body size, and application to salicylate intoxication; acute renal failure and some other disorders. Medicine (Baltimore) 45:1, 1966

140. Etteldorf JN, Dobbins WT, Summit RL, et al: Intermittent peritoneal dialysis using 5 percent albumin in the treatment of salicylate intoxication in children. J Pediatr 58:226, 1961

141. Schlegel RJ, Altstat LB, Canales L, et al: Peritoneal dialysis for severe salicylism: An evaluation of indications and results. J Pediatr 69:553, 1966

142. Summitt RL, Etteldorf JN: Salicylate intoxication in children—Experience with peritoneal dialysis and alkalinization of the urine. J Pediatr 64:803, 1964

143. Giacomini KM, Gibson TP, Levy G: Effect of hemodialysis on propoxyphene and norpropoxyphene concentration in blood of anephric patients. Clin Pharmacol Ther 27:508, 1980

144. Hayes CP, Metz EN, Robinson RR, et al: The use allopurinol (HPP) to control hyperuricemia in patients on chronic intermittent hemodialysis. Trans Am Soc Artif Intern Organs 11:247, 1965

145. Sherlock JE, Letteri JM: Effect of hemodialysis on methylprednisolone plasma levels. Nephron 18:208, 1977

146. Berlinger WG, Spector R, Flanigan MJ, et al: Hemoperfusion for phenylbutazone poisoning. Ann Intern Med 96:334, 1982

147. Frey FJ, Gambertoglio JG, Frey BM, et al: Nonlinear plasma protein binding and haemodialysis clearance of prednisolone. Eur J Clin Pharmacol 23:65, 1982

148. Flouvat B, Decourt S, Aubert P, et al: Pharmacokinetics of atenolol in patients with terminal renal failure and influence of haemodialysis. Br J Clin Pharmacol 9:379, 1980

149. Josseison J, Narang PK, Adir J, et al: Bretylium kinetics in renal insufficiency. Clin Pharmacol Ther 33:144, 1983

150. Finkelstein FO, Goffniet JA, Lindenbaum J: Pharmacokinetics of digoxin and digotoxin in patients undergoing hemodialysis. Am J Med 58:525, 1975

151. Holt DW, Traill TA, Brown CB: The treatment of digoxin overdosage. Clin Nephrol 3:119, 1975

152. van der Vijgh WJF, Oe PL: Pharmacokinetic aspects of digoxin in patients with terminal renal failure: On hemodialysis. Int J Clin Pharmacol 15:255, 1977

153. Iisalo E, Forsstrom J: Elimination of digoxin during maintenance haemodialysis. Ann Clin Res 6:203, 1974

154. Ackerman GL, Doherty JE, Flanigan WJ: Peritoneal dialysis and hemodialysis of tritiated digoxin. Ann Intern Med 67:718, 1967

155. Hoy WE, Gibson TP, Rivero AJ, et al: XAD-4 resin hemoperfusion for digitoxin patients with renal failure. Kidney Int 23:79, 1983

156. Sevka MJ, Matthews SJ, Nightingale CH, et al: Disopyramide hemodialysis and kinetics in patients requiring long-term hemodialysis. Clin Pharmacol Ther 29:322, 1981

157. Jacobi J, McGory RW, McCoy H, et al: Hemodialysis clearance of total and unbound lidocaine. Clin Pharm 2:54, 1983

158. Atkinson Jr AJ, Krumlovsky FA, Huang CM, et al: Hemodialysis for severe procainamide toxicity: Clinical and pharmacokinetic observations. Clin Pharmacol Ther 20:585, 1976

159. Gibson TP, Lowenthal DT, Nelson HA, et al: Elimination of procainamide in end stage renal failure. Clin Pharmacol Ther 17:321, 1974

160. Stec GP, Atkinson Jr AJ, Nevin MJ, et al: N-acetylprocainamide pharmacokinetics in functionally anephric patients before and after perturbation by hemodialysis. Clin Pharmacol Ther 26:618, 1979

161. Sica DA, Harford A, Small R: Procainamide utilization in chronic ambulatory peritoneal dialysis. p. 68A. American Society of Nephrology, 15th Annual Meeting. Chicago, Ill, 1982

162. Herrera J, Vurkovich RA, Griffth DL: Elimination of nadolol by patients with renal impairment. Br J Clin Pharmacol 7:227S, 1979

163. Lowenthal DT, Briggs WA, Gibson TP, et al: Pharmacokinetics of oral propranolol in chronic renal disease. Clin Pharmacol Ther 16:761, 1974

164. Bianchetti G, Graziani G, Brancaccio D, et al: Pharmacokinetics and effects of propranolol in terminal uraemic patients and in patients undergoing regular dialysis treatment. Clin Pharmacokinet 1:373, 1976

165. Woie L, Øyri A: Quinidine intoxication treated with hemodialysis. Acta Med Scand 195:237, 1974

166. Reimold EW, Reynolds WJ, Fixler DE, et al: Use of hemodialysis in the treatment of quinidine poisoning. Pediatrics 52:95, 1973

167. Chin TWF, Pancorbo S, Comty C: Quinidine pharmacokinetics in continuous ambulatory peritoneal dialysis. Clin Exp Dial Apheresis 5:391, 1981

168. Weigers U, Hanrath P, Kuck KH, et al: Pharmacokinetics of tocainide in patients with renal dysfunction and during haemodialysis. Eur J Clin Pharmacol 24:503, 1983

169. Hirakata H, Onoyama K, Iseki K, et al: Captopril (SQ 14225) clearance during hemodialysis treatment. Clin Nephrol 16:321, 1981

170. Hulter HN, Licht JH, Ilnicki LP, et al: Clinical efficacy and pharmacokinetics of clonidine in hemodialysis and renal insufficiency. J Lab Clin Med 94:223, 1979

171. Yeh BK, Dayton PG, Waters III, WC: Removal of alpha-methyldopa (Aldomet) in man by dialysis. Proc Soc Exp Biol Med 135:840, 1970

172. Vaziri ND, Saiki J, Barton CH, et al: Hemodialysability of acetazolamide. South Med J 73:422, 1980

173. Riva E, Fossali E, Bettinelli A: Kinetics of furosemide in children with chronic renal failure undergoing regular haemodialysis. Eur J Clin Pharmacol 21:303, 1982

174. Cutler RE, Forrey AW, Christopher TG, et al: Pharmacokinetics of furosemide in normal subjects and functionally anephric patients. Clin Pharmacol Ther 15:588, 1974

175. Schusziarra V, Ziekursch V, Schlmp R, et al: Pharmacokinetics of azathiaprine under haemodialysis. Int J Clin Pharmacol 14:298, 1976

176. Wang LH, Lee CS, Majeske BL, et al: Clearance and recovery calculation in hemodialysis: Application to plasma, red blood cell, and dialysate measurements for cyclophosphamide. Clin Pharmacol Ther 29:365, 1981

177. Gibson TP, Reich SD, Krumlovsky FA, et al: Hemoperfusion for methotrexate removal. Clin Pharmacol Ther 23:351, 1978

178. Ahmad S, Shen F-H, Bleger WA: Methotrexate-induced renal failure and ineffectiveness of peritoneal dialysis. Arch Intern Med 138:1146, 1978

179. Howell SB, Blair HE, Uren J, et al: Hemodialysis and enzymatic cleavage of methotrexate in man. Eur J Cancer 14:787, 1978

180. Black WD, Acchiarrdo SR: Acetohexamide hypoglycemia: Treatment by peritoneal dialysis. South Med J 70:1240, 1977

181. Graw RG, Clarke RR: Chlorpropamide intoxication: Treatment with peritoneal dialysis. Pediatrics 45:106, 1970

182. Glockner P, Lange H, Pfab R: Tolbutamidstoffwechsel bei Niereninsuffizienz. Med Welt Nr 52:2876, 1968

183. Kogan FJ, Sampliner RE, Mayersohn M, et al: Cimetidine disposition in patients undergoing continuous ambulatory peritoneal dialysis. J Clin Pharmacol 23:252, 1983

184. Abate MA, Hyneck ML, Cohen IA, et al: Cimetidine pharmacokinetics. Clin Pharm 1:225, 1982

185. Larsson R, Erlanson P, Bodemar G, et al: Pharmacokinetics of cimetidine and its sulfoxide metabolite during hemodialysis. Eur J Clin Pharmacol 21:235, 1982

186. Bjoeldager PAL, Jensen JB, Nielson LP, et al: Pharmacokinetics of cimetidine in patients undergoing hemodialysis. Nephron 34:159, 1983

187. Vaziri ND, Ness RL, Barton CH: Hemodialysis clearance of cimetidine. Arch Intern Med 138:1685, 1978

188. Hyneck ML, Murphy JF, Lipschutz DE: Cimetidine clearance during intermittent and chronic peritoneal dialysis. Am J Hosp Pharm 38:1760, 1981

189. Pizzella KM, Moore MC, Schultz RW, et al: Removal of cimetidine by peritoneal dialysis, hemodialysis, and charcoal hemoperfusion. Ther Drug Monit 2:273, 1980

190. McCoy HG, Cipolle RJ, Ehlers SM, et al: Severe methanol poisoning: Application of a pharmacokinetic model for ethanol therapy and hemodialysis. Am J Med 67:804, 1979

191. Freireich AW, Cinque TJ, Xanthaky G, et al: Hemodialysis of isopropanol poisoning. N Engl J Med 227:699, 1967

192. Keyvan-Larijarni H, Tannenberg AM: Methanol intoxication: Comparison of peritoneal dialysis and hemodialysis treatment. Arch Intern Med 134:293, 1974

193. Lee CS, Marbury TV, Perrin JH, et al: Hemodialysis of theophylline in uremic patients. J Clin Pharmacol 19:219, 1979

194. Kladjan WA, Martin TR, Delaney CJ, et al: Effect of hemodialysis on the pharmacokinetics of theophylline in chronic renal failure. Nephron 32:40, 1982

195. Brown GS, Lohr TO, Mayor GH, et al: Peritoneal clearance of theophylline. Am J Kidney Dis 1:24, 1981

196. Russo M: Management of theophylline intoxication with charcoal-column hemoperfusion. N Engl J Med 300:24, 1979

Index

Page numbers followed by *f* represent figures; numbers followed by *t* represent tables.